The Practicing Physician's Approach to Headache

2nd Edition

The Practicing Physician's Approach to Headache

2nd Edition

Seymour Diamond, MD

Assistant Professor of Neurology
Chicago Medical School and
Director, Diamond Headache Clinic, Ltd.
Chicago, Illinois

Donald J. Dalessio, MD

Head, Division of Neurology and
Chairman, Department of Medicine
Scripps Clinic and Research Foundation
La Jolla, California

The Williams & Wilkins Co. 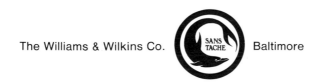 Baltimore

Made in the United States of America

Library of Congress Cataloging in Publication Data

Diamond, Seymour, 1925–
    The practicing physician's approach to headache.

    Bibliography: p.
    Includes index.
    1. Headache. I. Dalessio, Donald J., 1931– joint author. II. Title. [DNLM: 1. Headache. WL342 D537p]
RB128.D5 1978   616′.047   77-17126
ISBN 0-683-02502-3

    Reprinted April 1979
    Reprinted July 1979

Composed and printed at the
Waverly Press, Inc.
Mt. Royal and Guilford Aves.
Baltimore, Md 21202, U.S.A.

Dedicated to Our Wives and Our Parents

Preface to the Second Edition

This edition follows the first by approximately five years. In the interim, interest in headache has increased, and a plethora of new information on the subject makes this revision a necessity.

We have, however, attempted to keep the book simple, the drawings direct, and directions explicit, in short, a working text, as we like to term it. The reader may be assured that the authors have passed a great many patients with headache through their hands. This book is an attempt to set down and describe our experiences on this subject. We hope that the pages that follow will be of value to the person for whom they are intended, the practitioner of medicine.

S.D.
D.J.D.

Preface to the First Edition

Two important factors are paramount in the treatment and management of headache patients. The first is that perhaps half of them have been treated symptomatically—without regard to a diagnosis and with drugs used simply to relieve pain. There should be a logical sequence employed in investigating the problem. Many headache patients have not had a careful history or neurologic examination, nor has an adequate attempt been made to diagnose the type of cephalalgia from which they suffer. Even though the history and neurologic examination are the keys to the diagnosis, extensive testing procedures may have been performed without discrimination. It is the intention of the authors to promote and provide a logical understanding of the headache patient and the approach to the diagnosis and treatment of his problem.

To the patient who has suffered over a long period of time, his headache is most important, not "just a headache." He will travel from doctor to doctor and to large research and diagnostic centers. This brings us to our second important point. Diagnosis must be coordinated with continual treatment. The cephalalgic patient needs attention and treatment on a continuing basis, whether the diagnosis indicates psychogenic, vascular or organic causes. The follow-up treatment may be on the basis of trial and error until relief is afforded. Therefore, the patient must have full confidence in his physician and his approach to the problem. It is easier for one physician to mold this confidence rather than a continued series of consultants.

We should not, as physicians, be intolerant of the headache sufferer. It is easy to lose patience and lack concern for these people, especially those with persistent complaints. The simplest course is to blame the problem on a defective personality or the wish of the patient to avoid reality. Careful attention to symptoms and related details, however, will reveal the etiology and guide the subsequent treatment.

It is not the purpose of this book to be a reference text giving a multitude of information. Rather, we hope to demonstrate a definitive approach to both the diagnosis and treatment of headache. An attempt has been made to keep the text uncluttered, simple and easy to read and follow.

About the Authors

Seymour Diamond, MD, Assistant Professor of Neurology, the Chicago Medical School, and Director, Diamond Headache Clinic, Ltd., Chicago, Illinois, received his MD degree from the Chicago Medical School. His internship and residencies were spent in Little Rock University Hospital in Arkansas and White Cross Hospital, Columbus, Ohio. He is past president of the American Association for the Study of Headache and of the National Migraine Foundation. Dr. Diamond has published numerous articles on headache and is a frequent lecturer on this subject.

Donald J. Dalessio, MD, matriculated at Wesleyan and Yale, and trained in Neurology and Medicine at New York Hospital-Cornell Medical Center and at Yale. Formerly Professor of Neurology and Associate Dean for Clinical Affairs at the University of Kentucky, Dr. Dalessio is presently Head of Neurology Division, and Chairman, Department of Medicine, Scripps Clinic and Research Foundation, La Jolla, California. He was formerly editor of the journal *Headache* and author of *Wolff's Headache and Other Head Pain*.

Acknowledgments

We are particularly indebted to Judi Falk for illustrations for this work; to Joseph R. Kraft, MD, Chairman, Department of Clinical Pathology and Nuclear Medicine, St. Joseph Hospital, Chicago, Illinois, for his help with the scanning section of the book; Robert J. Borgerson, MD, Chairman, Radiology Department, St. Joseph Hospital, Chicago, Illinois, for the x-ray illustrations; Harvey Lee Meyers, Jr., MD, Associate Professor of Neurology, the Chicago Medical School, Chicago, Illinois, for his help with certain illustrative material; Bernard J. Baltes, MD, PhD, our co-worker in headache and Martin E. Bruetman, MD, Professor and Chairman, Department of Neurology, the Chicago Medical School, Chicago, Illinois.

We acknowledge our debt to others who work in this field, and whose names appear in the bibliography. In particular, the painstaking and careful work of the late Harold G. Wolff, MD, deserves mention.

Special mention should also be given to Mrs. Betty Stewart of Chicago and Mrs. Joan Bryan of Lexington for their help in the preparation of this manuscript.

For the 2nd edition, Catherine Dalessio has revised some of the drawings. We thank Mrs. Camille Mead, of La Jolla, for help with the manuscript preparation. Drs. Stanley Seat and James Usselman of Scripps Clinic have prepared new radiographs including computerized tomographic scans. Mrs. Ruby Richardson of Williams & Wilkins coordinated the project as Editor.

If a writer is so cautious that he never writes anything that cannot be criticized, he will never write anything that can be read. If you want to help other people you have got to make up your mind to write things that some men will condemn.

Thomas Merton
"Seeds of Contemplation"

Contents

1 **Classification and Mechanisms of Headache** . . **1**

From the Stone Age to industrial society, headache has ranked high on the list of man's complaints. But you can't prescribe treatment until you establish etiology. A simple classification system . . . pain mechanisms . . . and a review of migraine biochemistry provide clues to approach therapy.
SELF-ASSESSMENT EXAMINATION

2 **Taking a Headache History** **12**

An incisive and complete headache history is important. Concepts of diagnostic history-taking identifying various headache syndromes are illustrated.
SELF-ASSESSMENT EXAMINATION

3 **Physical and Neurologic Examination of the Headache Patient** **31**

Every headache patient should have a physical and neurologic examination—it can lead to a correct diagnosis and reassure the patient. Examination procedure is detailed.
SELF-ASSESSMENT EXAMINATION

4 **Additional Studies Are Sometimes Necessary in Investigating Headache** **39**

When standard evaluations don't turn up the cause of headache, specific indications may call for more elaborate techniques.
SELF-ASSESSMENT EXAMINATION

5 **Migraine Headache** **51**

How can you be sure the patient has migraine? Is there a "migraine personality"? Outlined in detail are clinical signs, symptoms and specific suggestions for therapy.
SELF-ASSESSMENT EXAMINATION

6 **Cluster Headache** **67**

"Cluster" is a term that describes a unique and specific type of vascular headache that occurs in bursts or clusters. It is sometimes diagnosed by the peculiar facial characteristics of the patient.
SELF-ASSESSMENT EXAMINATION

Classification and Mechanisms of Headache

Since all physicians may be called upon to treat patients with headache, it is important to have a simple classification which may give clues to appropriate therapy. We have separated headache into three main groups, rather than providing a series of disparate headache syndromes which may tax the memory. These groups are *vascular, muscle contraction* and *traction and inflammatory* (Table 1-1).

Vascular headache includes classic and common migraine, hemiplegic and ophthalmoplegic migraine, cluster headache, toxic vascular headache and hypertensive headache. Common to all these is a tendency to vascular dilation, which provokes the headache phase in each instance. Vasoconstriction may also occur and may be responsible for the painless sensory and motor phenomena occurring with some forms of vascular headache. Toxic vascular headache refers to that state evoked by a systemic vasodilation, and may be produced by fever, ingestion of alcohol, poisons, CO_2 retention, therapeutic agents such as the nitrates and the like. Hypertensive headache is related to elevation in the systemic arterial blood pressure.

Perhaps the most common form of headache is termed muscle contraction headache, characterized by persistent contraction of the muscles of the head, neck and face. This produces dull, bandlike, persistent pain, which may last for days, months or years. When the headache is incapacitating, persistent and not obviously vascular in nature, a disorder of mood, thought or behavior should be suspected. This complaint is frequently seen in the depressed patient, but is not exclusively associated with depression. Headache may also be a sign of chronic anxiety, or may present as a form of a contemporary conversion reaction.

Traction and inflammatory headache includes headache evoked by organic diseases of the skull or its components, including the brain, meninges, arteries, veins, eyes, ears, teeth, nose and paranasal sinuses. The term "traction headache" is used to describe the often nonspecific headache seen with mass lesions of the brain, including tumors, hematomas, abscesses, or brain edema for whatever cause. Traction and inflammatory headache of a particularly intense type occurs in subarachnoid hemorrhage. Traction and inflammatory headache is associated with inflammatory disease of the meninges, and intracranial or extracranial arteritis or phlebitis. Inflammatory headache may be associated with disease of the special sense organs and the teeth, and with disorders of the joints of the neck and the jaw. The major neuralgias are also listed here, in parentheses, since the neuritic pain which characterizes these

Table 1-1. Classification and Treatment of Headache

Vascular headache	Muscle contraction headache	Traction and inflammatory headache
Migraine Classic Common Hemiplegic $\rbrace$ complicated Ophthalmoplegic $\rbrace$ migraine	Depressive equivalents and conversion reactions	Mass lesions (tumors, edema, hematomas, cerebral hemorrhage)
Cluster (histamine)	Cervical osteoarthritis	Diseases of the eye, ear, nose, throat, teeth
Toxic vascular Hypertensive	Chronic myositis	Infection Arteritis, phlebitis (Cranial neuralgias) Occlusive vascular disease Atypical facial pain TMJ disease
Suggested treatment		
Ergot derivatives Sedation Methysergide Cyproheptadine Propanolol Clonidine Lithium Platelet antagonist Analgesics Antihypertensives Behavioral conditioning	Common analgesics Sedation Antidepressants Physical therapy Behavioral conditioning	Appropriate consultation Therapy of underlying disease Antibiotics Anticonvulsants Corticosteroids $\rbrace$ as indicated Miotics Surgery

conditions is associated with specific abnormalities of the function of the central nervous system.

The management of traction and inflammatory headache or the major neuralgias generally involves specific treatment for the associated underlying disease. The patient whose headache is classified in this group may require extensive investigation and numerous consultations with neurologists, neurosurgeons, ophthalmologists, otolaryngologists and dentists. Thus, treatment for this form of headache or facial pain is extremely varied, and may range from surgery to anticonvulsants. It is in this group that prompt and emergency treatment is often required; the headache or facial pain is considered a secondary phenomenon, which often responds to alleviation of the primary disease.

All the conditions mentioned above and listed in the classification of headache will be discussed in detail in subsequent chapters.

The Nature of Headache

Knowledge of headache and its variants is essential to the practitioner. Headache is a unique syndrome in medicine and has been termed the most common medical complaint of civilized man. Yet severe headache is only infrequently caused by organic disease. Hence, it may be inferred that for the most part headache represents an inability of the individual to deal in some measure with the uncertainties of life—that it is a symptom of wrong pace or wrong direction rather than a structural disease of the nervous system. Nonetheless, headache may also be the presenting complaint of catastrophic illness such as brain tumor, cerebral hemorrhage or meningitis, and to ignore the symptom in this context is to risk the life of the patient. Headache may be equally intense whether its source is benign or malignant. The problem is compounded further by the difficulties of studying the brain and its appendages, which are encased in the bony fortress of the skull and resist the usual efforts of diagnosis. It forces one to rely on peripheral methods of investigation.

Anatomic Substrate of Pain

What structures of the head are capable of causing pain? In a series of anatomic studies, performed for the most part on patients prepared for neurologic surgery, B. S. Ray and H. G. Wolff (1940) showed that the pain-sensitive structures of the head include the skin of the scalp and its blood supply and appendages, the head and neck muscles, the great venous sinuses and their tributaries, parts of the dura mater at the base of the brain, the dural arteries, the intracerebral arteries, at least the fifth, sixth and seventh cranial nerves and the cervical nerves. The cranium, the brain parenchyma, much of the dura and pia mater, the ependymal lining of the ventricles and the choroid plexuses are not sensitive to pain (Table 1-2).

In general, pain pathways for structures above the tentorium cerebelli are contained in the trigeminal nerve, and pain that is referred from these structures is usually appreciated in the frontal, temporal and parietal regions of the skull. Pain pathways for structures below the tentorium cerebelli are contained especially in the glossopharyngeal and vagus nerves, as well as the upper cervical spinal roots. Pain referred from these structures is usually felt in the occipital region of the head.

The Biochemistry of Migraine

In order to understand the roles of the vasoactive substances in migraine, a brief discussion of some mechanisms of inflammation is necessary. This is appropriate, since vasodilation in itself does not invariably produce headache. One does not usually complain of headache, for example, after severe exertion, or after sitting in a tub of hot water. Yet extracranial vasodilation is obvious at these times. Thus it has been suggested that the peripheral manifestations of migraine (or, as the patient describes it, the "pounding headache") are related to vasodilation associated with a sterile local inflammatory reaction. In other terms, it has been suggested that migraine is a clinical syndrome of self-limited neurogenic inflammation.

Vasodilation alone does not invariably produce headache. Probably, inflammation is involved also.

Furthermore, when one begins to study inflammation one must also study blood

Table 1-2. Pain Sensitivity of Cranial Tissues

	Pain sensitive		Insensitive to pain
Intracranial	Cranial sinuses and afferent veins	Intracranial	Parenchyma of the brain
	Arteries of the dura mater		Ependyma, choroid plexus
	Arteries of the base of the brain and their major branches		Pia mater, arachnoid membrane, parts of the dura mater
	Parts of the dura mater (in the vicinity of large vessels)		
Extracranial	Skin, scalp, fascia, muscles	Extracranial	Skull (periosteum slightly sensitive)
	Mucosa		
	Arteries (veins: less sensitive)		
Nerves	Trigeminal, facial, vagal, glossopharyngeal		
	2nd and 3rd cervical nerves		

clotting, the complement system and immune mechanisms, for all the systems are intertwined. Indeed, their separation is unnatural.

Inflammation begins with a series of cellular events. Usually a specific or nonspecific injury occurs, provoked by multiple factors including ischemia or injury, the deposition of immune complexes, activation of the Hageman factor, deposition of bacterial toxins and, possibly, stress and/or higher nervous activity. Vasoactive amines such as histamine and serotonin are released from platelets, basophils and tissue mast cells. Other tissues, when injured, may release slow-reacting substance of anaphylaxis (SRSA) and prostaglandins. All are vasoactive and increase vascular permeability. Serum components come in contact with extravascular proteins, modifying these proteins. The complement cascade is stimulated. Fixation of complement, for example to immune complexes, attracts polymorphonuclear leukocytes which localize in the area. Upon rupture of their lysosomal membranes, a series of enzymes are elaborated. Kinins are produced when the coagulation system is activated. Prostaglandins are released by antigen-antibody reactions and by bradykinin; prostaglandins themselves aggregate platelets, causing their disruption and so increasing the concentration of vasoactive substances.

Thus, present evidence implicates at least five and possibly more groups of vasoactive substances associated with inflammation, including

- catecholamines
- histamine and serotonin
- peptide kinins
- prostaglandins
- slow-reacting substance of anaphylaxis (SRSA), an acidic lipid.

All have potent biologic properties which differ with their structure and include, among other effects

- contraction and relaxation of smooth muscle

- constriction or dilation of arteries and veins
- induction of water and sodium diuresis
- fever
- wheal-and-flare reactions
- induction of pain, including headache

The migraine episode can be studied only in humans, and its study is limited by its relatively benign course and the lack of a suitable animal experimental model. Nonetheless, the following statements about vasoactive substances as they affect the migraine episode may be made:

- Serotonin levels fall at onset of migraine.

- Local accumulation of a vasodilator polypeptide occurs.

- Tyramine taken orally may evoke migraine.

- Temporal arteries of migrainous patients bind norepinephrine.

- Prostaglandins injected evoke vascular headache.

- Histamine levels are increased in cluster headache.

Serotonin levels of the plasma fall at the onset of a migraine attack and platelets of patients with migraine, incubated with serotonin, aggregate more readily than those of controls. Serotonin will constrict scalp arteries in man. An increase in the major metabolite of serotonin, 5-hydroxyindoleacetic acid (5HIAA), has been inconsistently demonstrated during a migraine attack.

S. V. Deshmukh, M.D. and J. S. Meyer, M.D. of Houston, Texas have investigated the pathophysiologic role of platelets in the pathogenesis of migraine. To determine the role of platelets in the pathogenesis of migraine, 27 patients with migraine were studied while off medication during the headache-free period. The migraineurs showed a significantly lower ($p < 0.002$) circulating microemboli index (CMI) and a higher aggregation response to adenosine diphosphate (ADP) ($p < 0.025$) when compared to 35 normals.

Platelet function tests were performed in 14 migraine patients during the headache-free period and repeated subsequently in 11 patients during the prodrome and in 11 patients during the headache phase. Platelet adhesiveness to glass beads and aggregation response to ADP, epinephrine, thrombin and serotonin increased during the prodrome. During the headache phase, however, adhesiveness increased significantly ($p < 0.01$) and aggregation in response to ADP and epinephrine decreased significantly ($p < 0.0$ and $p < 0.05$).

The increase in platelet aggregation during the prodrome and decrease during the headache phase parallel the reported increase in plasma serotonin level during the prodrome and subsequent decrease during the headache phase. Since platelets contain all the serotonin present in blood and release it during aggregation, it is possible that changes in plasma serotonin levels in migraine are secondary to changes in platelet aggregation.

M. Sandler, of Great Britain, has observed a platelet monamine oxidase deficiency in migraine. He noted that a transitory but highly significant decrease in platelet monoamine oxidase activity was seen during headache attacks in migrainous subjects and reverted to normal during attack-free periods. This was not the result of drugs used for the treatment of migraine. It is possible that decreased platelet monoamine oxidase and 5-hydroxytryptamine occur in response to release into the circulation of an unidentified substance during the headache and, perhaps, is responsible for it. Sandler draws attention to the biochemical relationship of migraine and depressive illness, an association well described in the past by others. (See Chapter 5.)

Local accumulation of a vasodilator polypeptide, akin to bradykinin, can be demonstrated in the subsurface tissues of patients with migraine.

Tyramine, a pressor amine found in certain foods, can evoke migraine in suscepti-

ble subjects. Tyramine liberates norepinephrine from tissues. A defect in the conjugation of tyramine has been reported in migraine patients, which has genetic implications, since migraine is at least a familial if not a genetic disorder.

Temporal arteries removed from humans during the painful stage of migraine have an increased capacity to take up norepinephrine. Conversely, infusions of norepinephrine can be used to treat migraine.

G. D. A. Lord, M.D. and J. W. Duckworth, M.D. of Sydney, Australia, have investigated the roles of the complement cascade and immunoglobulin patterns in migraine.

Serum complement components and immunoglobulins were measured in migraineurs. Patients were assigned to three groups: Group 1 (prodromal migraineurs), and Group 2 (nonprodomal). The latter group was subdivided into Group 2A (common) and Group 2B (with focal neurologic symptoms commencing after headache onset). In the immunoglobulin study: Group 1 had an elevated IgA level, Group 2A had elevated IgG and IgA and Group 2B had elevated IgG, IgA and IgM when compared with appropriate controls. The IgM in group 2B was significantly higher than in Groups 1 and 2A, supporting the division into two groups of patients with focal neurologic symptoms.

The complement study compared patients during headache and when headache-free. The "in headache" patients were further subdivided into early and late groups. The complement results are from patients in Group 2 only. During headache, samples were obtained from 18 migraineurs. In 9 patients headache-free specimens were collected, enabling paired analysis of results.

Reductions in levels of complement components C4 and C5 in the paired study, and lower levels of C4, C1s and C1(1) during early headache in the unpaired study are evidence of complement activation associated with migraine. Demonstration of complement breakdown products in 3 patients at least 3 hours before headache onset, and absence of difference in component levels between headache-free and late headache migraineurs indicate complement activation of short duration.

Elevated immunoglobulin levels and complement activation suggest a late-onset immune reaction of short duration. Such a mechanism provides an explanation of many of the features of nonprodromal migraine: platelet release of serotonin, basophil and mast cell degranulation, increased whole blood histamine during an attack, fluid retention, increased thrombotic tendency and increased cerebrospinal fluid (CSF) lactate and GABA (Gamma-Amino-Butyric Acid).

Prostaglandins have not been measured in humans with migraine, but injections of prostaglandins may produce headache in susceptible subjects.

In cluster headache, related to migraine, an increase in whole blood histamine levels has been demonstrated at the onset of an attack. Injection of histamine and other vasodilators may provoke an attack in susceptible subjects with cluster headache.

Medications

These observations and others have led to the therapeutic and prophylactic use of medications which inhibit the actions of some vasoactive substances, tend to stabilize membranes, reduce excessive vasomotor activity and interfere with the chemical mediators of inflammation. Examples follow.

Medications are used to inhibit the actions of vasoactive substances, stablize membranes and reduce vasomotor activity and inflammation.

Antihistamine and antiserotonin compounds will interfere with vasoactive amines, or inhibit their elaboration from their respective depots.

Nonsteroidal anti-inflammatory drugs, including aspirin and indomethacin, stabilize proteins and inhibit the formation of active prostaglandins from their precursors. Aspirin reduces platelet aggregation and indirectly affects the release of vasoactive substances.

Corticosteroids reduce inflammation at several levels, lower the complement titer and stabilize lysosomal membranes. Experimental evidence indicates that corticosteroids

- inhibit release of histamine from mast cells, normalize capillary permeability and reduce exudation

- stabilize cell membranes, enhance cell resistance to cytotoxins and interrupt the chain reaction to cell breakage

- stabilize lysosome membranes

- stabilize capillaries and inhibit emigration of neutrophils (polymorphonuclear leukocytes)

- inhibit granulation, fibrosis and collagen deposition

Some anti-inflammatory drugs interfere with kinin functions, or with the actions of prostaglandins.

Some drugs have multiple effects. Ergot, for example, is both a vasoconstrictor and an alpha-adrenergic blocker. Propranolol, a beta-adrenergic blocker, is used in migraine prophylaxis. No single drug will block or inhibit all components of inflammation. Effective therapy may require the use of several.

The relationship between the efficacy of strictly antiserotonin compounds and migraine prophylaxis is a complex one. It seems evident with each passing year, however, that the specific antiserotonin activity of this or that compound has little to do with its efficacy in migraine. It simply is not enough to block the peripheral actions of serotonin alone and expect adequate migraine prophylaxis to be accomplished. Cyproheptadine, which blocks both serotonin and histamine, comes closest to this therapeutic situation. Methysergide, advertised as a serotonin antagonist, has complex pharmacologic effects. It also blocks histamine indirectly by interfering with histamine liberators, at least in vivo. Furthermore, as suspected early on, it has significant vasoconstrictor properties. Recent studies in the dog make it evident that methysergide produces profound vasoconstriction of the external carotid artery.

This being the case, the question may be posed regarding the etiologic role of the indoleamine, serotonin, in the pathogenesis of migraine. The changes in the level of plasma serotonin observed prior to the onset of migraine may represent only one aspect of the genesis of migraine. Similarly, the importance of the changes of whole blood histamine prior to the onset of cluster headache is suspect. Other diseases in which there are great changes in blood histamine are not characterized by unilateral severe headache.

What seems more likely is that histamine, serotonin, the plasma kinins and perhaps other vasoactive substances participate in a sterile inflammatory reaction involving painful and distended blood vessels. They are, then, an integral but peripheral part of the migraine process and certainly one part of the process that can be measured and toward which therapy can be directed. But they are important primarily to that part of the migraine episode wherein *an increase in vascular permeability occurs.*

Central Process of Migraine

This has been a brief summary of the peripheral aspects of migraine and the possible relationship of biochemical processes and vasoactive substances. Let us turn now for a moment to the central processes of migraine, for it is generally accepted that in classic migraine the intracranial vessels are profoundly affected. Indeed, it has been shown by cerebral blood flow measurements, utilizing radioactive gas as a marker,

that the prodromes of migraine are associated with a profound reduction in blood flow to the cerebral cortex, sometimes focal, sometimes generalized.

John Edmeads, M.D. of Toronto, Canada, has described his study of cerebral blood flow in migraine. The results of these studies tend to confirm Wolff's hypothesis that cerebral blood flow is decreased during auras and increased during headaches. However, some findings were unexpected. The distribution in time and space of the blood flow changes did not always correlate with clinical features of the attack. Autoregulation of the cerebral blood vessels may be impaired in aura and in headache, and this is a key factor in intensifying and prolonging attacks.

The measurements of cerebral blood flow have made significant contributions to the pathogenesis and therapy of migraine. In terms of practical therapeutics, Edmeads' study shows that ergotamine does not affect cerebral blood flow even when it has clearly been effective in ablating headache. This is an important observation, since the immunity of the intracranial circulation to ergotamine suggests that the traditional prohibition of this drug to patients who have severe vasoconstrictive auras may be unnecessary, and that these patients may now receive the benefits of treatment at the onset of their aura, rather than waiting until the headache begins.

The theoretical implications of the blood flow studies are more far-reaching. They provide the additional evidence required to confirm Wolff's hypothesis regarding the vascular theory of migraine. Perhaps more important, these blood flow studies indicate that the Wolff theory, while correct, is also incomplete. The unexpected data on the frequent discrepancy between the spatial and temporal relationship of blood flow and the distribution of symptoms, and on the disordered cerebral vasoreactivity during attacks, will serve as a point of departure for further research into the mechanisms of migraine and the autonomic nervous system.

Dr. K. Welch of Houston has made biochemical comparisons between migraine and stroke. He measured gamma-amino-butyric acid (GABA) and 3',5'-cyclic adenosine monophosphate (cyclic AMP) in the CSF of patients with stroke and vascular headache of migraine type. GABA was elevated in CSF of patients with recent onset of thromboembolic occlusive cerebrovascular disese (CVD) and within 48 hours of an attack of vertebrobasilar ischemia (VBI). Similarly, GABA was elevated in CSF of all patients studied during a migraine attack but not in asymptomatic migraine patients or patients with muscle contraction (tension) headache. CSF cyclic AMP was also elevated in patients with recent onset of thromboembolic occlusive CVD and in patients studied during or within 48 hours of a migraine attack.

Since the biochemical abnormalities reported herein were common to occlusive CVD and migraine headache, it seems probable that they are due to the ischemia associated with both conditions and possibly related to the resultant disorder of cerebral energy metabolism.

In recent years interest has again focused on the role of the autonomic nervous system in the maintenance of cerebral vascular tone and blood flow. It is recognized that minute changes in the level of carbon dioxide in the blood significantly affect cerebral blood flow. This carbon dioxide regulating effect is more important than either hypoxia or hypoglycemia. And a sudden fall in systemic arterial blood pressure will also evoke vasodilation.

If all these variables are controlled, however, is it possible to alter cerebral blood flow through stimulation of the autonomic nervous system? There is an abundant network of autonomic nerves in contact with the basal and pial arteries of the brain. Electron microscopic studies have shown that these nerves terminate in contact with vascular smooth muscle. Stimulation of the cervical sympathetic nerves can, in animals, produce constriction of the carotid and vertebral arteries to the extent of affecting tissue perfusion. These arteries can be made to constrict after local application of catecholamines and these responses can be blocked by adrenolytic agents. After prolonged spasm, stores of norepinephrine in the perivascular nerves are reduced.

Control of Cerebral Blood Flow

J. Olesen (1972) proposes a useful hypothesis for the control for cerebral blood flow, which has clinical implications with respect to migraine. He divides the cerebral blood vessels into two systems, dependent upon their adrenergic nervous supply. One system comprises the large arteries at the base of the brain and the pial arteries, and is distinguished by its rich nerve supply and the responsiveness of the vessels to catecholamines (catecholamine responses can be blocked). The term "innervated vascular system" is suggested for these vessels. The other system, consisting of parenchymal vessels, has little or no autonomic innervation and responds only to the metabolic needs of the brain tissues to which it is closely approximated. These vessels are not responsive to application of catecholamines. The two systems of blood vessels are connected in series.

The character of the two systems relates structure to function. The blood vessels of the noninnervated system, being in close contact with brain tissue and regulated by their local metabolic needs, include the terminal high resistance arterioles. The innervated system, with its abundant nervous supply, regulates flow through the large arteries and is capable of reacting to external or nonlocal factors, thus protecting the parenchymal arteries in the brain from sudden increases or decreases in arterial pressure—for example, during active exercise. The dual system also allows maximum tissue blood flow if the systemic arterial blood pressure falls suddenly.

We suggest that, in migraine, the sudden neurogenic vasoconstriction of the great arteries of one internal carotid would lead to a temporary reduction in flow through the noninnervated system. The local metabolic demands of the brain would rapidly thereafter produce a focal acidosis and intracranial vasodilation, particularly of the noninnervated system, but also involving the innervated system, which might be mirrored in the extracranial subsurface scalp tissues and so produce the typical hemicranial headache.

There is some indirect evidence also to support these concepts. Methysergide has peripheral and central effects and the central effects are at least in part mediated through inhibition of central vasomotor responses. The concentration of brain serotonin is, in animals, intimately related to the functions of the central vasomotor centers. It has been proposed that the central vasomotor centers and the central autonomic nervous system perform a neuroregulatory role in the control of the vascular tone of the major blood vessels at the base of the brain.

Unified Theory of Migraine

Hence, a unified theory of migraine emerges—a neurogenic concept of migraine. Subsequent to some stress or nonspecific or specific stimulus, the series of nervous reflexes which initiate the migraine

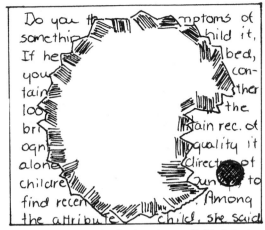

Fig 1-2. *A typical migrainous field defect.*

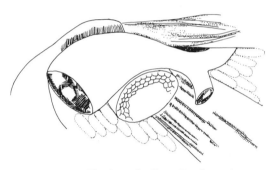

Fig 1-3. *Vasodilation. Ordinarily there is one-sided throbbing pain associated with dilation of intracranial and extracranial blood vessels.*

process occurs. The preheadache vasoconstrictor phenomenon represents neurogenic vasospasm of the innervated vascular system at the base of the brain and the pial arteries (Fig 1-1). This vascular activity represents the initial vector of vascular reaction in migraine. The vasoconstriction produces a relative reduction in local cerebral blood flow, with the consequent local metabolic tissue abnormalities including acidosis and anoxia (Fig 1-2). The noninnervated parenchymal arteries, responsive to local metabolic demands, next dilate and if vasodilation is sufficiently great, the cranial arteries on the outside of the head also expand (Fig 1-3). The alteration in tone of the extracranial arteries provokes the liberation of multiple local chemical and vasoactive substances as described above, pro-

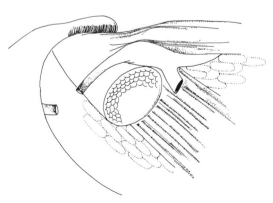

Fig 1-1. *Clinical features of migraine vasoconstriction. The head pain is preceded by painless preheadache phenomena, particularly visual field defects. Other symptoms include speech difficulties, dizziness or weakness.*

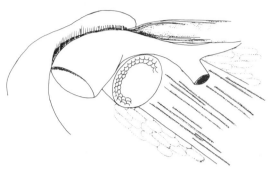

Fig 1-4. *The edema phase. In this stage the headache becomes persistent and steady, associated with vascular edema, nausea, vomiting and general malaise.*

ducing edema, a lowering of pain threshold and, eventually, pounding headache (Fig 1-4). Since the initial vasoconstrictor phase may be focal or unilateral, so also the subsequent headache may be hemicranial. A suggestion is therefore provided for the enigma of the hemicranial aspect of migraine.

Summary

In summary, migraine can be viewed as a form of relatively benign vasospasm, usually unilateral. It is an episodic disorder produced by the interactions of the central and peripheral autonomic nervous systems, and the extra- and intracranial blood vessels. It involves both central and peripheral vasomotor mechanisms, combined with a sterile inflammatory reaction, neurogenically induced.

Migraine can be viewed as a form of relatively benign vasospasm.

SELF-ASSESSMENT EXAMINATION

1 Headache associated with brain tumor is always more severe than migraine. True or False

2 Headache may be classified into three groups, including vascular, muscle contraction, and traction and inflammatory. True or False

3 The brain parenchyma is itself exquisitely sensitive to touch and pain. True or False

4 Pain pathways for structures above the tentorium cerebelli are contained in the glossopharyngeal and vagus nerves. True or False

5 Migraine is characterized by vasodilation of extracranial blood vessels. True or False

6 Vasoactive amines reduce vascular permeability. True or False

7 Vasoactive amines are implicated in the migraine attack, in addition to extracranial vasodilation. True or False

8 Present evidence implicates the following vasoactive substances as being associated with inflammation: (a) nitroglycerine; (b) peptide kinins; (c) prostaglandins; (d) serotonin; (e) histamine; (f) angiotensin

9 Vasoactive substances may have, among others, the following properties: (a) wheal-and-flare reactions; (b) induction of pain; (c) induction of major hemorrhage; (d) all of the above; (e) none of the above

10 Some characteristics of vasoactive substances, as they apply to migraine, are (a) serotonin levels in plasma rise at the onset of migraine; (b) tyramine provokes histamine release; (c) a vasodilator polypeptide is released into the general circulation during migraine; (d) all of the above; (e) none of the above

11 In the prophylaxis of migraine the following medications may be useful, based on their interaction with vasoactive substances: (a) antiserotonin compounds; (b) nonsteroidal anti-inflammatory drugs; (c) corticosteroids; (d) quinine; (e) diphenylhydantoin

12 Corticosteroids reduce inflammation by (a) inhibiting release of histamine from mast cells; (b) stabilizing lysosomal membranes; (c) suppressing pituitary growth hormone; (d) inhibiting granulation and fibrosis

13 The central manifestations of migraine (a) may produce painless preheadache experiences; (b) are associated with a reduction in blood flow to the cerebral cortex; (c) affect the intracranial vessels

14 Modern concepts of migraine include (a) migraine is considered as a form of benign vasospasm; (b) both central and peripheral autonomic nervous systems are involved; (c) the process includes extracranial and intracranial blood vessels; (d) a sterile inflammation is evoked

ANSWERS:

1—False; 2—True; 3—False; 4—False; 5—False; 6—True; 7—True; 8—b, c, d, e; 9—a, e; 10—e; 11—a, b, c; 12—a, b, d; 13—a, b, c; 14—a, b, c, d

2

Taking a Headache History

A detailed and relevant history geared to the headache patient is the most important factor in making a correct diagnosis. By carefully questioning and directing the inquiry, a specific headache profile evolves which makes the diagnosis in many instances, for the majority of patients with headache have negative neurologic and physical examinations. The essentials of a headache history should be set down in a short, concise manner so that a pattern will evolve and the clinician will be able to identify the kinds of headache that are present.

Headache outlines at the end of this chapter depict the form used for the headache history. We start the headache history by asking the patient for a precise description of headache; it is quite common for a patient to have two or three separate types of headache. The charting of the headache frequency by the patient for a month or two (the headache calendar) often gives clues to the type of headache present. Table 2-1 shows a headache calendar kept by a migraine patient; Table 2-2 depicts migraine with depression.

Onset

We are interested in the specific time of life when the headaches began. Headaches that start in childhood, in adolescence and in the second and third decades of life are often vascular in nature, such as migraine. Headaches which occur later in life suggest an organic etiology or may be due to psychogenic ills such as depression. The occurrence of a headache after a traumatic episode such as a death of a loved one, a serious financial loss, etc., may be a key to an underlying depression. Headaches due to high blood pressure are usually present on awakening and often disappear as the day goes on. Migraine can awaken a patient at three or four o'clock in the morning but, more often, cluster headaches occur at night and frequently awaken the patient several hours after going to sleep. Sinus headache usually begins gradually in the morning and increases in severity during the day. Headache related to anxiety without an obvious depressive component often follows upon a specific stressful incident (for example, the patient whose headache starts with the death of a brother from a brain tumor). Under the general heading of *onset* we also ask about the length of illness. Many migraine or depressive sufferers will give a 20-, 30- or 40-year history of the headache. The chronicity of their headache suggests that we are not dealing with a progressive neurologic lesion. Conversely, the sudden onset of severe headache and diagnostic neurologic signs is much against a self-limited headache syndrome.

Location

It is important to know whether the cephalalgia is generalized over the entire head or whether it is localized on one side. It is

Table 2-1. Headache Calendar

Patient's Name:
Date Started: Oct. 13, 1972

DATE	TIME ONSET ENDING (Insert hr. and am/pm)		(*1) SEVERITY OF HEADACHE	(*2) RELIEF OF HEADACHE	MEDICATION TAKEN AND DOSAGE	(*3) PSYCHIC AND PHYSICAL FACTORS	(*4) FOOD AND DRINK EXCESSES
10-13							
10-14	12 ⁰⁰ noon	4 P	8	3	Cafergot - 2	# 19	
10-15							
10-16							
10-17							
10-18							
10-19							
10-20							
10-21	10 A	12 N	6	3	Cafergot 1		J
10-22							
10-23							
10-24							
10-25							
10-26							
10-27							
10-28							
10-29							
10-30							
10-31							
11-1							
11-2	2 P	3 P	3	2	Cafergot 1	# 15	
11-3							
11-4	4 P	7 P	7	5	Cafergot 3	# 15	L
11-5							
11-6							
11-7							
11-8							
11-9							

also important to know whether the pain switches from one side of the head to the other, for migraine frequently acts in this way. Generalized head pain may indicate psychogenic disease, in the absence of increased intracranial pressure. Focal pain on one side of the head may be migraine but can also be due to organic disease. Pain localized to the eye alone should make one suspicious of their ocular disease or cluster headache. The "hatband" distribution of head pain speaks for muscle contraction headache.

Frequency

Migraine may occur at sporadic intervals during a lifetime. By the time medical advice is sought an identifiable pattern is often ascertained. Commonly, in women there is an association with the menstrual

Headache Keys for Tables 2-1 & 2-3

HEADACHE KEYS

(*1) SEVERITY SCALE

1---⊦---⊥---⊦---5--⊦--⊦--⊦--⊦---10
None   Mild   Moderate   Severe

(*2) RELIEF SCALE

1--⌐---⊦---⊥---5--⊥--⊥--⊥--⌐---10
Complete   Moderate   Mild   No Relief

(*3) PSYCHIC & PHYSICAL FACTORS

1 – Emotional Upset/Family or Friends
2 – Emotional Upset/Occupation
3 – Business/Reversal
4 – Business/Success
5 – Vacation Days
6 – Weekends
7 – Strenuous Exercise
8 – Strenuous Labor
9 – High Altitude Location
10 – Anticipation Anxiety
11 – Crisis/Serious
12 – Post-Crisis Period
13 – New Job/Position
14 – New Move
15 – Menstrual Days
16 – Physical Illness
17 – Over-sleeping
18 – Weather
19 – Other _____

(*4) FOOD & DRINK EXCESSES

A – Ripened Cheeses (Pizza)
B – Herring
C – Chocolate
D – Vinegar
E – Fermented Foods (pickled or marinated)
                 (sour cream/yogurt)
F – Freshly Baked Yeast Products
G – Nuts (Peanut Butter)
H – Monosodium Glutamate (Chinese Foods)
I – Pods of Broad Beans
J – Onions
K – Canned Figs
L – Citrus Foods
M – Bananas
N – Pork
O – Caffeinated Bev. (Colas)
P – Avocado
Q – Fermented Sausage (Cured Cold Cuts)
R – Chicken Livers
S – Wine
T – Alcohol
U – Beer

cycle. Often there is an absence of the headache pattern during vacations and after the third month of pregnancy, but some headaches appear only during periods of relaxation. Cluster headache may be seasonal and often occurs in the spring and fall in bouts lasting from 1 to 2 weeks to 4 or 5 months. Rarely, cluster headache is chronic. The character of muscle contraction headache is one of chronicity and lasts for years, or a lifetime.

Duration

If the headache is due to organic causes, it is usually constant and continuous and progressively increases in intensity. The headache due to migraine is episodic and lasts anywhere from 6 hours to 3 days or even longer. Cluster head pain can last anywhere from several minutes to less than 4 hours. As mentioned above, muscle contraction headache is often persistent.

Severity

The severity of the pain in migraine is often described as intense. Characteristically, it is pulsating or throbbing, rather than a constant pain. The pain of cluster headache is also throbbing, but it is frequently described as deep, boring and very severe. Tic douloureux is a shocklike, transient, stabbing pain, typically neuritic in character. Pain of muscle contraction headache is often dull, nagging and persistent, with occasional exacerbations of more severe pain.

The warning signs of migraine are usually ocular in nature.

Table 2-2. Headache Calendar

Patient's Name:
Date Started: Dec. 30, 1972

DATE	TIME ONSET (Insert hr. and am/pm)	TIME ENDING	(*1) SEVERITY OF HEADACHE	(*2) RELIEF OF HEADACHE	MEDICATION TAKEN AND DOSAGE	(*3) PSYCHIC AND PHYSICAL FACTORS	(*4) FOOD AND DRINK EXCESSES
12/30/72	7 AM	11 A	5	4	Fiorinal x 2	10	
	2 P	8 P	6	4	Fiorinal x 2	10	
12/31/72	6 P	12 AM	8	3	Fiorinal x 4		m, s
1/1/73	10 AM	3 P	9	5	Fiorinal x 4	17	
1/2/73	11 AM	8 P	9	4	Fiorinal x 2	1	
1/3/73	8 P	1 A	9	5	Fiorinal x 3		N
1/4/73	8 AM	11 A	4	3	Fiorinal x 1	8	
1/5/73	6 PM	10 P	10	10	Fiorinal x 4 / Cafergot x 2	11	
1/6/73	11 P	1 A	5	3	Fiorinal x 3	12	
1/7/73	8 A	11 P	4	4	Fiorinal x 2		C
	4 P	9 P	6	8	Fiorinal x 2	1	C
1/8/73	8 A	11 P	8	4	Fiorinal x 4	1	
1/9/73	8 P	12 A	5	3	Fiorinal x 4	6	S
1/10/73	10 A	4 P	4	3	Fiorinal x 2	17	
1/11/73	9 A	11 A	6	4	Fiorinal x 3	2	
1/12/73	6 P	8 P	2	1	Fiorinal x 1	7	
1/13/73	8 A	7 P	10	10	Fiorinal x 4 / Cafergot x 3	15	
1/14/73	9 A	5 P	9	8	Fiorinal x 4	15	
1/15/73	9 A	1 P	6	4	Fiorinal x 2	15	
1/16/73	8 P	12 A	9	7	Fiorinal x 3	15, 1	
1/17/73	8 A	11 A	5	3	Fiorinal x 2	6	U
1/18/73	6 P	9 P	6	4	Fiorinal x 3	17	
1/19/73	8 A	1 P	8	7	Fiorinal x 3 / Cafergot x 1	1, 18	
1/20/73	4 P	9 P	10	10	Fiorinal x 4	1	S
1/21/73	8 A	11 A	4	3	Fiorinal x 2		F
1/22/73	1 P	3 P	3	2	Fiorinal x 1	18	
1/23/73	8 A	2 P	7	6	Fiorinal x 4	6, 18	
1/24/73	4 P	6 P	3	2	Fiorinal x 1		G
1/25/73	10 A	5 P	6	5	Fiorinal x 3	10	

Prodromata

Prodromata, or warning signs, are most common with migraine and are most usually limited to visual symptoms (Table 2-3). It is believed that both the positive and negative eye prodromes originate in the visual cortex portion of the occipital lobe. The metamorphopsias indicate a disturbance of function in the optic radiation of the posterior temporal zone. Other aura may take the form of paresthesias, defects in mobility and, rarely, a disturbance of the sense of smell. Tumors and angiomas of the occipital lobe can also cause teichopsia, or fortification spectra, but they occur more persistently than in migraine.

Associated Symptoms

The migraine attack may include a wide variety of symptoms occurring in associa-

Table 2-3. Ocular Prodromata of Migraine

Positive	Teichopsia, or fortification spectra
	Zig zags
	Flashing lights and colors
Negative	Scotomata
	Hemiopia
Metamorphosia	Illusions of distorted size, shape and location of fixed objects

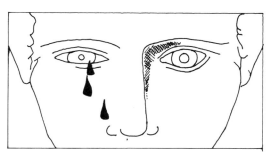

Fig 2-1. *Horner syndrome and cluster headache: enophthalmos, ptosis of the eyelid, myosis of the pupil, lacrimation.*

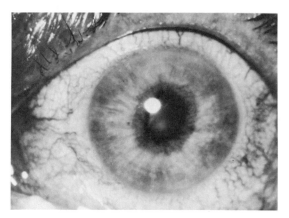

Fig 2-2. *Steamy cornea indicates overt glaucoma.*

tion with the pain. Photophobia, nausea, vomiting and urinary and focal neurologic changes may be seen. With cluster headache, a modified Horner's syndrome may appear, including ptosis and constriction of the pupil (Fig 2-1). Lacrimation, a flushing of the face and a mucoid discharge from the nostril on the side of the headache are often present with the cluster headache. Overt glaucoma is characterized by a steamy cornea and difficulty in seeing (Fig 2-2). If subarachnoid hemorrhage has occurred, meningeal signs will appear rapidly. Sudden loss of power in the arms or legs with associated headache suggests a stroke, either thrombotic or hemorrhagic. Be alert to unilateral tinnitus or diplopia, which may be evidence of an intracranial mass. Associated epilepsy is usually an ominous sign.

Sleep Habits

Difficulty in falling asleep is indicative of anxiety. The doctor should look for an environmental stress syndrome, or psychologic factors which may be producing the problem. If the patient has frequent and early awakening, depression is suggested and questioning should be directed toward a possible depressive illness. Migraine patients can be awakened by severe headache during the night, but are usually helped by sleep. Cluster headache patients are frequently awakened by their severe head pain and the intensity of the pain forces them into ceaseless activity until the attack subsides.

Precipitating Factors

Among the multiple factors which precipitate migraine are fatigue, loss of sleep, stress, menstruation, bright sunlight and foods and drugs containing tyramine and other vasoactive materials. Less common factors include alcohol, prolonged hunger and high humidity. Cough headache, contrary to popular belief, is not always associated with an intracranial tumor, can often be benign and may occur as a part of a vascular headache syndrome.

Emotional Factors

The patient's relationship to his family, occupation, social life, environmental stresses and sexual habits should all be ascertained by the interviewer in detail. Emotional factors such as these have special relevance to his headache. Careful questioning about other physical, emotional and psychic symptoms may uncover an underlying psychologic illness that has been masked by the cephalalgic patient. Overt depression will be obvious to the interviewer. It is possible to uncover a stressful situation with associated anxiety by doing a simple inventory of the factors mentioned above.

Relationship to Occupation

Emotional factors and stress on the job are common headache causatives. There are certain specific occupations, however, that have a built-in predisposition to head pain. Those dealing with the public in the provision of services are particularly susceptible. Abattoir workers are subject to Q fever, with intense headache as one of the symptoms. The nitrites to which munitions workers are exposed cause vasodilatation of the cerebral vessels and mimic vascular headaches. Mechanics and others who work in poorly ventilated areas can get headaches from the carbon monoxide in their atmosphere.

Some environmental exposures will cause headaches.

Family History

Migraine is a familial illness, while cluster headache is not. Depression also is frequent in families. Studies suggest a hereditary relationship of migraine. If both parents have had migraine, there is a 70% chance that the children will also have migraine; if only one parent has had migraine, the chances are reduced to about 45%. If neither parent has had migraine, but there is a history of migraine in other family members, it will occur in perhaps 25% of the children.

Seasonal Relationship

Cluster headaches are more common in the spring and fall. Depression with chronic headache often occurs during happy periods of the year, such as Christmas.

Menstrual and Obstetric Factors

A common type of migraine occurs with the onset of menses. It tends to disappear by the third month of pregnancy only to return after the birth of the child. Migraine in women often disappears with onset of menopause. The administration of hormones in the postmenopausal period can prolong the headache syndrome. Conversely, migraine which reappears at the time of the menopause may be improved by ingestion of estrogens.

Medical History

Questions should always be asked regarding recent or remote head trauma. Subdural hematomas may occur after trivial blows. A recent spinal tap done for reasons of anesthesia or diagnosis may cause a self-limited headache. A low spinal fluid pres-

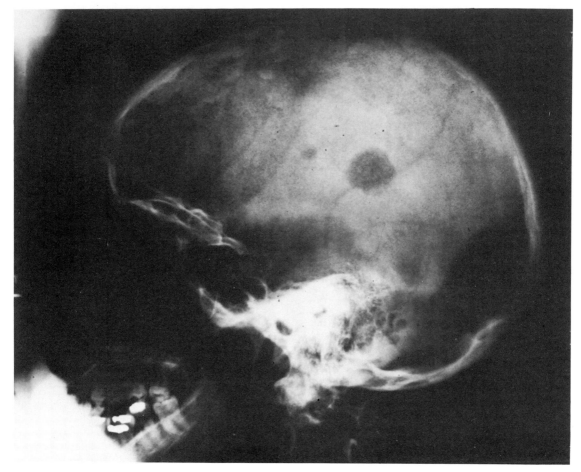

Fig 2-3. *Multiple lucencies in a patient with previous carcinoma of the breast complaining of nonspecific headache.*

sure syndrome has been described, which can be associated with a chronic subdural hematoma. A history of seizures, one-sided headache and neck stiffness should make one question whether there is an aneurysm or angioma present with a slow leak.

Surgical History

If a person has had surgery on a mole or other tumor it may follow that the tumor has metastasized to the brain, producing headache (Fig. 2-3). A past history of tuberculosis may have significance as to possible spread to the brain. Obviously, any previous cranial surgery will alert the physician to previous head trauma, tumor,

aneurysm or other brain disease of significance.

Systems Review

A complete, careful review of the systems should be done in all headache work-ups. Disease of the eyes, ears, nose, throat, teeth and neck should be emphasized, for all may produce local head pain.

Allergy

The relationship of headache to seasonal allergy should be sought. Patients may experience increased headaches accompanying their hay fever or seasonal allergy symp-

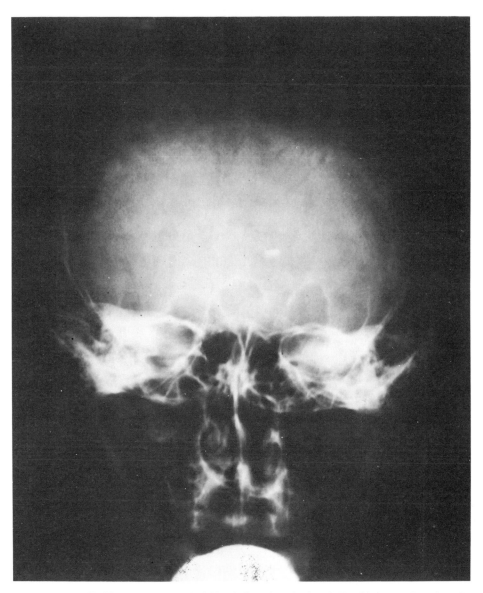

Fig 2-4. *Routine skull films may reveal shift of the pineal gland. In this case the pineal gland is significantly shifted to the left, suggesting a mass in some part of the right hemisphere, or atrophy on the left. Further neurologic diagnostic studies would be indicated.*

toms, as a part of an increased capacity for vasomotor activity. We have not been able to show, however, that migraine or other forms of headache result from a specific antigen-antibody reaction.

Previous Tests for Headache

We see countless patients who have had repeated, sophisticated work-ups, including angiograms and pneumoencephalograms. The age and adequacy of these studies, considered with the history and current physical findings, dictate whether or not these studies should be repeated. Headache may be associated with metabolic diseases, such as hypothyroidism, or with significant anemia. There is, therefore, no substitute for an adequate medical survey. However, if the patient has had an adequate work-

Chemical Factors

Certain headache patients have a chemical sensitivity to tyramine-containing foods and other vasoactive substances. Below is a diet used at the Diamond Headache Clinic:

Avoid:

Ripened cheeses (cheddar, emmentaler, gruyere, stilton, brie, and camembert)

(Cheeses Permissible: American, cottage, cream and Velveeta)

Herring

Chocolate

Vinegar (except white vinegar)

Anything fermented, pickled or marinated

Sour cream, yogurt

Nuts, peanut butter

Hot fresh breads, raised coffeecakes and doughnuts

Pods of broad beans (lima, navy and pea pods)

Any foods containing large amounts of monosodium glutamate (Chinese foods)

Onion

Canned figs

Citrus foods (no more than 1 orange per day)

Bananas (no more than ½ banana per day)

Pizza

Pork (no more than 2–3 times per week)

Excessive tea, coffee, cola beverages (no more than 4 cups per day)

Avocado

Fermented sausage (bologna, salami, pepperoni, summer and hot dogs)

Chicken livers

Avoid all alcoholic beverages, if possible. If you must drink, no more than two normal size drinks.

Suggested drinks: Haute sauterne
                    Riesling
                    Seagram's VO
                    Cutty Sark
                    Vodka

up previously and you have no neurologic or historic reasons to do any further tests, it is prudent to avoid repeating expensive and potentially dangerous studies.

Past Medications and Their Effectiveness

This can be a key to the diagnosis as well as the treatment. For example, if we know that ergotamine tartrate has helped a patient previously, we can assume that we are probably dealing with migraine. If the patient has had a trial on antidepressants with some success, the likelihood of a depression is increased. Therefore, a history of past medications and their successes and/or failures acts both as a diagnostic and therapeutic clue to management of this patient.

A patient may be taking medications that cause headaches.

Present Medications and Their Effectiveness

You should also ascertain the medications currently employed by the patient. We see many a migrainous or depressed person taking reserpine, which tends to promote both conditions. Migraine may be increased in severity and frequency by birth control pills. We know that nitrates can activate migraine in certain susceptible people. Indomethacin is another drug that can on occasion cause chronic head pain. The physician should pursue with vigor the drug history of the patient (see Chapter 11).

Case Histories

Headache 1: Migraine
(Figs 2–5, 2–6)

Mr. D. F. is 38 years old and describes episodic headaches involving one side of

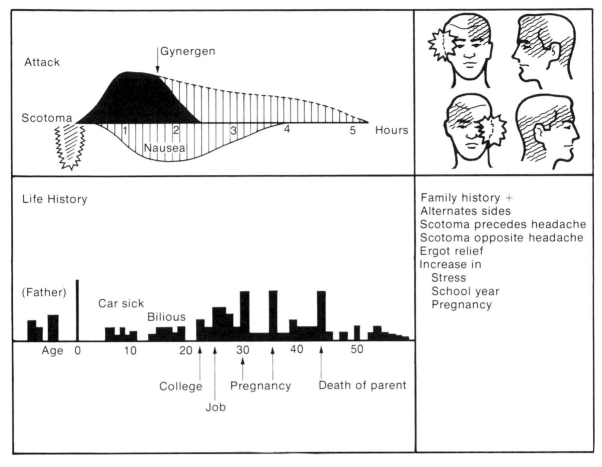

Fig 2-5. *Classic migraine. [Adapted with permission of Graham J: Seven common headache profiles. Neurology **13**:3, Part 2, 16–23, Copyright New York Times Media Company.]*

his head. His father and his only son have a similar problem. As a child he was easily carsick, found it difficult to play twirling games and had recurrent episodes of unexplained vomiting without diarrhea, which puzzled the family pediatrician. His headaches began at age 15 and have continued to the present. They appear perhaps four to six times a year, and often begin in mid morning. He notes initially a slight loss of vision in part of his visual field, following which he sees twinkling lights and a series of jagged lines which he can sometimes draw on paper. These visual images appear in both eyes. Promptly thereafter, as the visual images cease, his headache begins. It is localized to one side of the head but with different episodes may shift from side to side. The pain is severe and pounding, increases with bending over or straining, and is not particularly relieved by lying down. Shortly after the pain begins, he experiences significant nausea and vomiting and may vomit repeatedly. Bright lights and sound bother him—he must leave work and return home, where he retires to his bedroom, pulls the blind and tries to sleep. If he can get to sleep he may waken free of headache. After approximately 24 hours the headache begins to wane and is usually gone by 48 hours; then he is left depleted, with a feeling of exhaustion. His physician has diagnosed his problem as migraine and has given him ergot derivatives for treatment. If D. F. takes these early in the course of the headache, he can sometimes abort the episode.

D. F. is recognized by his co-workers to

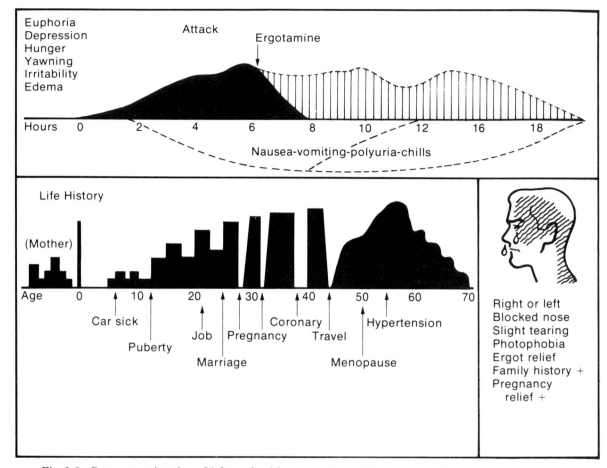

Fig 2-6. *Common migraine. [Adapted with permission of Graham J: Seven common headache profiles. Neurology **13**:3, Part 2, 16–23, Copyright New York Times Media Company.]*

be extremely competent and meticulous to a fault. He is compulsive about details and consistently checks the work of subordinates carefully. He tends to be grim and unsmiling but, after a few drinks, loosens up and has an excellent sense of humor. His superiors recognize him as a man of talent and have marked him for rapid advancement to an executive position.

Headache 1 Outline

Types	One
Onset	At age 15
Location	Unilateral
Frequency	Once every two months
Duration	One to two days
Severity	Severe
Aura	Twinkling lights, jagged lines
Associated symptoms	Nausea and vomiting, photosensitivity; sound bothers him; pain is better lying down
Sleep pattern	Not affected
Emotional status	Perfectionist … compulsive … likes to get things done
Family history	Father and son with headaches
Seasonal	Not related
Allergy	None—no foods bring on headaches

Headache 2: Migraine With Depression

E. B. is a homemaker, aged 37, who enjoys good health with the exception of incapacitating headaches. She started having one-sided headaches at age 18 which were diagnosed as migraine but were helped by the ingestion of Ergomar® tablets given her by the family doctor.

These migraine-type headaches occurred almost once weekly and lasted 2 to 3 days, accompanied by an aura of flashing lights about ½ hour before the headache. The patient also noted that she has severe headaches with her periods and that the migraines seem worse since she started taking birth control pills. When the headache is severe she also has nausea and vomiting and occasionally sees black spots before her eyes. E. B. has a very neat house with everything in its place and always finishes her housework and other projects. She notices that chocolate will bring on headaches, and remembers that her grandmother also had headaches.

Three years ago, E. B. started having another type of headache which was present on both sides of her head and included the cervical spine. Upon questioning, E. B. revealed that she and her husband have been having marital problems for the past 4 years. This second type of headache is always present upon awakening. She has problems falling asleep but is always awake early in the morning, usually by 4:30 or 5:00 AM. E. B. feels depressed due to her headaches; she is losing interest in her home and children. She tries to sleep to escape, and usually feels fatigued. She states she cannot tolerate the pain much longer as it lasts all day and sometimes into the night. E. B. was placed on Bellergal® Spacetabs®, b.i.d.; Ergomar® p.r.n., and Elavil® 50 mg h.s. Birth control pills were discontinued. After 3 weeks she began to show some improvement and is being followed carefully now in the headache clinic.

Headache 2 Outline

Types	Two, (A) and (B)
Onset	(A) At age 18
	(B) Three years ago
Location	(A) Usually left side; starts behind left eye and spreads to entire left side
	(B) Bilateral—including cervical spine
Frequency	(A) Once weekly
	(B) Daily
Duration	(A) Two to 3 days
	(B) All day
Severity	(A) Always severe
	(B) Moderate to severe
Aura	(A) Flashing lights ½ hour before headache
	(B) None
Associated symptoms	(A) Nausea and vomiting; occasionally sees black spots
	(B) None
Sleep pattern	Difficulty falling asleep. Stays asleep. Occasional early awakening at 5 AM for no known reason
Emotional status	Some depression for 3 to 4 years due to martial problems . . . tries to get things done . . . perfectionist
Family history	Maternal grandmother had migraines
Seasonal	Not related
Menses	Gets left-sided headaches with periods. On Ovral® birth control pills
Medical history	Negative
Surgical history	Negative
Allergy	None to medications or foods; chocolate brings on a headache
Tests	None
Medications	Plain Darvon® 65 mg, p.r.n. (no help); Ergomar®, p.r.n. (helps relieve migraines); Valium® 5 mg, q.i.d. (no help)

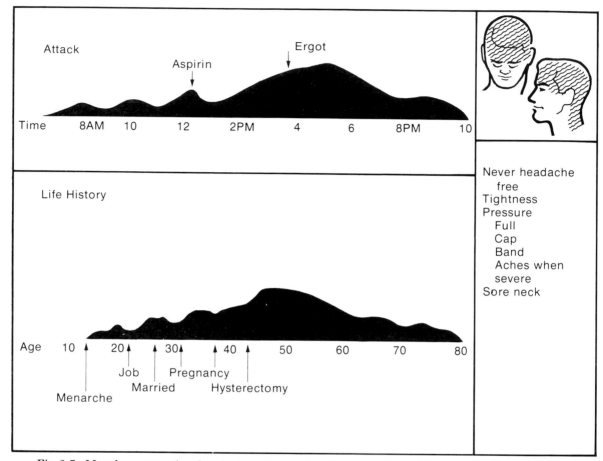

Fig 2-7. *Muscle contraction headache. [Adapted with permission of Graham J: Seven common headache profiles.* Neurology **13**:3, *Part 2, 16–23, Copyright New York Times Media Company.]*

Headache 3: Muscle Contraction (Fig 2-7)

W. B. is aged 59 and has complained of headaches for 20 years. They occur almost daily. They are not well localized but he often describes a band of pain about his forehead that waxes and wanes. Sometimes he notes pain in the neck and lower part of the head. He takes large amounts of over-the-counter medications, switching from one to another, seemingly dependent upon the vagaries of the latest television headache commercials. By his own admission he is an aspirin-popper. He has been to many physicians and has been subjected to examinations and testing, but no cause

for these headaches has been found. In addition to headache, he describes chronic fatigue, which is not relieved by rest. Indeed, he sleeps poorly, has problems getting to sleep and often wakes early in the morning. He often has a vague sense of being unwell. He has withdrawn from many social activities; they tire him and are too much trouble besides. He would rather stay at home now. He has lost his appetite for sex. He is irritable, has trouble concentrating and has a "short fuse." He is more emotional than formerly, feeling at times that he might weep without reason.

He recently reported to his physician and another unsuccessful neurologic survey was done. His physician then wisely referred

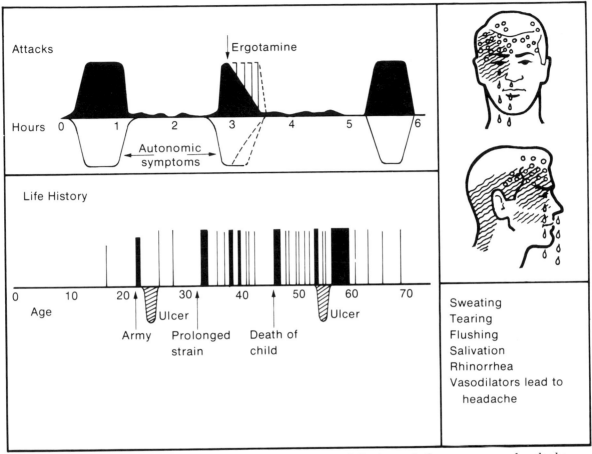

Fig 2-8. *Cluster headache. [Adapted with permission of Graham J: Seven common headache profiles.* Neurology **13:**3, Part 2, 16–23, Copyright New York Times Media Company.]

W. B. to a clinical psychologist where psychologic testing was performed. This revealed a marked masked depression expressed particularly as body complaints. After a period of antidepressant therapy and counseling he is somewhat improved and his headaches are better though not entirely relieved. He continues to consume rather large amounts of aspirin regularly.

Headache 3 Outline

Types	One
Onset	At age 39
Location	Pain about forehead; occasional pain in cervical spine and occiput
Frequency	Almost daily
Duration	Daily
Severity	Severe
Aura	None
Associated symptoms	None
Emotional status	Feels unwell, irritable, nervous and depressed
Sleep pattern	Problems getting to sleep; often has early awakening
Family history	None
Seasonal	Not related

Headache 4: Cluster (Fig 2-8)

R. B., aged 45, is a successful contractor who has always enjoyed good health. He was a former athlete but in recent years has exercised little and has gained 30 pounds in the last decade. He smokes heavily, and on occasion drinks to excess. About 2 years ago he had a series of excruciating, usually nocturnal, headaches, which began suddenly, lasted 3 weeks, and then ceased spontaneously. His physician was contacted at that time but offered no explanation for these episodes.

One month ago the nocturnal headaches began again. They often waken him at 3 AM, and are localized to and above the left eye. The left eye waters copiously with the onset of headache. The left side of the nose is plugged initially and then runs later. His left eye becomes very red, perhaps because he rubs it. The pain is steady and intense, severe enough to make this stolid man cry for help. The pain usually lasts 45 minutes and then rapidly clears; thereafter, he feels perfectly well. He has noticed, however, that even small amounts of alcohol can reproduce this set of symptoms and so he has stopped drinking completely in the last month. His physician was contacted again and advised R. B. that he was working too hard and was too tense. He went away for a week's vacation but the headaches continued. He began to worry that he might have a brain tumor. In the last several days, however, the headaches have again begun to disappear and are no longer so intense. He has not responded to any of several pain medications provided by his physician.

Headache 4 Outline

Types	One
Onset	Two years ago
Location	Above left eye
Frequency	Nightly
Duration	45 minutes
Severity	Severe
Aura	None
Associated symptoms	Left eye tears; nose stuffy
Allergy	None; alcohol brings on headache
Sleep pattern	Not affected
Emotional status	None
Family history	None
Seasonal	Spring and fall

Headache 5: Subarachnoid Hemorrhage (Fig 2-9)

J. S., a 29-year-old man, was in his usual state of good health. He maintained his weight at moderate levels and practiced abstemious habits. A recent complete physical examination had been within normal limits. He had never complained of headache. Two weeks ago, while jogging, he experienced a sudden and severe head pain involving his entire head; the pain did not wax and wane and was not relieved by rest. He became ill and vomited, and found no relief from aspirin, codeine or an ice pack applied to his head by his wife. Shortly thereafter he became sleepy and was not easily roused. His wife recognized immediately that a serious illness had occurred, and brought him to the emergency room of a hospital close by, but he could not walk from the car to the examining room. On admission he was restless and moaning in pain, and could not give an adequate history. One pupil had become dilated but other signs of neurologic damage were not prominent. He was not paralyzed. He had developed slight stiffness of the neck. A spinal tap was done within the hour and the spinal fluid obtained was bloody. After consultation among several specialists, angiograms were done which showed a leaking aneurysm of one of the brain arteries. This was eventually clipped successfully by a neurosurgeon and J. S. is now recovering rapidly.

Headache 5 Outline

Types	One
Onset	Age 29; two weeks prior to first visit

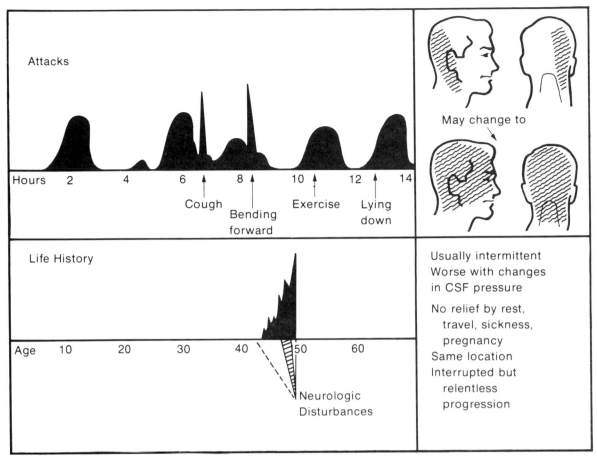

Fig 2-9. *Aneurysm and angioma. [Adapted with permission of Graham J: Seven common headache profiles.* Neurology **13**:3, Part 2, 16–23, Copyright New York Times Media Company.]

Location	Entire head; occurred while jogging	Medical history	Negative
Frequency	One—the initial attack	Surgical history	Negative
Duration	Constant and unrelenting		
Severity	Severe	Allergy	None to medications or food
Aura	None		
Associated symptoms	Vomiting, gradually became drowsy and comatose, dilation of one pupil, slight stiffness of the neck	Tests	No previous examinations done
		Medications	Aspirin, codeine; no relief
Sleep pattern	Not affected		
Emotional status	None related		
Family history	None with headaches		
Seasonal	Not related		

Headache 6: Brain Tumor (Fig 2-10)

L. R., aged 60, began to note difficulty with his vision. He stated that his vision to the right was impaired. He found it difficult to

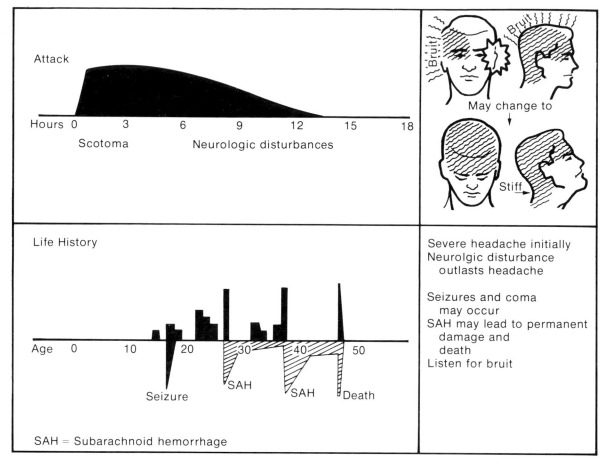

Fig 2-10. *Brain tumor. [Adapted with permission of Graham J: Seven common headache profiles. Neurology* **13:**3, *Part 2, 16–23, Copyright New York Times Media Company.]*

read. He was bumping into objects on the right side of his environment. He saw an ophthalmologist who performed visual fields and elicited a field defect, although the patient's cooperation was not optimal.

L. R. has a long history of chronic frontal and temporal headaches which he associates with hay fever and sinusitis. He says that this has not increased, but during the course of the interview and examination he later states that he has more pain in the left side of the head which is relatively constant and now not easily relieved by medications. He describes great turmoil recently associated with problems with the Internal Revenue Service. These business difficulties have been very trying and he blames many of his current complaints on them. He takes large amounts of medication, including a sleeping pill, a tranquilizer, and an antihistamine, and he uses cigarettes and alcohol liberally.

When examined, he had a significant loss of visual acuity with a definite visual field cut on the right. His recent memory was poor. His speech was slow and suggested sedation. There was minimal weakness of the right leg. The patient followed directions poorly and seemed confused.

He was admitted to a hospital where appropriate studies were done and a mass lesion was found in the left temporal and occipital area of the brain. He was transferred to a neurosurgical facility where a well-circumscribed and encapsulated tumor was removed. The patient has made an excellent recovery, is now free of headaches and is no longer confused, but still has a slight right visual field defect. He continues to complain of difficulties with the Internal Revenue Service.

Headache 6 Outline

Types	One
Onset	One year
Location	Frontal and temporal areas
Frequency	Constant
Duration	All day and night
Severity	Moderate to severe
Aura	None
Associated symptoms	Vision impaired; speech slowed; some confusion
Sleep pattern	Has trouble falling asleep
Emotional status	Irritable
Family history	None
Seasonal	Not related

Headache 7: Brain Tumor

Mrs. W. T., aged 29, had complained for 2 months of "spin-outs," a sensation of unsteadiness and unreality associated with the feeling she might fall. She has had mild headaches in the left frontal area and above the left ear, but these have been relieved by aspirin until recently. Now, however, she notes an increase in headache, particularly when she coughs. She describes early morning nausea and loss of appetite. Her speech has slowed appreciably and has recently seemed slurred at times, and she sleeps often. She is forgetful. Her husband notes that her handwriting appears sloppy. He has also commented on intermittent twitching of the right side of her face and right hand. These complaints have progressed rapidly and inexorably.

When examined by her physician there were signs of increased pressure in the head, with weakness of the right arm and hand. She was admitted to a hospital where x-rays of the skull were done, which were normal, but the electroencephalogram and brain scan showed a mass lesion in the left frontal area of the brain. Operation was attempted, but the tumor which was found was too large to be removed. It did not respond to radiation therapy after surgery. Six months after the onset of symptoms, Mrs. W. T. was dead.

Headache 7 Outline

Types	One
Onset	Left frontal area—above left ear
Duration	All day
Frequency	Daily
Severity	Moderate to severe
Aura	None
Associated symptoms	Vertigo; nausea and loss of appetite; speech slurs; forgetful; handwriting sloppy; twitching of right face and head
Sleep pattern	Headache keeps her awake
Emotional status	Agitated since headaches started
Family history	None
Seasonal	Not related
Menses	Not related

SELF-ASSESSMENT EXAMINATION

1 Migraine often begins in childhood. True or False

2 Headache appearing after emotional trauma may be related to depression. True or False

3 The "hatband" distribution of head pain is common in migraine. True or False

4 Cluster headache frequently appears in bouts or clusters, interspersed with periods free from headache. True or False

5 Pain of vascular headache is often described as throbbing. True or False

6 Tic douloureux is a chronic nagging pain in the face. True or False

7 The visual prodromata of migraine most often originate in the occipital cortex. True or False

8 Migraine is sometimes associated with the following signs and symptoms: (a) photophobia; (b) nausea; (c) vomiting; (d) paresthesias; (e) defects in motility

9 Disturbances of sleep are often associated with (a) cluster headache; (b) depression; (c) migraine; (d) cerebral aneurysms and angiomas

10 Tyramine, a vasoactive substance, is contained in (a) cheese; (b) herring; (c) chocolate; (d) all of the above; (e) none of the above

11 The family history of headache is an important diagnostic clue in (a) temporal arteritis; (b) cluster headache; (c) migraine; (d) subdural hematoma; (e) trigeminal neuralgia

12 Migraine associated with menstrual cycles often (a) disappears with pregnancy; (b) is increased during pregnancy; (c) is less frequent after the menopause; (d) may be exacerbated by ingestion of estrogens

13 Allergic symptoms (a) are always associated with migraine; (b) bear a direct relationship to the appearance of cluster headache; (c) all of the above; (d) none of the above

---

ANSWERS:

1—True; 2—True; 3—False; 4—True; 5—True; 6—False; 7—True; 8—a,b,c,d,e; 9—a,b,c; 10—a,b; 11—c; 12—a,c,d; 13—d

Physical and Neurologic Examination of the Headache Patient

Every headache patient, after an all-inclusive history, deserves a complete physical and neurologic examination. Often there will be no significant findings, but this cannot be assumed, even if the medical history suggests a specific diagnosis. An outline of the examination covers

- general survey and physical examination
- mental state
- head
- cervical spine
- cerebellar functions
- cranial nerves
- motor functions
- sensory functions
- pathologic reflexes

General Survey and Physical Examination

The facial characteristics and overall actions of a headache patient may give clues to the diagnosis. Depressed patients are frequently easy to spot by the down-turning of the corners of their mouths and their generally sad appearance (Fig 3-1). The migraine patient may have her clothes neatly folded and will often fold her paper examination gown upon completion of the examination. Meticulous attention to personal appearance is a clue to the migrainous subject. Lists of symptoms and medications and careful documentation of headache frequency are other characteristics of the migraine patient (Fig 3-2).

The cluster patient may, during an attack, exhibit a complete or partial Horner's syndrome with ptosis, a constricted pupil of the affected eye and flushing of the face; eye and nasal lacrimation may also occur. J. R. Graham (1968) has described, and we have confirmed, the typical facial characteristics seen in a cluster patient: flushed appearance, square jaw, accentuated glabellar creases, thick chin and well-chiseled lower lip. Careful examination of the skin reveals telangiectases, coarse cheek skin (peau d'orange) and accentuated skin folds (Figs 3-3, 3-4).

Sometimes the diagnosis of facial pain is obvious, for example as in postherpetic neuralgia where there are trophic changes in the skin related to the antecedent viral infection (Fig 3-5). Evidences of neurofibromatosis, with more than five accompanying brownish disk lesions of the skin (cafe-au-lait spots), may indicate an increased predilection for intracranial tumors, particularly neuromas and meningiomas (Fig 3-6). Angiomata of the skin makes one suspicious of intracranial angioma. External evidences of hypothyroidism, including puffy, dry skin, brittle hair and loss of hair, can be associated with headache. We have seen several patients with hypothyroidism and bizarre chronic headache of an uncertain type. Pituitary deficiency with smooth skin, lack of body hair and testicular atrophy may also be an infrequent cause of chronic headache, if a pituitary tumor is present.

One should question the headache patient carefully regarding surgical scars, since these can be a clue to cerebral metastases, especially from lesions such as melanomas.

The general physical examination may reveal many disparate illnesses which can cause headache. Hypertension, coarctation of the aorta and abnormalities of the cervical spine are but a few.

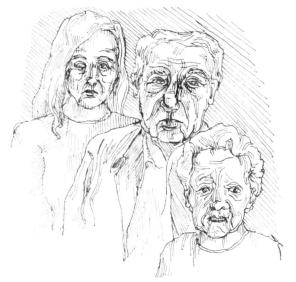

Fig 3-1. *Depression.*

Physical examination may reveal many illnesses causing headache.

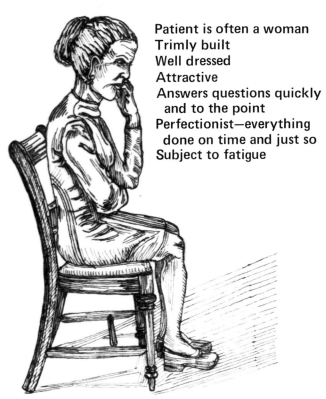

**Patient is often a woman
Trimly built
Well dressed
Attractive
Answers questions quickly
  and to the point
Perfectionist—everything
  done on time and just so
Subject to fatigue**

Fig 3-2. *Frequent characteristics of migraine patients.*

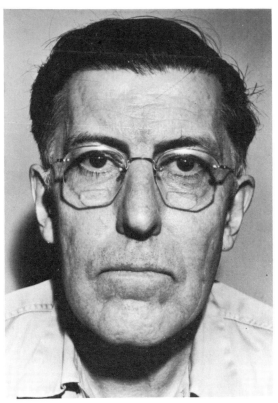

Fig 3-3. *Patient exhibits typical facial characteristics of cluster headache.*

A reflex "autonomic headache" can be caused by a distended bladder and should be sought in the general physical examination. Although headache caused by distended bladder is most common in paraplegics, it can occur in others.

Mental State

This subject has been covered in part during the gathering of the history, but can be further assessed during the physical examination. Examine orientation, memory, intelligence and speech. Obvious indications of either anxiety or depression may be present. Agitation and ceaseless activity may be evident. Failure to carry out the necessary tasks of the examination suggests inattention or dementia. Aphasia and other disorders of speech occurring in a right-handed person indicate a lesion of the left hemisphere. Memory impairment for re-

cent events and failure to remember relevant details discussed only a few minutes before should alert the examiner to early dementia which, if accompanied by chronic headache, will require intensive neurologic investigation.

Head

A careful examination of the head is required in all patients suffering cephalalgic pain. Evidence of local infection, hardened temporal arteries (temporal arteritis), a trigger point (tic douloureux), dysfunction of the temporal mandibular joint with spasm of muscles of mastication and crepitus, and tenderness over one of the sinus areas should be carefully sought in all patients. One should perform auscultation of the head and neck, searching for bruits which may be a clue to a possible aneurysm,

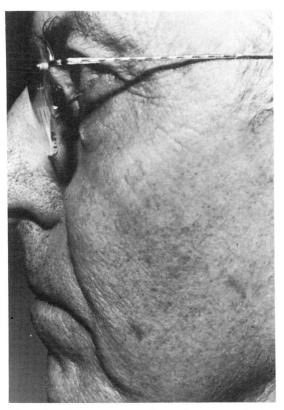

Fig 3-4. *Closer examination of same patient reveals telangiectasis, peau d'orange and accentuated skin folds.*

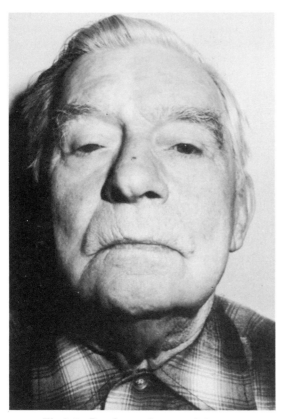

Fig 3-5. *Postherpetic neuralgia.*

carotid stenosis or angioma. Headache which occurs with coughing or with to-and-fro movements of the head may indicate a midline lesion, such as a cyst of the third ventricle.

Cervical Spine

Muscle spasm, rigidity and reduced range of motion of the cervical spine can be indicative of muscle and/or spinal disease of the neck as a cause of chronic head and neck pain. Cervical spondylosis with headache is common in the elderly.

Cerebellar Functions

Cerebellar tumors, primary or metastatic, cerebellopontine angle tumors and large acoustic neuronomas may produce dyscoordination and signs of truncal ataxia with associated difficulties in equilibrium and steady movement. A wide-based gait is a common early manifestation of cerebellar disease. Abnormal finger-to-nose and/or heel-to-knee tests are often indications of cerebellar dysfunction. Headache is relatively uncommon in cerebellar disorders unless increased intracranial pressure develops.

Cranial Nerves

Olfactory Nerve (I)

Loss of sense of smell is most often due to local pathology in the nose and its accessory structures. A head injury or a tumor of the olfactory nerve in the olfactory groove may cause a unilateral disturbance of smell. If there is accompanying mental confusion, a frontotemporal tumor is suspected.

Tests may indicate cranial nerve dysfunction causing headache.

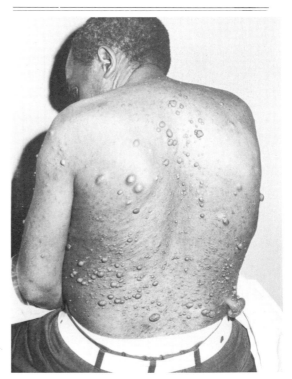

Fig 3-6. *Neurofibromatosis.*

Optic Nerve (II)

An eye examination is most important and must be included in the study of every headache patient. Simple observation may reveal the "steamed cornea" so typical of overt glaucoma. Testing of the pressure with the fingers can also elicit a difference in pressure between the two eyes. This should be confirmed with a tonometer. Gross examination of the visual fields should be performed and, if the exam is in any way abnormal, the visual fields should be plotted. Examination of the fundi is imperative since evidence of papilledema, optic atrophy, hemorrhages or exudates may indicate an organic brain lesion, hypertension or diabetes, among other things.

Oculomotor Nerve (III), Trochlear Nerve (IV)

A patient who complains of sudden pain behind the eye, with an accompanying third nerve palsy, should be evaluated for an expanding aneurysm. If the pupil on one side shows progressive enlargement, progressive compression of the oculomotor nerve is suggested. Herniation of the temporal lobe through the tentorium should be suspected (Table 3-1).

Abducens Nerve (VI)

Lesions, such as a lateral sinus thrombosis, may produce a unilateral sixth nerve paralysis. Bilateral sixth nerve paralyses may occur in acute hydrocephalus or cerebral edema.

Trigeminal Nerve (V)

The face and mucous membranes of the head should be examined for the trigger points of trigeminal neuralgia. Corneal testing should be performed with a wisp of cotton. Motor function of the trigeminal nerve is tested by opening the jaw against resistance.

Facial Nerve (VII)

This nerve is evaluated by testing the motor power of the facial muscles. Evidences of a residual stroke or facial palsy may be elicited.

Remember that the upper part of the face is bilaterally innervated, and that the lower part of the face is contralaterally innervated. There are four possible levels of facial nerve dysfunction on a peripheral basis, as follows, from above downward:

1 A lesion at or proximal to the geniculate ganglion will lead to loss of tearing of the ipsilateral eye, hyperacusis, paralysis of the facial muscles and loss of taste of the anterior two thirds of the tongue.

2 A lesion above the origin of the muscle to the stapedius gives rise to all of the findings mentioned above, but loss of tearing of the ipsilateral eye will not be noted.

Table 3-1. Clinical Manifestations of Temporal Lobe Herniation

Compressed structure	Clinical manifestations
1. Third cranial nerve	Dilated pupil ipsilateral to herniation
2. Midbrain	
Physiologic transection	Decerebrate rigidity
Reticular formation	Impairment of consciousness progressing to coma
Ipsilateral cerebral peduncle (direct compression)	Contralateral hemiparesis progressing to hemiplegia
Occlusion of aqueduct of Sylvius	Headache due to acute hydrocephalus
Contralateral cerebral peduncle (displaced against the sharp free edge of the tentorium)	Hemiparesis ipsilateral to herniation (false localizing sign)
3. Posterior cerebral artery as it crosses the tentorial edge to reach the occipital lobe (calcarine cortex)	Contralateral homonymous hemianopsia, false localizing sign

3 Involving the facial nerve in the facial canal above the origin of the chorda tympani gives rise to the lesions mentioned above, excluding hyperacusis and loss of tearing of ipsilateral eye.

4 Involving the facial nerve at the stylomastoid foramen or below produces weakness of the facial muscles. Taste, hearing and tearing are unaffected.

With a suprasegmental facial paresis, the lower part of the face is more profoundly affected than the brow, since the brow is bilaterally innervated.

The face may also be affected in lesions of the basal ganglia as in Parkinson's disease. Here lack of movement of the face is primarily noted.

Auditory Nerve (VIII)

Both cochlear and vestibular functions should be tested. Simple tests of hearing should be done. Procedures such as calorics and rotational tests may be necessary. Unilateral tinnitus and deafness should always be investigated, to rule out an acoustic neuroma. Posterior fossa myelography and angiography may be necessary.

Glossopharyngeal, Vagus, Accessory and Hypoglossal Nerves (IX, X, XI, XII)

Most often involvement of these structures is not associated with serious headache problems. Lingual pain may occur in cranial arteritis. Bilateral absence of the pharyngeal reflex may be a hysteric phenomenon, but disease of the brainstem should also be ruled out.

Motor Functions

Basically there are three motor systems. These include:

1 The pyramidal or corticospinal system. Lesions of this system produce paralysis or weakness, spasticity and hyperactive deep tendon reflexes.

2 Lesions of the extrapyramidal system produce instability of posture and disorders of muscle tone, as well as slowness of movement in nonparalyzed limbs.

3 The cerebellar system involves primarily accuracy of movements of the trunk and limbs. The cerebellum can be divided into two basic functional parts. The vermis is related to movements of the trunk, while the hemispheres serve especially coordination of the extremities, particularly the arms. It is also important to remember that the cerebellar tracts cross twice so that a lesion involving the right cerebellar hemisphere gives difficulty with the right arm and right leg.

Lower motor neuron disease is characterized by wasting, weakness, atrophy and loss of deep tendon reflexes, depending upon the extent of the lesion.

Sensory Functions

Central or peripheral lesions of the nervous system can be uncovered by careful sensory testing. Two-point discrimination is particularly important in assessing cortical sensation. A disturbance of astereognosis, or failure to recognize the size or shape of objects, can be the only sign of a parietal lobe tumor.

Remember that the basic sensory pathway consists of a three-neuron pattern. The primary sensory neuron has its cell body outside the central nervous system, usually in the dorsal root ganglia. The second neuron must cross the midline. The third neuron must have its cell body in the opposite thalamus and radiates thence to the cortex. A large proportion of the sensory cortex is taken up by sensation from the face, especially the mouth and tongue, and by the hand, especially the thumb and first finger. This may in part be responsible for the common complaints of abnormalities of head and neck sensation, especially head and neck pain.

The integrity of the parietal lobes is always responsible for normal perception of the body image. If there is loss of parietal function, extinction may occur. The patient will deny appreciation of sensation of the body subserved by the diseased parietal lobe when bilateral sensory testing is performed.

Reflexes

It is important to remember the concepts of upper motor neuron and lower motor neuron disease. The upper motor neuron system organizes groups of muscles to mediate movement of body parts. The lower motor neuron system organizes individual muscles.

By testing the deep tendon reflexes as well as the superficial reflexes, one can sample the influences of both the upper motor neuron and the lower motor neuron on the reflex arcs. Beginning from the lower extremities and proceeding proximally, the plantar response depends on the intactness of the L-5 and S-1,2 segments. If the plantar response is extensor it indicates that the corticospinal pathway serving the L-5, S-1,2 segments has been disturbed.

> **Deep Tendon Reflexes and Superficial Reflexes**
> Achilles reflex: S-1,2
> Quadriceps reflex: L-2, 3,4
> Low abdominal: T-11, L-1
> Upper abdominal: T-6, T-9
> Hoffman reflex: C-7, C-8, and T1
> Brachioradialis reflex: C-5,6
> Biceps reflex: C-5, C-6
> Triceps reflex: C-67,8
> Jaw reflex: midpons
> Those numbered segments underlined indicate the dominant or main spinal segments involved.
> If present, pathologic reflexes are a sign of organic brain or spinal cord disease.

Conclusion

In conclusion, an adequate history, a thorough physical examination and a competent neurologic examination usually enable the physician to make a correct headache diagnosis and do much toward reassuring the patient.

SELF-ASSESSMENT EXAMINATION

1 Migrainous patients are always characterized by neatness and compulsive attention to details. True or False

2 Horner's syndrome may appear during cluster headache. True or False

3 Patients with cluster headache are characterized by a thin, delicate facial appearance. True or False

4 Occipital headache of the elderly, with associated stiff neck, should suggest cervical spondylosis. True or False

5 Loss of sense of smell always suggests an olfactory bulb tumor. True or False

6 A single cafe-au-lait spot is strongly suggestive of neurofibromatosis. True or False

7 In hypothyroidism, a classical migraine syndrom frequently appears. True or False

8 Examination of the head in a patient with headache should include: (a) palpation of the skull; (b) auscultation of the head and neck for bruits; (c) evaluation of possible trigger zones; (d) auscultation of the temporomandibular joint; (e) all of the above; (f) none of the above

9 In cerebellopontine angle tumors (a) headache is common in the early stages of tumor growth; (b) headache never occurs; (c) headache frequently appears with increased intracranial pressure

10 A third nerve palsy may be related

to (a) ophthalmoplegic migraine; (b) an expanding aneurysm; (c) herniation of the temporal horn through the tentorium; (d) diabetes mellitus; (e) trigeminal and glossopharyngeal neuralgia

ANSWERS:

1—False; 2—True; 3—False; 4—True; 5—False; 6—False; 7—False; 8—a,b,c,d,e; 9—c; 10—a,b,c,d

4

Additional Studies Are Sometimes Necessary in Investigating Headache

Many headache patients have had extensive diagnostic studies, particularly if their complaints are persistent and chronic, if they have responded poorly to prescribed therapy and if they have visited in many consultation rooms. Often such procedures have been done for what seem to be weak indications. But it is unwise to be too critical of others, for even when the attending physician has the best of intentions, patients with headache may be overtested, especially if the historic data hint at some form of obscure disease as a basis for their complaints. It is unfortunately true that some diagnostic studies, particularly arteriograms and pneumoencephalograms, may increase the patient's headache and more permanently fix in his mind the concern that serious organic disease of the brain is present.

Some diagnostic studies may increase the patient's headache.

Yet, on occasion, headache can be the first symptom of organic disease. If the patient is being seen for the first time for this complaint, some work-up is indicated, unless history is crystal clear. We advise that skull films be performed on all patients with headache and, if the symptoms warrant it, computerized axial tomography (CAT) and an electroencephalogram. This constitutes a baseline work-up and is usually adequate to rule out organic disease. We proceed to more invasive studies including arteriography only if a specific indication for these procedures is present. Chronic complaints of pain are *not* a specific indication.

It is important to disturb the patient as little as possible by your examinations and to reassure him by informing him when the tests are negative. If further investigations are indicated, make your patient understand the reasons for these studies and the risks involved, and obtain his consent for them.

Some Diagnostic Points of Importance

Plain Skull Films

This procedure, although sometimes castigated as overused or unnecessary, does provide a large amount of clinical evidence, both positive and negative, of obvious and significant importance to the clinician caring for the patient with headache. It is first necessary to make certain that the alignment of the films has been satisfactory. For example, on the lateral view, the orbital plates and the mandibular rami should be superimposed, and on the anterior-posterior view, the distances from the orbital rim to the outer bony table should be the same. The outer and inner table of the skull should be examined, as well as the lines and sutures, character and density of the bones, the shape and size of the sella turcica, unusual calcifications (especially the pineal calcification) (Fig 2-4), the soft tissues of the skull, and the craniocephalic index and the general vault-to-base relationships. The basal angle should be calculated, and signs of basilar impression should be sought.

The clinician should learn to identify, among other abnormalities,

fractures

splitting of the sutures

increased digital markings suggesting increased intracranial pressure

normal and pathologic vascular markings

shifts of the calcified pineal gland

other intracranial calcifications

the abnormal range of sellar size (maximal internal AP diameter is 17 to 18 mm, average AP diameter is 10 mm)

— erosion of the sella

Metastatic disease (Fig 2-3)

Some findings, such as subgaleal hematomas, can be recognized on skull films as benign, and will usually disappear slowly without intervention.

Spinal Puncture

This should be done only if there is a specific indication. If you are suspicious of a slowly leaking aneurysm, or there is neurologic evidence of a subdural hematoma, then this study should be considered. In the latter case, there may be xanthochromic

Table 4-1. A View of the Headache "Work-up"

General
  History and physical
    examination
  Skull films
  EEG
If focal disease, mass lesions or hydrocephalus
    is suspected
  EMI scan and/or
  Brain scan
If arterial disease is suspected
  Angiograms
If infection, aneurysm or angiomatous rupture
    is suspected
  Lumbar puncture, immediately
If temporal arteritis is suspected
  Sedimentation rate
  Temporal artery biopsy, anti-nuclear antibody (ANA)
Also, occasionally indicated in special situations
  X-rays of the temporomandibular joints—for
  chronic facial pain
  Pneumoencephalo-) for   mass   lesion
    grams   } and/or hydroceph-
  Ventriculograms   ) alus
If disease of cervical spine is suspected
  Cervical spine films
  EMG   for signs of radiculo-
  Myelography, rarely   pathy or spinal cord
                       compression

fluid or blood in the spinal fluid. If the patient's neck is rigid and he is running a febrile course, a spinal puncture is mandatory to rule out intracranial infection. An increase of spinal fluid pressure is often present with a brain tumor and the spinal fluid pressure should be taken before any spinal fluid is withdrawn. Herniation of the brainstem into the foramen magnum and sudden death can occur if fluid is rapidly removed, if a brain tumor is present with associated increase in intracranial pressure. In general, if a brain tumor is seriously suspected as a cause of headache, spinal puncture is *best avoided*.

Electroencephalogram, Echoencephalogram

In some instances, an electroencephalogram may reveal a specific focal lesion, or dysrhythmia, suggestive that further studies should be done. If you are suspicious of a focal lesion or of organic disease of the brain, a negative electroencephalogram may be misleading. Echoencephalograms are used to assess the state of the midline structures. Lesions such as a unilateral subdural hematoma may shift the midline to the side opposite the lesion. If, however, bilateral lesions are present, the midline structures may not be shifted and this factor should be appreciated, particularly if there is a history of head trauma.

Computerized Axial Tomography (The CAT Scan)

Most authorities agree that the CAT scan, also termed the EMI scan, is the greatest advance in diagnostic medicine in the last several decades. This noninvasive technique uses a computer coupled with a special x-ray device to produce vividly detailed cross-sectional pictures of the body's interior. A narrow x-ray beam scans the patient's head in a series of 1-cm-wide slices. A total of 28,800 absorption readings are produced in 5 minutes. The readings are processed by a mini computer that calculates 6,400 absorption values of the material in each slice from the simultaneous 28,800

equations. The technique discloses variations in tissue density which aid in detecting many pathologic conditions.

The technique gives information about the brain and its appendages which could previously not be obtained, or was obtained only with the greatest difficulty, using techniques such as pneumoencephalography, cerebral angiography, ventriculography or radioisotope scanning. In many cases hazardous procedures such as pneumoencephalograms and cerebral arteriograms can now be avoided.

The CAT scan makes it possible to differentiate hemorrhage from tumor, to follow multiple brain lesions, to monitor chemotherapy, and the accuracy in diagnosing supratentorial lesions is above 90%. Furthermore, the testing can almost always be done on an outpatient basis, is rapid and does not overexpose the patient to irradiation.

In evaluation of the patient with headache, the CAT scan is of particular value. It allows us to exclude conditions including brain tumors, chronic subdural hematomas and hydrocephalus which result in chronic recurrent headaches which at times simu-

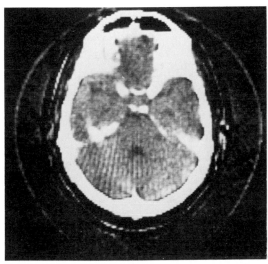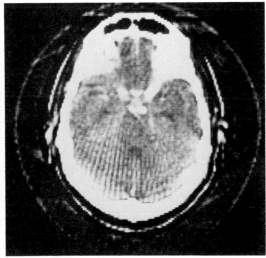

Fig 4-1. *A 70-year-old man with a history of recurrent vertex headaches, of moderate severity, often relieved by common analgesics. More troublesome was a history of recurrent episodes of severe sweating which were termed "male menopause." The CAT-scan demonstrates a pituitary tumor with contrast enhancement. The patient has been treated with radiation. A specific tissue diagnosis has not been obtained.*

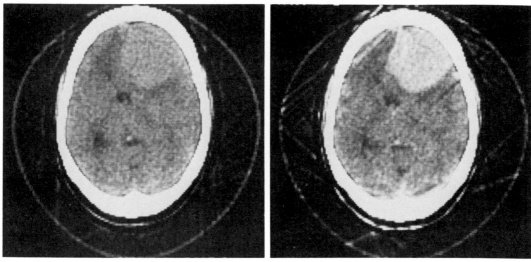

Fig 4-2. *A young girl of 18 years with a strong family history of vascular headache, with recent onset of increasingly severe headaches for the last 3 months. No alteration with position or activity. No papilledema was present. The EMI scan demonstrates a large tumor with contrast enhancement in the right frontal area. Pathological diagnosis was meningioma.*

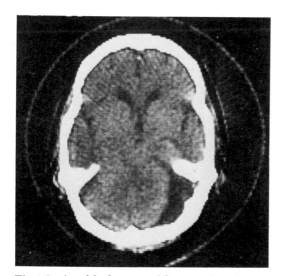

Fig 4-3. *An elderly man with a previous history of bilateral subdural hematomas, occurring 3 years prior to the onset of nonspecific occipital headaches, increasing somnolence and disorientation. The EMI scan demonstrates a recurrent posterior subdural hematoma which was easily evacuated.*

late migraine. Also, for the first time, the CAT scan has enabled us to recognize transient morphologic changes such as cerebral edema in the cerebral parenchyma after an acute attack of migraine, especially in cases of complicated migraine of the hemiparetic variety.

In a small percentage of patients with complicated migraine, abnormalities will appear in CAT scans including cerebral edema, which is transient, lasting only a few days, and, in addition, in patients with repeated severe attacks, enlargement of the cerebral ventricles and cerebral cortical atrophy have been reported.

The indications for the use of the CAT scan in patients with recurrent headache are as follows:

- ■ if the neurological exam or clinical history makes one suspect an intracranial lesion

- ■ in cases of complicated migraine including hemiparetic and vertebral basilar varieties, where there is a question of a structural lesion

- ■ in patients with brain tumor phobia, as a method of reassurance

See Figures 4-1, 4-2, 4-3, 4-4, 4-5 and 4-6.

Radioisotope Scanning

Radioisotope scanning (brain scanning) has become the most frequently performed pro-

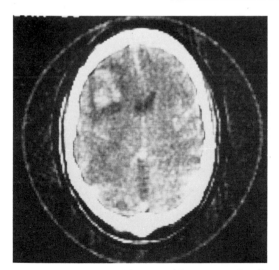

Fig 4-4. *A 27-year-old man with a strong family history of migraine referred because of increasing headaches, termed by his physician-father as migrainous. Note the large defect in the left frontal area with contrast enhancement. Pathological diagnosis was an astrocytoma Grade III.*

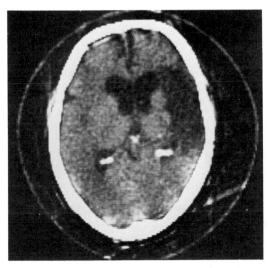

Fig 4-5. *A 54-year-old man complaining of nonspecific frontal and occipital headaches with a previous history of a cerebrovascular accident and a persistent left hemiparesis. The EMI scan shows a large lucent area in the right hemisphere compatible with the previous cerebral infarction.*

cedure in most nuclear medicine laboratories. The popularity of radioisotope brain scanning is related to the utilization of ^{99m}Tc and other short-lived agents introduced in the mid-1960s.

This allowed a greater dose in millicurie amounts to be administered than before, with a subsequent shortening of the examination time as well as a reduced radiation dose to the patient.

In the brain scan, what is imaged is everything around the brain and abnormalities appear as areas of isotope uptake.

The brain scan is really a nonbrain scan. The isotope does not go to the brain sub-

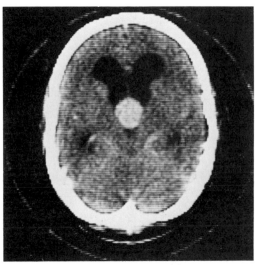

Fig 4-6. *J. W., a 36-year-old male, noted the onset of severe headaches in November of 1974, with associated fatigue, lack of energy and weight loss in early 1975. In the past he had taken "handfulls" of aspirin for minor headaches but recently the headaches had become more severe and occurred several times per week, radiating from the occipital region to the frontal area. They were non-throbbing but were associated with a sensation of pressure. Neurological examination was normal. The discs were sharp. He appeared depressed.*
The initial EMI scan shows massive dilation of the lateral ventricles with the fourth ventricle of normal size. There is a mass density present in the region of the foramen of Monro. At operation this proved to be a colloid cyst of the third ventricle. His postoperative course was complicated by persistent hydrocephalus, and a ventriculo-peritoneal shunt was placed, subsequent to which he improved. He has remained relatively asymptomatic to the present time.

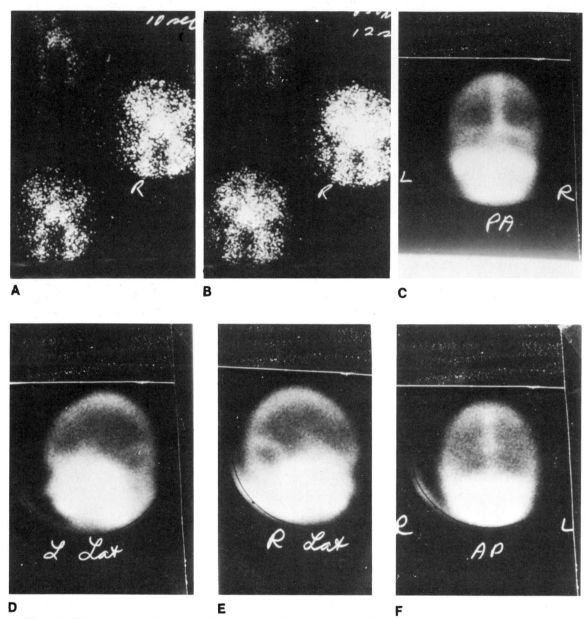

Fig 4-7. *Normal gamma camera imaging and brain scan. (A, B) Gamma imaging; (C) PA scan; (D) left lateral scan; (E) right lateral scan; (F) AP scan.*

stance but is selectively kept out by the blood-brain barrier, consisting of tight intercellular junctions which preclude the entrance of macromolecules into the cerebral substance. What is imaged is actually everything around the brain. The anatomic structures one sees include scalp vascularity, facial and nasal structures, salivary glands, the superior sagittal and transverse sinuses and other vascular structures. If the barrier or microvascular anatomy is broken down by injury, tumor, inflammation, etc., the abnormality in the brain will appear as an area of isotope uptake. Abnormal appearance of isotope within the hemispheres is positive evidence for a lesion but does

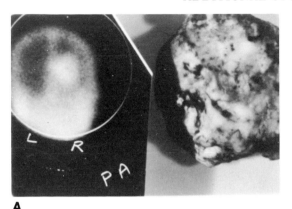
A
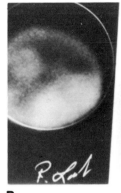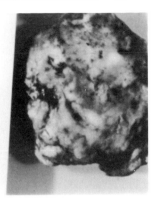
B

Fig 4-8. *Meningioma—PA and lateral scan (surgical specimen). (A) PA scan; (B) right lateral scan.*

not give the etiology. An abnormal isotope finding in two or more views, which is necessary to diagnose the scan as positive, locates the lesion.

Accuracy of Brain Scanning

The overall accuracy of brain scanning in primary brain tumors is 80–85%, with the best returns being in highly vascular and poorly differentiated tumors located in the midhemispheres above the tentorium.

The poorest returns are in the small and/or well-differentiated slowly growing lesions and/or lesions near the base of the brain and/or lesions in the posterior fossa, which may become masked in the normal tissue background.

Brain scans are of value in many nonneoplastic conditions.

Brain scans are of value in many nonneoplastic conditions such as subdural hematomas and in cerebrovascular disease. Most strokes will give positive scans in the 2nd and 3rd week and only rarely in the 1st week. Given the usual acute onset of signs and symptoms occurring in a stroke and the slow progression of symptoms seen with a tumor, the similarity of positive scans in

these conditions can be minimized with careful attention to the history (Figs 4-7–4-13).

Myelography

This may be employed in headache patients by a radiologist to spot acoustic neurinomas or other lesions of the posterior fossa. Myelography may also be of value in the investigation of headache associated with cervical spondylosis.

Ventriculography

Either with air or contrast media, ventriculography is done by a neurosurgeon with very specific indications, most often if a brain tumor is suspected.

Angiography

This is performed by a neuroradiologist, a neurosurgeon or a vascular surgeon and depicts aneurysms, angiomas, hematomas and pathologic circulation in tumors. It can be highly effective in localizing tumors, but the procedure is not without risk and should be used only when there is definite suspicion of an organic lesion. Angiography should be avoided, if possible, during episodes of migraine.

Pneumoencephalography

This procedure commonly produces severe but self-limited headache. It has the value of showing both the ventricles and the sub-

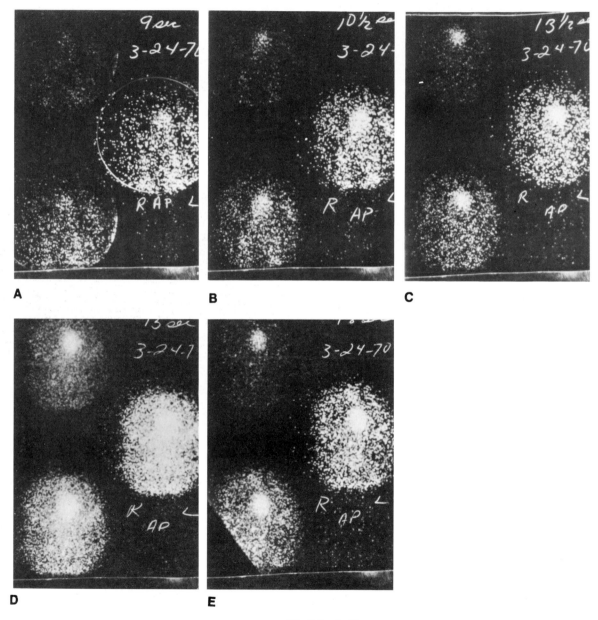

Fig 5-9. A–E

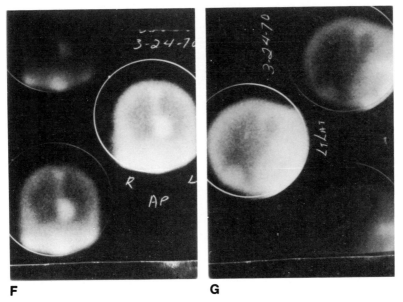

Fig 4-9. *Hemangioma. (A–E) Gamma camera imaging; (F) AP brain scan; (G) lateral (left) brain scan.*

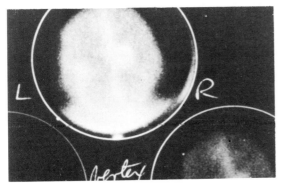

Fig 4-10. *Metastatic lesions, brain scan vertex view.*

arachnoid spaces. It is useful in the investigation of hydrocephalus, hydrocephalic dementia and new growths. Again, it is rarely done in a patient complaining of headache without a specific indication.

Conclusion

The laboratory and radiologic investigation of a patient with headache, without any definite neurologic signs or symptoms, is often unprofitable. Extensive testing of these patients, without indications, is unwise, unrewarding for the physician and may subject the patient to undue risk. It is difficult to give specific advice regarding the extent of the diagnostic work-up in a headache patient. Much will depend upon the diagnostic acumen of the examiner. In general, however, arteriography and pneumoencephalography should be avoided unless there are specific indications for these procedures beyond the subjective complaint of head pain.

SELF-ASSESSMENT EXAMINATION

1 All patients with headache deserve an extensive laboratory work-up. True or False

2 If subarachnoid hemorrhage is suspected, xanthochromia in the cerebrospinal fluid should be sought. True or False

3 In general, if a brain tumor is seriously suspected, lumbar puncture is best avoided. True or False

4 The clinical suspicion of meningitis

and/or encephalitis is a specific indication for examination of cerebrospinal fluid. True or False

5 Negative or normal electroencephalograms always imply absence of a focal cortical lesion. True or False

6 The state or position of the midline structures is assessed by echoencephalography. True or False

7 Echoencephalography is particularly helpful in evaluating recent head trauma. True or False

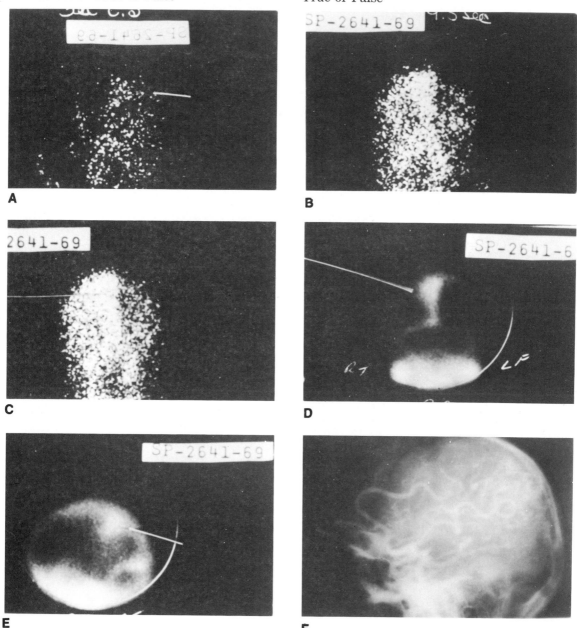

Fig 4-11. *Arteriovenous malformation. The carotid-cerebral flow reveals the AV malformation which concurred arteriographically and surgically. Without the dynamic imaging the positive scan is only a positive scan and nonspecific. Shown are (A) 6.5-second gamma camera imaging; (B) 9.5-second gamma camera imaging; (C) 11-second gamma camera imaging; (D) right lateral brain scan; (E) PA brain scan; and (F) arteriogram.*

8 In isotope scanning, the following structures take up isotope (a) the brain parenchyma; (b) blood vessels including great venous sinuses; (c) scalp; (d) salivary glands; (e) facial and nasal structures

9 Myelography is of value in evaluating the headache patient (a) only rarely; (b) if a posterior fossa lesion is present; (c) if cervical spondylosis is associated with oc-

cipital head pain; (d) if discogenic root disease is present

10 Angiography (a) should always be done in investigating chronic headache; (b) should never be done in investigating chronic headache; (c) is helpful if brain tumor is suspected; (d) may be extremely valuable in pursuing the source of subarachnoid hemorrhage; (e) is, on occasion,

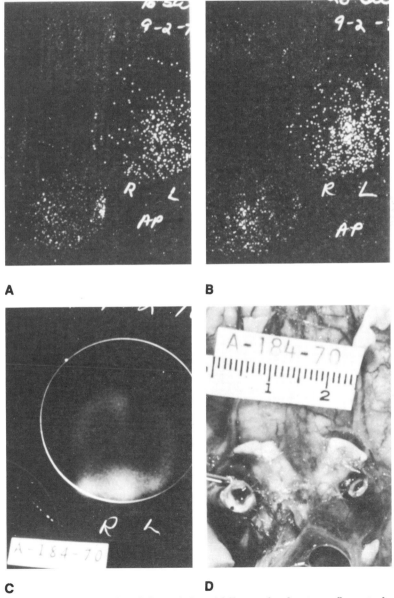

A   **B**

C   **D**

Fig 4-12. *Negative scan with positive defect, right middle cerebral artery; flow study and autopsy reveal thrombosis. (A) 16-second AP gamma camera imaging; (B) 20-second AP gamma camera imaging; (C) AP brain scan; (D) pathology specimen showing cerebral artery thrombosis.*

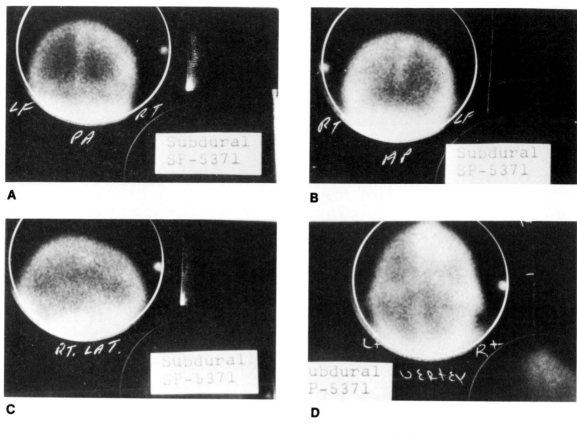

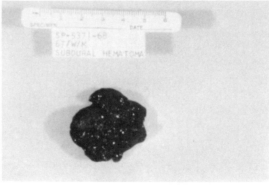

Fig 4-13. *Subdural hematoma. (A) PA brain scan; (B) AP brain scan; (C) right lateral brain scan; (D) vertex scan; (E) surgical pathology specimen.*

associated with unpleasant side effects, including strokes

11 Headache following pneumoencephalography implies (a) a disaster has occurred; (b) self-limited discomfort usually short-lived in nature; (c) a headache requiring specific treatment; (d) a headache relieved by recumbency, and increased by sitting or standing; (e) air has been retained in the brain

ANSWERS:

5

Migraine Headache

It has been estimated that from 8 to 12 million Americans suffer from migraine. The term migraine comes from the French and is derived from the Greek word *hemicrania* which means "half a head." This describes many of the migraine attacks in which pain is limited to one side of the head, although the headache is not always unilateral. It may be bilateral or shift from side to side. In general, however, migraine headache is usually a recurrent, throbbing, unilateral head pain, separated by pain-free periods. Nausea and emesis often appear during the attack. A family history of similar attacks is consistently obtained. Preheadache warnings occur in some cases. Patients with migraine are described as compulsive, rigid and perfectionist in character. Not all of these traits are present in all migraine sufferers, but they occur with frequency in the majority of patients and thus make the diagnosis fairly simple (Fig 5-1). But one should avoid describing a "typical migraine personality."

Different Forms of Migraine

Migraine includes classic and common migraine and hemiplegic and ophthalmoplegic migraine. Common to all these is a tendency to vascular dilation, which represents the headache phase of the migraine attack. Initial vasoconstriction may also occur and produce painless preheadache experiences. This serves to separate classic from common migraine. In classic migraine, prehea-

dache experiences are described. In common migraine, they do not occur, or at least are not readily recognized by the patient. Hemiplegic migraine and ophthalmoplegic migraine are considered to be more severe forms of classical migraine. If recurrent migraine becomes associated with permanent neurologic residual damage to the nervous system, the term "complicated migraine" is used. All forms mentioned above will be discussed in detail in this book.

Sex Distribution

Migraine is more common in women than in men. Estimates have varied but most experts agree that 60% of sufferers are women.

Age Distribution

Migraine may appear in childhood. Usually migraine begins before the age of 40 and most commonly in the second and third decades of life. An occasional patient shows his first symptoms in the fifth and sixth decades, although migraine tends to decrease with advancing age. Many patients may have the prodromal preheadache symptoms persist even when their headaches disappear.

Family History

Migraine patients frequently can relate a history of their disorder in a close blood

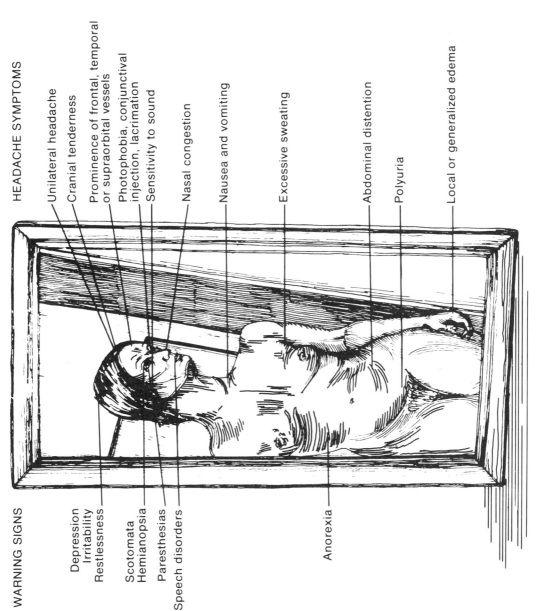

HEADACHE SYMPTOMS

Unilateral headache

Cranial tenderness

Prominence of frontal, temporal or supraorbital vessels

Photophobia, conjunctival injection, lacrimation

Sensitivity to sound

Nasal congestion

Nausea and vomiting

Excessive sweating

Abdominal distention

Polyuria

Local or generalized edema

WARNING SIGNS

Depression
Irritability
Restlessness

Scotomata
Hemianopsia

Paresthesias

Speech disorders

Anorexia

Fig 5-1. Clinical features of migraine.

relation. Whether the problem is hereditary or familial is conjectural, but a positive family history is obtained in some 70% of the individuals affected by migraine.

Factors Influencing Attacks

Stress and Fatigue

We have found many but not all migraine sufferers to be obsessive, compulsive and rigid. They keep long lists of their attacks and treatment and medications (Fig 5-2). The stress situations of life, such as menopause, puberty and change of school or job, seem to paralyze their adapting mechanisms. This inability to adapt creates anger and resentment and has been described as the repressed hostility of the migraine patient. Physicians who deal with headache need to emphasize that a patient's migrainous attacks may not represent the essence of the problem at hand. Consider the remark of a woman who said angrily, "Doctor, will you stop talking about my headache and discuss my other symptoms: my tendency to fatigue, my inability to keep up with my husband and the social and work tasks I set up for myself." An attack will occur more frequently when the patient is excessively tired. Migraine patients as a whole tend to build for themselves lives with too many environmental demands. They are extremely sensitive to overload. They may suffer situational anxieties in addition to those caused by deeper subconscious conflicts.

Dietary Migraine

No clinical problem is more perplexing to the practicing physician than the relationship of foods and beverages to the production of migraine. A great deal of folklore surrounds the subject and little scientific work has been done to clarify the issue. Furthermore, various misconceptions about diet and migraine are given impetus by articles in the popular press. Thus, the physician may encounter patients who have constructed elaborate diets in the hope of escaping recurrent migraine attacks. Occasionally these diets assume ridiculous extremes; for example, one may find that a patient is living primarily on scallions or bananas or onions. The purpose of this section is to make some sense out of a confusing clinical dilemma and, at the least, to stress those facts which seem conclusive.

Diet and Vascular Headache

Alcohol

Unquestionably some ingested substances will provoke vascular headaches in susceptible individuals. Alcohol, for example, produces a vascular headache in migraine patients, particularly if they are in a migraine phase. Patients with cluster headache are notoriously sensitive to even small amounts of alcohol and they learn to avoid alcohol during the period of cluster headache recurrence. Alcohol is a nonspecific vasodilator, which probably accounts for its precipitation of the vascular headache process. The vasodilation is assumed to be the result of depression or alteration of the central vasomotor centers, since the direct action of alcohol on blood vessels is insignificant. Moderate amounts of alcohol do not affect cerebral blood flow but severe intoxication causes a significant increase in cerebral blood flow with diminished cerebrovascular resistance.

Tyramine

Foods which contain tyramine, a vasoactive amine, may precipitate headache, particularly in patients who are treated with monoamine oxidase inhibitors. Tyramine-rich foods include strong or aged cheeses, pickled herring, chicken livers, canned figs and the pods of broad beans. Tyramine acts as a sympathomimetic amine, both directly and through the release of norepinephrine. It is theorized that the release of norepinephrine from tissues results in selective cerebral vasoconstriction; when tissue

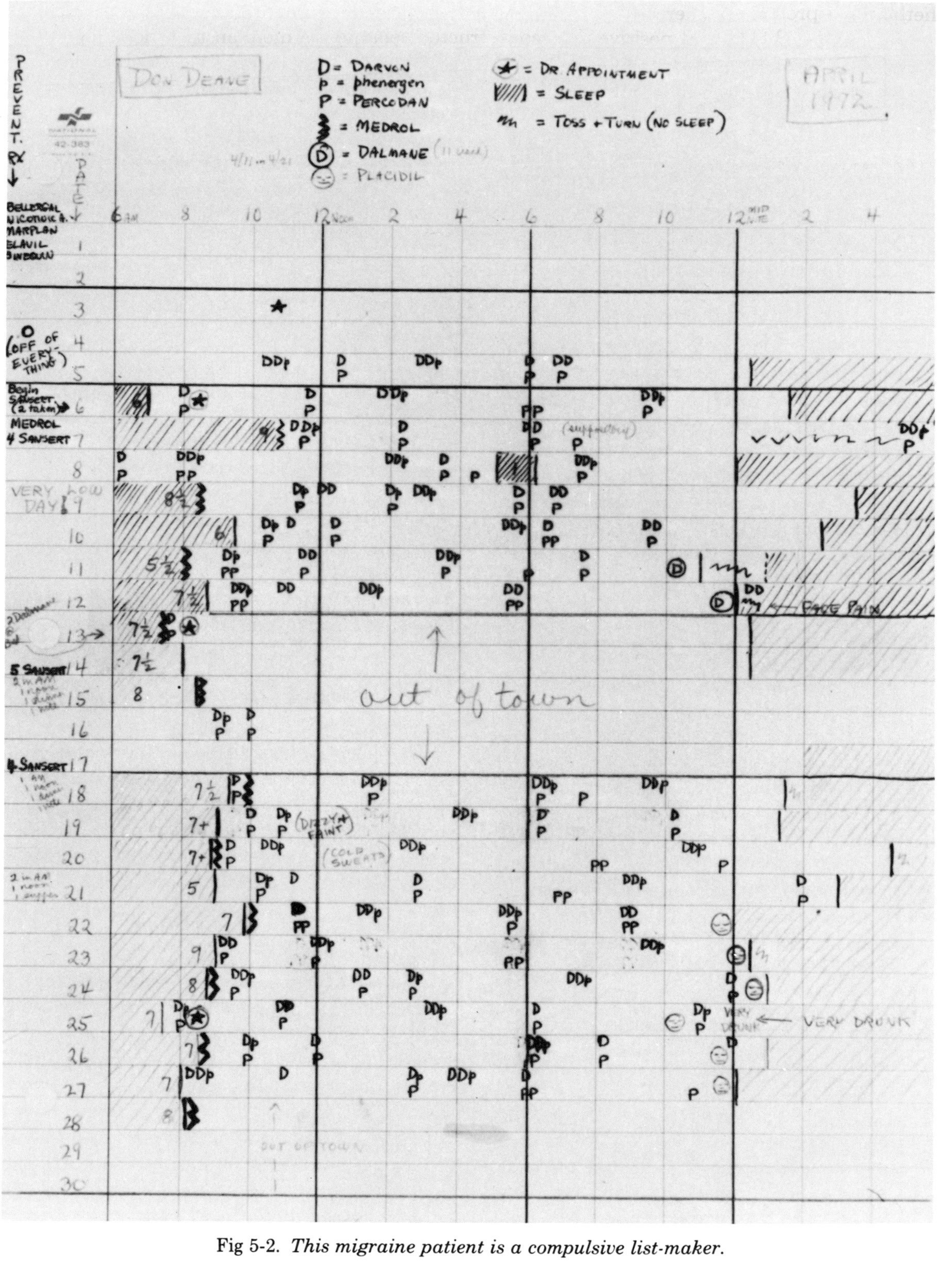

Fig 5-2. *This migraine patient is a compulsive list-maker.*

stores of norepinephrine are exhausted, rebound dilation of the extracranial vessels occurs, producing headache. Patients with migraine appear to metabolize tyramine in a different manner from normal controls; in a study conducted by English investigators, dietary migraine patients excreted less conjugated tyramine, both before and after an oral load of that substance, than did normal subjects.

Cured Meats

Recently Henderson and Raskin reported an unusual sensitivity to sodium nitrite in a patient who noted the onset of moderately severe headaches after the ingestion of cured meat products, such as hot dogs, bacon, ham and salami.

The cured meat products contain sodium nitrite, which maintains the red coloring of these foods by reacting with myoglobin and hemoglobin to form red nitroso-compounds. Henderson and Raskin were able to demonstrate that the small amounts of sodium nitrite found in cured meats (about 5 to 10 mg) produced headaches in a susceptible patient. This is another example of vasoactive substance producing headaches and not a true allergic reaction.

Elimination Diets

Our own approach to this problem has been to eliminate from the diets of patients with migraine those foods and beverages which have been shown to have vasoactive qualities. Thus, our recommendations include avoidance of alcohol, particularly some wines which contain large amounts of histamine, aged or strong cheese, pickled herring, chicken livers, chocolate and canned figs. We do not suggest avoidance of milk products. Large amounts of monosodium glutamate (MSG) may produce a generalized vasomotor reaction which may include headache ("the Chinese restaurant syndrome"). Use of excessive amounts of monosodium glutamate is unwise.

If the patient persists in his contention that a specific substance is provoking headaches, we usually suggest that he partici-

pate in an experiment that is performed in the laboratory. An appropriate amount of the suspected substance is prepared in pow-

---

Diet for the Headache Patient
Avoid:
Ripened cheeses (cheddar, emmentaler, gruyere, stilton, brie and camembert)
(Cheeses permissible: American, cottage, cream and Velveeta)
Herring
Chocolate
Vinegar (except white vinegar)
Anything fermented, pickled or marinated
Sour cream, yogurt
Nuts, peanut butter
Hot fresh breads, raised coffeecakes and doughnuts
Pods of broad beans (lima, navy and pea pods)
Any foods containing large amounts of monosodium glutamate (Chinese foods)
Onions
Canned figs
Citrus foods (no more than 1 orange per day)
Bananas (no more than $\frac{1}{2}$ banana per day)
Pizza
Pork (no more than 2–3 times per week)
Excessive tea, coffee, cola beverages (no more than 4 cups per day)
Avocado
Fermented sausage (bologna, salami, pepperoni, summer and hot dogs)
Chicken livers
Avoid all alcoholic beverages, if possible. If you must drink, no more than two normal size drinks.
Suggested Drinks: Haute Sauterne
                Riesling
                Seagram's VO
                Cutty Sark
                Vodka

dered form to put into capsules so that ingestion of this substance can be compared, in a double-blind study, to consumption of a similar amount of lactose. After a control period of about 1 week, the experiment is set into motion. The patient ingests the capsules for 2 weeks and the code is then broken. Invariably we find that patients experience just as much headache from lactose ingestion as from the "offending" substance.

Hypoglycemia

A word should be said about the quality and amount of food consumed by the patient with migraine. Hypoglycemia exerts a profound effect on the tone of the cranial blood vessels. If the sugar content of the blood is reduced by insulin or by other means, conspicuous cerebral vasodilation occurs. Headache is a prominent symptom of insulin shock, for example. Furthermore, in migraine patients, the relative hypoglycemia produced by fasting may evoke typical vascular headaches. Even reactive hypoglycemia occurring after ingestion of an excessive carbohydrate load may precipitate vascular headache in a susceptible person. For these reasons, we suggest that the patient with migraine eat three well-balanced meals a day and avoid an overabundance of carbohydrates at any single meal. An avoidance of oversleeping on weekends is also recommended. Excessive sleep may alter the body's normal blood sugar level and thus precipitate headaches when a rigid schedule of awakening is not kept.

Hormonal Changes

Approximately 70% of the women seen with migraine say that some of their attacks occur prior to, during, or at the end of their menstruation. By the 3rd month of pregnancy, most women are free of their migraine except for a very small number who get their first attack with pregnancy.

The oral contraceptives and postmenopausal hormonal therapies usually increase the severity and frequency of migraine attacks. Migraine patients appear to have an extremely labile vascular system and are subject to complications such as stroke from the use of the oral contraceptives.

Allergy, Epilepsy and Migraine

We do not believe that there is any relationship between migraine and allergy or epilepsy. Migraine patients may note an increase in headache during or following an allergic episode, related to increased vasomotor activity. Presumably, also, the vasoconstrictive phase of migraine can set off seizure activity in one predisposed to seizures, but this series of events must be rare. EEG changes have been reported in migraine patients but their importance is conjectural. An occasional migraine patient with a significant dysrhythmia may respond to anticonvulsant agents.

Medina and Diamond have presented their studies on migraine and atopy. They determined serum IgE levels in 116 patients with headache by the radioimmunoassay technique. A second group consisted of 504 patients who were seen at a headache clinic during a period of 2 months. Elevation of the serum IgE was noted in 5.7% of the migraine population, approximately the same as the incidence of elevated serum IgE in the normal population. This incidence is far below that seen in atopic disorders. In the second group of 504 patients, the prevalence of atopic disorders in migraine patients and their relatives was approximately the same as the prevalence in patients with chronic muscle contraction headaches. The numbers are close to the prevalence of atophy in the normal population or their relatives and are not statistically significant. There is, therefore, no increase in the prevalence of atopy in the relatives of patients suffering from migraine headaches. This study casts further doubt on any supposed relationship between atopy, allergy, elevation of the serum IgE and migraine. It now seems evident, from this and other careful studies, that migraine is not an allergic phenomenon, and is not related to the atopic diseases.

Site and Character of Headache

The most frequent history obtained is that of a dull ache, progressively worsening and finally developing into a throbbing or pulsating pain. The headache as it becomes stabilized may again become constant and nonthrobbing. About 70% of migraine is unilateral and frequently affects the frontal and temporal regions but may settle behind the eye. The pain can radiate across the head and to other regions of the face and neck surrounding the primary pain site.

Number, Duration and Onset of Attacks

The number of attacks can vary, with the most severe cases having attacks every few days to those only having an attack once or twice a year. Most frequently, patients report two to four attacks monthly. Most migraine episodes last longer than 4 hours, and usually for a day or two. A severe attack can last up to 6 days. The onset can occur at any time and may be precipitated by various factors. It is not uncommon for a migraine patient to wake up with a headache.

The Attack

In the initial phase of migraine, during the prodromal phase, there is vasoconstriction, followed by vasodilatation, during which the headache occurs. In about 35% of cases, the patient has the typical classic migraine described above. The patient notes an aura (most often visual) which may precede the attack by 10–20 minutes. Then the typical one-sided, pulsating headache occurs with its associated symptoms. Nonclassic migraine does not have preheadache prodromes.

Prodromes in Order of Frequency

The prodromes in order of frequency are

1 Scotomata, or blind spots
2 Teichopsia, or fortification spectra—a zigzag pattern resembling a fort (Fig 5-3).
3 Flashing of lights (photopsia) light-colored
4 Paresthesias
5 Visual and auditory hallucinations; Alice in Wonderland syndrome described by Lewis Carroll, a sufferer from migraine, who saw the distorted figures of "Alice" as part of his migraine attack (Fig 5-4).

Other Rare Prodroma

Diplopia, ataxia, vertigo, syncope and hyperosmia may occur. The prodromata usu-

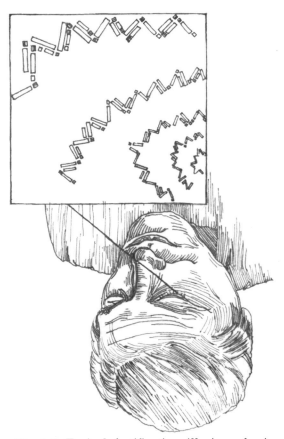

Fig 5-3. *Typical fortification illusion of migraine.*

ally resolve before each attack but can, on occasion, remain permanent. As a migraine sufferer grows older he may note only the prodrome without the subsequent headache.

Symptoms Accompanying Migraine Attacks

■ Photophobia—Undue sensitivity to light, preferring darkened room. Noise can also increase discomfort.

■ Nausea and emesis—Occurs in 90% of migraines. Rarely, diarrhea ensues. Dehydration may occur if recurrent emesis persists.

■ Arteries (vascular changes)—Cold hands and feet, tenderness over the superficial vessels over the part of the head where the headache occurs and pale skin of the face are often noted.

■ Other body changes—During attack there is most often an increase of weight with sodium retention and an oliguria. As the patient improves, diuresis often occurs. Hyperesthesia of the scalp is a frequent complaint of the migraine patient.

Special Types of Migraine

An occasional patient with migraine will note neurologic manifestations which persist beyond the immediate headache period. Such complications include hemiparesis, hemisensory defects, occlusion of the retinal artery, and ophthalmoplegia. We assume that these complications are related to the prolonged vasoconstriction or vasodilation occurring as a part of the migraine process. If the brain becomes sufficiently ischemic during these vasoactive changes, permanent damage may ensue related to cerebral infarction. This situation is termed "complicated migraine."

The incidence of complicated migraine is uncertain, but the best studies suggest that less than 1–2% of patients with mi-

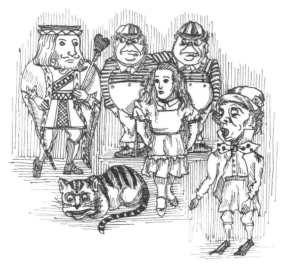

Fig 5-4. *Distorted figures of Alice in Wonderland.*

graine experience episodes which could be characterized as complicated migraine.

Ophthalmoplegic migraine is associated with a third nerve or other ocular nerve palsy. This is usually transient but may become permanent. The occurrence and recurrence of this problem suggests the diagnosis, as opposed to an intracranial aneurysm, producing a third nerve palsy.

Hemiplegic migraine is associated with motor (and sensory) changes of hemiplegia. It may persist for days or weeks. This is a rare form of migraine, in which the family history is usually positive.

Migraine Therapy

Therapy may be either prophylactic or abortive (Table 5-1). If the headaches occur only occasionally, once a month or once every 2 months, abortive therapy is preferable.

Two groups of agents are used to treat migraine, those given for symptomatic relief of the acute attack, and those given prophylactically.

Ergot alkaloids are vasoconstrictor agents, and specifically counteract the episodic dilation of certain extracranial arteries and arterioles, primarily the branches of the external carotid artery, which are affected in migraine. Ergotamine tartrate is the most consistently effective drug for the treatment of acute attacks and has the most prolonged effect. Relief of headache after intermuscular injection of 0.5 mg of ergotamine tartrate is almost conclusive evidence that the headache is of vascular origin. Dihydroergotamine (DHE 45®) may also reduce or abolish the headache without inducing nausea or vomiting. However fewer patients respond to dihydroergotamine than to ergotamine, and since the drug is approximately half as active as ergotamine tartrate, twice as much must be given. The other available ergot alkaloids including ergonovine and methylergonovine are used principally as oxytocic agents, though they may be used for chronic vascular headache.

If ergotamine is to be effective in migraine, it should be administered soon after onset and in adequate dosage to obtain relief. Since it does not have effects upon the intracranial circulation, it can be used during the painless preheadache phenomena which may herald the onset of migraine.

The usual dose, given either subcutaneously or in intramuscular fashion, in adults is 0.25 to 0.5 mg at the start of the attack. This may be repeated in 1 hour. The maximum total dose in 1 week given parenterally should be no more than 1 to 2 mg. The drug can also be used sublingually, given 2 mg at the start of an attack, followed by 2 mg every 30 minutes if necessary but no more than 6 mg in 24 hours and 12 mg in 1 week.

If given orally one may prescribe 1 to 2 mg at the start of an attack, followed by 1 to 2 mg every 30 minutes up to a total of 6 mg in 24 hours. The maximum dose in 1 week is 12 mg. Children over 5 years of age may take up to 1 mg daily with a maximum daily dose of 2 mg.

The drug is also available by inhalation. A single inhalation contains 0.36 mg of ergotamine tartrate. Inhalation may be repeated at intervals of no less than 5 minutes up to a total of six in 24 hours. Overdosage should be carefully avoided.

Only occasionally is the drug used intravenously, employing 0.25 mg initially, but not more than 0.5 mg should be given in 24 hours by this route.

For dihydroergotamine the same doses apply, except that this drug is always given either intramuscularly or intravenously. One begins with 1 mg at the start of an attack, repeating at hourly intervals up to a total of 3 mg. Intravenously, 1 mg is given for rapid effect, and this may be repeated in 1 hour.

If ergonovine or methylergonovine are used for acute attacks, the usual dose is 0.2 to 0.4 mg initially, repeating the dose every 2 hours to a total of not more than 1.6 mg in 24 hours. The maximum dose in 1 week is 12 mg.

Methysergide maleate is also a form of ergot, and is discussed below.

There are adverse reactions and precautions to be followed when using ergot. If given in large doses ergot compounds may cause nausea, vomiting, epigastric discomfort, diarrhea, paresthesias of the extremities and cramps and weakness of the legs. Angina may be provoked in patients with coronary artery disease. Severe vasoconstriction and endarteritis may occur after long-term and uninterrupted use of these agents. Gangrene of the extremities may result but is rare (1 in 10,000 patients) when ergot alkaloids are given in recommended doses and in the absence of peripheral vascular disease and other contraindications.

Fibrotic changes in the retroperitoneal, pleural, pulmonary and cardiac tissues have been noted in patients receiving methysergide but not with other ergot alkaloids.

The ergot preparations should not be used in patients with significant peripheral vascular disease including Raynaud's disease, Buerger's disease, thrombophlebitis or marked arteriosclerosis. They should be avoided in patients with severe hypertension or ischemic heart disease, or history of anginal pain after exertion. They should

Table 5-1. Migraine Therapy Chart*

Class	Type	Treatment	Route	Drug	Dosage
Vascular	Migraine Classic Nonclassic	Prophylactic	Oral	Ergotamine tartrate (Gynergen®)	1 mg twice daily—skip 1 day a week
				Ergotamine, phenobarbital and belladonna	
				Bellergal Spacetabs®	1 tablet twice daily
				Bellergal®	1 tablet four times daily
				Methysergide maleate (Sansert®)	2 mg three times daily
				MAO Inhibitors	
				Phenelzine sulfate (Nardil®)	15 mg three times daily—reduce gradually
				Isocarboxazid (Marplan®)	10 mg four times daily—reduce to maintenance dose in 1 month
				Cyproheptadine (Periactin®)	4–16 mg daily as tolerated
				Propranolol (Inderal®)	20 mg t.i.d. and increase as required
				Amitriptyline (Evalil®)	50–100 mg h.s.
				Clonidine (Catapres®)	0.1 mg t.i.d.
				Platelet inhibitors (see p. 61)	
		Abortive	Oral	Ergotamine tartrate (Gynergen®)	1 tablet immediately—repeat every $1/2$ hour, if necessary, to a minimum of 6 tablets per attack
				Ergotamine, caffeine, phenacetin, belladonna (Wigraine®) Ergotamine and caffeine (Cafergot®)	2 stat—repeat 1 every $1/2$ hour to a maximum of 10 per week
				Ergotamine tartrate, cyclizine and caffeine (Migral®)	2 tablets at onset. May repeat 1 tablet every $1/2$ hr up to 6 per day, 10 per week
				Isometheptene mucate, dichloralphenazone and acetaminophen (Midrin®)	Two capsules at once followed by 1 capsule every hour until relieved, up to 5 capsules in 12-hour period

* Recommended dosages of drugs do not conform with FDA approved package circulars but have proven effective in our management of headache patients with minimal side effects.

Table 5-1. Migraine Therapy Chart*

Class	Type	Treatment	Route	Drug	Dosage
			Sub-lingual	Ergotamine (Ergo-mar®, Ergostat®)	1 tablet immediately, under the tongue— repeat at $1/2$ hour intervals if necessary, but not more than 3 tablets in any 24-hour period
			Inha-lation	Ergotamine (Medi-haler-Ergotamine®)	One dose immediately—repeat every 5 min to a maximum of 6 per day, if necessary
			Intra-mus-cular	Ergotamine tartrate (Gynergen®)	$1/2$ to 1 cc immediately and no more than 3 cc per week
				Dihydroergotamine (DHE 45®)	1 cc at hourly intervals, up to 3 cc per day, if necessary
			Rectal	Ergotamine and caffeine (Cafergot®, Cafergot-PB®)	Insert 1 suppository in rectum immediately—repeat in 1 hour, if necessary
				Ergotamine, caffeine, phenacetin and belladonna (Wig-raine®)	

be used with caution in patients with peptic ulcer, renal or hepatic disease and in patients with recent infections. Ergotism is particularly likely to occur where there are signs of septicemia. Ergot preparations have oxytocic properties, particularly ergonovine and methylergonovine, and therefore they are best avoided during pregnancy.

Methysergide

Our studies with this material date back to the early 1960s. It should be recognized that the compound is a lysergic acid derivative, and is closely related to the naturally occurring ergot alkaloids.

There are several blood vessel responses to methysergide. It is capable of producing a permanent state of vasoconstriction, primarily noted as a side effect. It potentiates the pressor effects of catecholamines and other vasoconstrictor agents. It has an additive effect on blood pressure when combined with catecholamines. In animals, the pressor response to the injection of norepinephrine is potentiated by methysergide, and the responses of the nictitating membrane of the cat to both norepinephrine and cervical sympathetic stimulation are strikingly augmented by methylsergide.

The drug has mild anti-inflammatory effects. It is capable of reducing cutaneous inflammation produced by a variety of irritants in both animals and man.

The drug also has effects on unstable vasomotor functions which may play a role in the pathophysiology of migraine. It tends to dampen the activity of the conjunctival blood vessels, when those blood vessels are stimulated to react during periods of oliguria and diuresis. It alters the pressor response during repeated cold pressor tests in man. In animals, the pressor response produced by unilateral carotid occlusion or by direct stimulation of the pressor area of the hypothalmus is inhibited by methysergide.

Saxena has also investigated the mechanism of action of methysergide in vascular headache. He found that methysergide caused a dose-dependent decrease in blood flow almost exclusively in the common and internal carotid arteries, employing the external carotid artery of dogs for the study. Blood pressure was not appreciably changed by the drug, and thus vascular resistance in the carotid region was increased. There was no alteration in vascular resistance in other areas including the femoral, superior mesenteric, renal and vertebral arteries. Evidence was also found for the depression of central vasomotor loci by methysergide in the higher dose ranges.

Methysergide was not very effective in antagonizing the vasoconstrictor action of serotonin in the carotid vessels. Saxena suggested that selective carotid vasoconstriction, and not peripheral antiserotonin action, was most relevant to the antimigraine action of the drug.

Methysergide maleate (Sansert®) is administered orally in divided daily doses of 4 to 6 mg. This drug must be used with caution because of possible side effects. For example, it has been shown to produce retroperitoneal fibrosis as well as fibrotic changes in the heart. The drug should be discontinued for 6 to 8 weeks after 6 months of use. It is believed that this will allow any toxic effect to reverse itself. The patient should be followed with electrocardiograms and intravenous pyelograms while he is receiving the drug.

Cyproheptadine (Periactin®), an antihistaminic with mild-to-moderate antiserotonin activity, also affords headache prophylaxis. The usual oral dosage is 4 mg four times a day, although this may be increased as required to a maximum divided daily dose of 32 mg. No fibrosis has been reported after the use of this drug, but the patient may experience dry mouth (xerostomia), drowsiness and appetite stim-

ulation. (Note: This regimen has not yet been approved by the FDA.)

Lance has shown that the long-term treatment of patients with intractable migraine with the monoamine oxidase (MAO) inhibitor, phenelzine sulfate (Nardil®), reduces the severity and frequency of the attacks to less than half the original number. Patients are given an oral regimen of 15 mg phenelzine or 10 mg isocarboxazid (Marplan®) three times a day. After 10 to

---

Foods to Avoid When Taking Monoamine Oxidase Inhibitors

- liquor
- wine
- cheese, except cottage cheese
- herring
- nuts
- excessive amounts of caffeine and chocolate
- vinegar, except white vinegar
- yogurt
- sour cream
- fresh baked breads
- pods of broad beans
- chicken livers
- anything marinated
- generally, anything fermented

Also, do not take any other medications without advice, including Contact®, Dristan®, Sinutabs® and nose drops.

Tranquilizers may be used concomitantly with MAO inhibitors. But narcotics, especially meperidine (Demerol®), are known to produce hypotensive episodes when given in association with MAO inhibitors and should be avoided.

14 days, this is reduced to a maintenance dose. Patients must be cautioned about consuming any foods or drugs containing tyramine since hypertensive crises have been noted after such stimulation.

Propranolol has been proposed as prophylactic treatment for migraine by many investigators since the original suggestion was made by Weber and Reinmuth in 1972. It is theorized that beta-blocking drugs such as propranolol prevent cranial vasodilation and in this way provide headache prophylaxis. Usually a starting dose of 20 mg twice or three times daily is given, increasing by 20 to 40 mg every 3rd or 4th day until control is achieved. The peak plasma levels of propranolol are reached approximately 90 minutes after oral intake. Some of the reports from Scandinavia suggest that very large doses of the drug need to be employed, up to 240 mg per day. They do not report serious side effects with propranolol, but the experienced clinician will recognize that the drug has widespread effects, and should be employed with extreme caution in patients with cardiac disease, particularly conduction defects, congestive heart failure, and in those atopic individuals who may be predisposed to bronchial asthma. One can monitor the effect of propranolol by observing the pulse rate. The pulse rate should not be depressed below 60 beats per minute in a healthy individual with migraine with this medication.

Amitriptyline may also be used in the prophylaxis of migraine. Couch, Ziegler and Hassanien demonstrated that amitriptyline would improve migraine more than 50% in 72% of patients, and more than 80% in 57% of patients. Depression was absent in 40 patients, borderline in 53 and moderate to severe in 17. Overall depression ratings improved minimally with therapy and there was a weak relationship between improvement in depression and improvement in migraine. Their study suggests that amitriptyline is effective in migraine prophylaxis and it appears to have a primary effect on migraine that is relatively independent of its antidepressant action.

Use of Platelet Antagonists in the Treatment of Migraine

If one accepts the premise that vasoactive materials are important in the vascular permeability which characterizes migraine, then obviously the role of the platelets is critical to the cascade schema of sterile inflammation which accompanies the migraine attack. Studies performed at the Scripps Clinic have clarified the roles of vasoactive amines in inflammation, using an animal model of immune complex arteritis. Briefly, immune complexes can be made to deposit in the blood vessels of rabbits by simultaneous infusion of agents which increase vascular permeability or which liberate vasoactive amines from their storage sites. Conversely, antagonists of vasoactive amines given prior to the appearance of circulating immune complexes are generally effective in limiting the deposition of the complexes. The prophylaxis of migraine has come to depend on precisely those drugs employed in reducing vascular injury in immune complex disease in the experimental model. These include methysergide, combinations of antihistamines, cyproheptadine and corticosteroids. In addition, platelet depletion, which reduces the amounts of vasoactive amines present in storage sites, is also effective. These data suggest that vascular permeability related to injury of any type, including neurogenic injury, may be evoked by the release of vasoactive substances from their reservoirs in the circulation, particularly from the platelets.

Nonsteroidal anti-inflammatory drugs, including aspirin and indomethacin, stabilize proteins and inhibit the formation of active prostaglandins from their precursors. Aspirin will also reduce platelet aggregation and thus indirectly affects the release of vasoactive substances, particularly serotonin.

Recent studies suggest that there is chronic aggregation of platelets in migraine patients which may be unrelated to the type or severity of the migraine attack.

There also appears to be a significant increase in platelet adhesiveness during the headache phase of migraine, and this parallels the increase in plasma serotonin level during the headache prodromata, and the subsequent decrease during the headache phase. It seems likely that the alterations in platelet aggregation are responsible for the observed changes in the plasma serotonin levels, since, at least in humans, platelets contain virtually all of the total plasma serotonin.

Platelet antagonists, currently employed in the treatment of ischemic vascular disease, may also be useful in migraine. These include particularly aspirin, sulfinpyrazone (Anturane), and dipyrimadole (Persantine). Generally these drugs lengthen the survival time of platelets, and inhibit their adherence to various materials such as collagen in vitro. Therapeutic doses are aspirin, one tablet three times daily, sulfinpyrazone 200 mg two to four times daily, and dipyrimadole 100 to 400 daily, in divided doses.

Preliminary studies on the effects of platelet antagonists in the prophylaxis of migraine suggest that sulfinpyrazone may be particularly effective in reducing the intensity and frequency of headache attacks, in much the same manner that it alters the frequency of transient ischemic attacks. The well established use of aspirin in various headache syndromes may in part be related to its effects upon platelets although it is, in addition, an analgesic drug. It seems evident that substances which interfere with platelet aggregation provide yet another avenue for therapy of recurrent vascular headache, particularly for the prophylaxis of vascular headache, and large-scale trials on the efficacy of these medications in this situation are now indicated.

Abortive Treatment—Other Practical Considerations

The drugs used to abort migraine headache are most commonly ergot derivatives and their varied formulations. A few contain only ergotamine tartrate. Several are a combination of ergotamine with caffeine and other materials, such as antispasmodics and sedatives. Almost all routes of administration are included in these medications. Ergotamine tartrate, alone or in combination, may be given orally. These are fixed-dose medications, both as a single compound and in combination. With Cafergot®, Migral® or Wigraine®, two tablets should be administered at the onset of the headache, followed by one tablet every $\frac{1}{2}$ hour, up to a maximum of six tablets if no relief is obtained. Rectal suppositories should be administered at the onset of the attack and repeated in 1 hour if necessary. Ergotamine (Ergomar®, Ergostat®) should be placed under the tongue at the first sign of a headache and should be repeated at $\frac{1}{2}$-hour intervals if necessary, but not more than three tablets in any 24-hour period. Ergotamine may also be inhaled by means of a metered-dose device (Medihaler-Ergotamine®) at the onset of the aura or pain; it can be repeated as necessary every 5 minutes, up to six doses. The most rapid relief of migraine headaches can be achieved by parenteral administration of the ergotamine preparations. A compound containing isometheptene mucate, dichloralphenazone and acetaminophen (Midrin®) is effective in aborting migraine. It is especially useful for people who cannot tolerate ergotamine. In pregnancy, any migraine medication treatment should be avoided. However, if treatment is absolutely necessary, Midrin® may be used with care. During an attack, sedatives and pain-relieving drugs are often used to help the patient's symptoms. Phenothiazines, such as chlorpromazine (Thorazine®), given as rectal suppositories, may help the nausea and vomiting that accompany an acute attack. When a migraine headache lasts for over 24 hours, there is quite often a sterile inflammation around the enlarged vessel. The use of steroids, dexamethasone (Decadron-LA®), 16 mg intramuscularly, will sometimes hasten the end of a prolonged migraine.

Newer Drugs and Other Treatments for Migraine

BC-105 (Sandomigran®), a tricyclic drug, is now being used in Europe for treatment of migraine, primarily as a prophylactic agent. There have also been encouraging reports from Europe about the use of clonidine (Dixarit®), an antihypertensive drug. However, a double-blind study of clonidine and placebo used in the prophylactic treatment of migraine was reported by the Drs. Ryan and Seymour Diamond of the United States. They described 150 migraine patients who were placed on a double-blind cross-over study using clonidine and placebo, done at two different headache centers. The results of this study showed little effect of clonidine on the prophylaxis of migraine. The authors could not recommend continued use of the drug in this situation. Stensrud and Sjaastad of Oslo also reported on a double-blind study with clonidine in patients after long-term treatment with the drug. This was a double-blind cross-over study with clonidine and placebo carried out in 29 patients with migraine. The placebo and clonidine were each given for 7 weeks, and the headache days and headache indices during the last 5 weeks in each period were used for statistical evaluation. The authors concluded that there was no statistically significant difference between placebo and clonidine.

SELF-ASSESSMENT EXAMINATION

1 Almost all severe headaches are migraine. True or False

2 Migraine is derived from the Greek word *hemikrania,* meaning "half a head." True or False

3 Migraine may be unilateral, bilateral or may shift from side to side during an attack. True or False

4 Migraine never appears in childhood. True or False

5 A positive family history can be obtained in 70% of migraine patients. True or False

6 Migraine always occurs during periods of stress and never on vacations or during periods of relaxation. True or False

7 Multiple foods and environmental factors can provoke migraine. True or False

8 Increasing severity of migraine may occur during oral contraceptive therapy. True or False

9 Migraine, allergy and epilepsy are (a) commonly associated with each other; (b) linked by a common etiologic background; (c) characterized by similar electroencephalographic (EEG) changes; (d) all of the above; (e) none of the above

10 Migraine is characterized by (a) a tendency to unilateral head pain which may become generalized; (b) a tendency to throbbing or pulsating pain; (c) an initial vasoconstrictor phase; (d) extracranial vasodilation; (e) all of the above; (f) none of the above

11 The prodromata of migraine include, among other signs and symptoms, (a) scotomata, or blind spots; (b) teichopsia, or fortification spectra; (c) paresthesias, or defects in mobility; (d) episodes of depersonalization; (e) the dyscontrol syndrome

12 Complicated migraine is the term used to describe (a) small strokes associated with a migraine attack; (b) neurologic manifestations which persist beyond the headache period; (c) a peculiar type of abdominal paroxysmal pain; (d) headache associated with an expanding berry aneurysm; (e) a rare form of severe migraine affecting about 1% of migraine patients

13 When employing ergot therapy in migraine, (a) the total weekly dose should be limited to 12 mg; (b) the total daily dose is inconsequential; (c) abortive therapy should be employed if headache is infrequent; (d) multiple delivery forms (oral, sublingual, parenteral, rectal etc.) may be used; (e) associated vascular disease may be ignored

14 Methysergide (a) is used in acute migraine therapy; (b) is used in headache prophylaxis; (c) is a potent serotonin antagonist; (d) may be associated with retroperitoneal fibrosis if used chronically

15 If monoamine oxidase inhibitors are used in headache therapy, (a) patients should be cautioned about eating tyramine-containing foods, especially aged cheese; (b) patients should be cautioned about employing proprietary cold remedies; (c) patients should be cautioned about using vasoconstrictor nose drops; (d) all of the above; (e) none of the above

---

ANSWERS:

1—False; 2—True; 3—True; 4—False; 5—True; 6—False; 7—True; 8—True; 9—e; 10—e; 11—a,b,c; 12—a,b,e; 13—a,c,d; 14—b,c,d; 15—a,b,c,d

6

Cluster Headache

Cluster headache is a descriptive term for a type of headache classified by various authors as Horton's histamine cephalalgia, erythromelalgia of the head, greater superficial petrosal neuralgia and migrainous neuralgia. We prefer the term cluster headache, introduced by E. C. Kunkle, which at least hints at the occurrence of this form of headache in paroxysms, bursts, or "clusters."

Incidence, Onset and Sex Distribution

Since the diagnosis is often missed, or misclassified as migraine, the incidence of cluster headache cannot be realistically determined. Cluster headache, as opposed to migraine, occurs primarily in males in a ratio of about 5 to 1. Cluster headache appears at any age, although the majority occur between the years of 20 and 40.

Hereditary History and Other Factors

As opposed to migraine, there is only an infrequent hereditary history of cluster headache. The occasional woman with this complaint will observe no relationship to menses and no decrease of symptoms during pregnancy. There is an increased incidence of peptic ulcer in cluster headache patients. Some authors have reported an improvement of angina attacks with the occurrence of cluster headache. The attacks can occur with some seasonal regularity, most often in the spring or fall. However, the attacks can also become chronic and these are most difficult to treat.

Sadjadpour of the United States has presented a study on cluster headache, particularly the role of cigarette smoking and the incidence of oculosympathetic palsy. He described 36 patients, all males, ranging in age from 28–68 years, who had typical cluster headaches and had been examined and interviewed by the author since 1968. Of these 36 patients, 13 had partial oculosympathetic palsy when examined within hours or a day or two after their last headache. With a few exceptions a history of chronic and/or heavy cigarette smoking for many years was obtained, the smoking often starting in their teens and continuing to the time of their examination. The author suggests that cigarette smoking in particular may be etiologically related to this type of headache.

L. Kudrow of the United States has studied plasma testosterone levels in cluster headaches. These values were obtained by radioimmunoassay method from two groups of cluster headache males at separate laboratories. In each group the mean testosterone levels were compared with normal control and cluster headache patients in active remission. Significantly lower values were consistently obtained from cluster headache patients during the active phase of their illness when compared either to cluster headache patients in remission or to normal controls. Kudrow suggests that there may be a possible association of lowered plasma testosterone levels with the active phase of the cluster headache syndrome. Kudrow further reported on the prevalence of disorders in a cluster headache population. He surveyed 140 patients with cluster headache and two control groups, regarding the prevalence of migraine, ulcer disease, coronary heart disease and hypertension. Women with cluster headache were shown to have a significantly higher incidence of migraine than women of either control group. Although migraine was more prevalent among cluster headache males, the difference when compared to males of the U.S. population was not significant. Also, peptic ulcer disease among males with cluster headache was significantly more prevalent than in the control groups. In the female population the difference was not significant. Coronary heart disease was more commonly found among cluster headache males than in the control males, but not significantly so. None of the cluster women showed signs of cor-onary heart disease. The occurrence of hypertension in the cluster headache group was less than in either control group, although the difference was not significant. Thus, patients with cluster headache, particularly men, appeared to have more ulcer disease than control groups, may have more coronary artery disease than controls, but demonstrate less hypertension than controls.

Clinical Picture

The clinical features of cluster headache are shown in Fig 6-1. The pain described in cluster cephalalgia is of short duration. The attacks last from a few minutes to several hours, most often 30–45 minutes. Rarely is the pain present longer than 4 hours. The pain is severe, and burning and always one-sided; although an attack can vary from side to side, it almost never occurs on both sides at the same time. The pain is so severe that the patient feels better

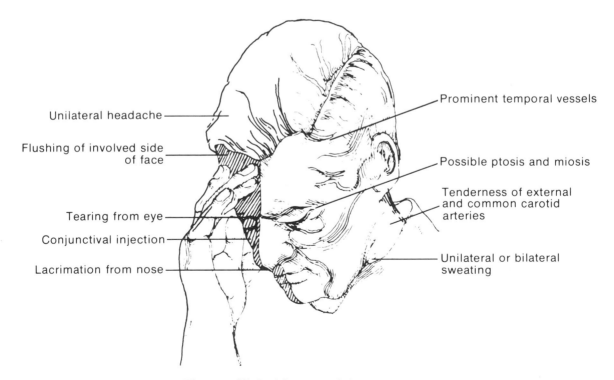

Fig. 6-1. *Clinical features of cluster headache.*

getting up and walking around, as opposed to migraine, where a patient is usually helped by lying down. Most frequently, the attacks occur at night, waking the patient from a sound sleep. There is no aura, as there is with migraine, and nausea and vomiting rarely occur. The location of pain most often described is behind or around the eye. Some patients will exhibit one or more signs of Horner's syndrome during an attack. Ptosis and meiosis may be noted. They may demonstrate flushing of the face, injection of the conjunctiva, nasal congestion and/or rhinorrhea. However, these signs do not have to be present for a diagnosis of cluster headache to be made. The attacks tend to appear in groups or clusters, lasting up to several weeks or several months. Provocative factors which may precipitate attacks include ingestion of alcohol or other vasodilating substances such as nitroglycerin. J. R. Graham has described the peculiar facial characteristics associated with cluster headache. Patients may have thick furrows in their forehead, vertical creases accentuated at the glabella, telangiectases, coarse cheek skin ("peau d'orange"), a square, thickly upholstered chin with a sharp crease between it and a well-chiseled lower lip (Figs 3-3, 3-4). Similar facial characteristics are also present in women. Graham also observed that a similar profile may be found in patients with the carcinoid syndrome.

Cluster headaches occur most frequently at night and may be precipitated by ingestion of vasodilating substances.

Etiology

The etiology of cluster headache remains an enigma. The recurrent symptoms, occurring almost exclusively in males who smoke heavily, at least suggest some possible precipitating factors. We have been unable to demonstrate, however, any unusual reactivity to tobacco or its products, as tested with intradermal challenge. Nor do these patients have unusual or exaggerated signs of histamine release. The Lewis triple response to stroking of the skin is not increased and the response to substances which provoke the release of histamine is no different from those of normal controls. Although it has been reported elsewhere that increased amounts of histamine are found in the blood of patients with cluster headache, our own attempts to confirm this finding using a sensitive bioassay technique have not been successful.

We are impressed, however, with the role of the sphenopalatine ganglion in this syndrome. This ganglion, located deep in the pterygopalatine fossa, receives parasympathetic efferents from cells of the superior salivary nucleus via the glossopalatine nerve, the greater superficial petrosal nerve, and the vidian nerve through the vidian canal. It receives sympathetic branches from the internal carotid plexus via the deep petrosal nerve which joins with the superficial petrosal nerve to form the vidian nerve. It receives afferent sensory fibres from the maxillary nerve particularly, enervating the lacrimal glands, the nose, the palatine membranes, and the periosteum of the orbit. When the sphenopalatine ganglion is electrically stimulated, a syndrome much like that of cluster headache is produced. It is our presumption that in heavy smokers the sphenopalatine ganglion is consistently irritated and eventually becomes hyperactive, usually on one side. Repetitive and nonspecific, disparate stimuli may thereafter set off attacks of typical pain.

Urgency of Symptoms

It is important to note that the pain can be severe enough for the patient to attempt suicide and, therefore, there should be active efforts made at pain alleviation.

Laboratory and Other Diagnostic Methods

Although the patient should be worked up, since glaucoma and vascular abnormalities can rarely mimic cluster headache, the laboratory or x-ray is usually of little help in establishing the diagnosis. B. T. Horton (1956) has described a provocative test employing subcutaneous histamine. Horton and other investigators have used the sublingual administration of 1.3 mg of nitroglycerine to precipitate attacks during cluster periods. We have rarely found it necessary to resort to that test.

Treatment

In any disease in which there is spontaneous remission, evaluation of treatment scientifically proves difficult. (See Table 6-1.)

Most drugs used in treating cluster headache are also used in treating migraine headache.

Treatment should be prophylactic rather than abortive. Acute attacks are difficult to treat since prodromal symptoms are frequently lacking, the pain may awaken the patient from sleep, and the pain rapidly attains its maximum intensity and is short-lived. Medications which reduce vascular activity and inhibit the elaboration of vasoactive amines, or their actions, are effective. Frequently we use methysergide 2 mg three times daily and cyproheptadine 8 mg at bedtime. Foods and alcohol containing vasoactive substances should be avoided in the diet. If these medications are not effective, corticosteroids should be added to the regimen. The rationale for the use of corticosteroids is not clear but is probably related to their multiple effects on inflam-

mation. Prednisone 30 mg every other day have or Triamcinolone 4 mg four times/day have been effective if given for 10 to 14 days. As the headache period ends, the medications are gradually reduced and discontinued. In an occasional patient *chronic* cluster headaches appear and represent a treatment problem of significance. Methysergide should not be used for prolonged periods of time because of its tendency to produce fibrosis. Cyproheptadine may be employed.

Recent reports by Ekbom, Kudrow and Mathew have suggested that, in *chronic* cluster headache, lithium prophylaxis may be an effective treatment. The results from all series are similar. More than half of the chronic cluster headache patients showed improvement with lithium. A small minority derived no benefit whatever, and several had partial improvement. Persistence of autonomic symptoms without accompanying headache was noted in several patients during the initial weeks of therapy.

The method of action of lithium is not fully understood, but it has been suggested that it alters electrical conductivity in the central nervous system. Lithium does affect sodium, calcium and magnesium metabolism, inhibits the action of the antidiuretic hormone, and reduces rapid eye movement stage of sleep (REM).

The drug is completely absorbed in 6 to 8 hours following oral administration and its ordinary half life in the plasma is 24 hours. It is excreted by the kidneys, is distributed in total body water and, after a steady state has been reached, the cerebrospinal fluid contains approximately 40% of serum lithium.

The dose should be individualized, but in general, 900 mg per day can be used for cluster headache patients. To prevent toxicity, the drug should be maintained in a narrow critical range and serum lithium levels should be obtained at least monthly. The levels should not be permitted to exceed 2.0 mEq/1. Generally we suggest that the serum lithium be kept within the range

Table 6-1. Cluster Therapy Chart*

Class	Type	Treatment	Route	Drug	Dosage
Vascular	Cluster	Prophylatic	Oral	Methysergide maleate (Sansert®)	2 mg three times daily
				Triamcinolone (Aristocort®)	4 mg four times daily
				Methylprednisolone (Medrol Alternate Day Therapy Pac®)	16 mg every other day
				Cyproheptadine (Periactin®)	4 mg four times daily
				Ergotamine tartrate (Gynergen®)	1 mg twice daily—skip 1 day a week
				Ergotamine, phenobarbital and belladonna	
				Bellergal Space-tabs®	1 tablet twice daily
				Bellergal®	1 tablet 3–4 times daily
				Lithium (Eskalith®) (See p. 70)	900 mg per day
		Abortive	Oral	Ergotamine tartrate (Gynergen®)	1 tablet immediately—repeat every ½ hour if necessary to a maximum of 6 tablets per day
				Ergotamine, caffeine, phenacetin, belladonna (Wigraine®) Ergotamine and caffeine (Cafergot®)	2 stat—repeat 1 every ½ hour to a maximum of 10 per week
				Ergotamine tartrate, cyclizine and caffeine (Migral®)	2 tablets at onset. May repeat 1 tablet every ½ hour up to 6 per day, 10 per week
			Sublingual	Ergotamine (Ergomar®, Ergostat®)	1 tablet immediately under the tongue—repeat at ½-hour intervals if necessary, but not more than 3 tablets in any 24-hour period
			Inhalation	Ergotamine (Medihaler-Ergotamine®)	One dose immediately—repeat every 5 min to a maximum of 6 per day, if necessary
			Intramuscular	Ergotamine tartrate (Gynergen®)	½ to 1 cc immediately and no more than 3 cc per week
				Dihydroergotamine (DHE 45®)	1 cc at hourly intervals, up to 3 cc per day, if necessary
			Rectal	Ergotamine and caffeine (Cafergot®, Cafergot-PB®) Ergotamine, caffeine, phenacetin, belladonna (Wigraine®)	Insert 1 suppository in rectum immediately—repeat in 1 hour, if necessary

* Recommended dosages of drugs do not conform with FDA approved package circulars but have proven effective in our management of headache patients with minimal side effects.

of 0.7–1.2 mEq/l during maintenance therapy. The blood samples for serum lithium determinations should be drawn 8 to 12 hours after the previous dose when lithium concentrations are relatively stable.

Transient and mild adverse reactions will usually appear in most patients who have serum lithium levels of 1.5 mEq/l and include thirst, polyuria, fatigue and tremor. With more serious side effects, persistent nausea and vomiting, blurred vision and fasciculations may occur, progressing to choreoathetoid movements and convulsions. Unfortunately there is no specific antedote for lithium poisoning but if serum levels reach or are above 2 mEq/l, the lithium should be discontinued and fluid and electrolyte replacement begun. The excretion of lithium can be facilitated by the administration of osmotic diuretics such as urea and mannitol and by alkalization of the urine, using an infusion of sodium lactate. Occasionally peritoneal dialysis and/or hemodialysis may be indicated if renal function is impaired. These problems should rarely occur if the physician is vigilant and if adequate means for measuring serum lithium are available to him. Certainly the drug should not be used at all unless serum lithium levels are easily and immediately obtainable.

A word should be said regarding the surgical treatment of cluster headache. With typical cluster headache this is almost never necessary, but if the problem becomes chronic, then local infiltration of the sphenopalatine ganglion with cocaine can be attempted twice or three times weekly, so long as symptoms persist. If this procedure consistently relieves the patient's complaints of pain, an occasional patient may benefit from cryotherapy of the sphenopalatine ganglion.

Histamine desensitization is difficult to evaluate and is not currently employed as a method of treatment by most headache clinicians. In patients refractive to all other types of therapy, this method can occasionally be of help.

Upper and Lower Cluster Headache Syndromes

Ekbom's recent monograph on cluster headache provides a concise and clear description of this difficult problem. Ekbom makes the point that two clinical forms can be distinguished, which he terms upper and lower syndromes. These differ with respect to the age of onset, as well as radiation of pain from the eye. He notes that in the upper syndrome the maximal pain has an orbital or supraorbital localization, radiating from the eye to the forehead and to the temple. The lower syndrome was characterized by an infraorbital radiation of pain, ipsilateral partial Horner syndrome and ipsilateral hyperhydrosis of the forehead, but absence of clinically visible swelling of the superficial temporal artery. Ekbom suggests that the upper syndrome is associated with dilation of the external carotid artery and that the lower syndrome is characterized primarily by dilation of the internal carotid artery.

Ekbom also reports on carotid angiography in cluster headache, with observations made during an attack of headache. Four of 18 patients had generalized ectasia of all cerebral arteries. In the remaining patients the findings on carotid angiography were essentially within normal limits. One patient was examined before and during an attack. Localized narrowing of the extradural part of the internal carotid artery was observed distal to its exit from the carotid canal. The ophthalmic artery was markedly dilated. When the headache had diminished, another injection of contrast medium was made. This showed that narrowing of the artery had spread to the upper portion of the carotid canal. It is suggested that edema with or without a spastic contraction of the arterial wall characterized the headache attack in this patient.

On the basis of a clinical comparison with 40 consecutive migraine patients, Ekbom made the following observations. Visual prodromes are invariably lacking in cluster headache patients, whereas they occur commonly in patients with migraine. The intensity and character of the pain in cluster headache are usually different from that described in migraine. There is a lower incidence of migraine among close relatives of patients with cluster headache compared to those of migraine subjects. Ekbom concludes that, from a clinical point of view, cluster headache is not merely a variant of migraine headache.

Chronic Paroxysmal Hemicrania

Sjaastad has described this syndrome with strictly unilateral headache, never changing sides, unaccompanied by nausea or vomiting. The most characteristic clinical finding, however, is the frequency of the attacks, 6–18 attacks occuring per 24 hours. These patients are benefited by salicylates and the pain attacks disappear completely on continuous indomethacin medication.

SELF-ASSESSMENT EXAMINATION

1 Cluster headache occurs predominantly in women. True or False

2 Often a strong family history of cluster headache is obtained. True or False

3 Cluster headache is chronic and rarely paroxysmal in character. True or False

4 Cluster headache is frequently prolonged and lasts 24 hours. True or False

5 Cluster headache is often, but not always, nocturnal. True or False

6 Ingestion of alcohol and other vasodilators may provoke headache attacks. True or False

7 Angiography is of value in establishing the diagnosis of cluster headache. True or False

8 Medications employed in cluster headache include (a) methysergide; (b) cyproheptadine; (c) prophylactic ergot therapy; (d) corticosteroids; (e) diphenylhydantoin

9 A provocative test for cluster headache may employ (a) parenteral histamine; (b) oral vasodilators such as nitroglycerine; (c) methysergide; (d) ergotamine tartrate; (e) prostaglandins.

10 Facial characteristics of patients with cluster headache may include (a) coarse cheek skin; (b) deep furrows of face and brow; (c) telangiectases; (d) multiple facial nevi; (e) café-au-lait spots

11 Clinical characteristics of patients with cluster headache include, among others, (a) partial or complete Horner's syndrome; (b) rhinorrhea; (c) lacrimation; (d) flushing of the face; (e) malocclusion of the teeth

ANSWERS:

1—False; 2—False; 3—False; 4—False; 5—True; 6—True; 7—False; 8—a,b,c,d; 9—a,b; 10—a,b,c; 11—a,b,c,d

7

Rare Forms of Migraine and Other Vascular Headaches

Unusual Types of Migraine and Other Vascular Headaches

Visual Field Defects

In Chapter 5 we cited the ophthalmic prodromes of classic migraine such as scotomata, colored spectra, flashing lights and fortification spectra. Rarely do these persist over an hour, and usually they will disappear as the headache begins. More careful investigation is warranted when a visual field defect does persist. Angiomas or other vascular malformations should be ruled out by careful neurologic examination, and appropriate studies. The absence of a cranial bruit, bloody spinal fluid, or history of epilepsy is evidence against a vascular defect. In this situation, computerized axial tomography with contrast enhancement should be employed.

A recent study from England suggests that computerized axial tomography (CAT) in patients with severe migraine may demonstrate pathologic changes where none were suspected. Cerebral atrophy and cerebral infarction were the two principal types of abnormalities seen on CAT scans in patients with or without permanent neurologic sequelae. One could argue that atrophy was related to age and not to the se-

verity of migraine and that the changes, when generalized, were only mild to moderate. On the other hand, perhaps of greater significance was the frequency of focal atrophy and associated infarction. The significance of these findings remains to be determined. The reader is reminded that CAT scans may be normal for some patients with life-long severe migraine, and that there is no obvious association between abnormalities seen on the CAT scan and persistent treatment with ergot derivatives.

Ophthalmoplegic Migraine

Most often the third cranial nerve is involved, but the fourth and sixth nerves can also become involved. The patient usually describes his headache as surrounding his eyeball and complains of symptoms of diplopia, ptosis and strabismus which occur as the headache begins to clear. The ophthalmoplegia can persist from a few days to 3 months. Some cases, after many attacks, can become permanent.

Hemiplegic Migraine

Rarely, patients may develop motor paralysis and/or sensory disturbance as a complication of their migraine. The findings are unilateral and may also include vertigo, dysphasia and ophthalmic symptoms. It is suggested that in hemiplegic migraine prolonged vasoconstriction occurs with associated cortical anoxia. The headache may begin after the neurologic symptoms have persisted 10–90 minutes. With the appearance of the headache, the neurologic signs usually disappear. Rarely, the symptoms of paralysis or sensation persist up to several days and, even more rarely, remain permanently. Some authors have reported a familial occurrence of hemiplegic migraine.

Glista and associates have described 10 members of one family with hemiplegic migraine. The typical attack was stereotyped from member to member and three of the 10 members had hemiplegic migraine attacks associated with minor head traumata. One person had persistent neurologic signs after an episode of hemiplegic migraine. The authors suggest that focal edema of the brain associated with initial vasoconstriction and subsequent vasodilatation produces the neurologic changes. They suggest further that propranolol appears to reduce the intensity and frequency of familial hemiplegic migraine attacks.

Basilar Artery Migraine

The symptoms are uncommon, but the patients report vertigo, diplopia, ataxia, dysarthria and incoordination as preheadache phenomena. Some may have a history of fainting or loss of consciousness. The symptoms usually precede the headache but can persist after the headache subsides, for several days.

Toxic Vascular Headache

This category includes all of the diseases and conditions which produce headache of a vascular nature as part of their overall symptomatology (Table 7-1). The most common nonmigrainous vascular headache is produced by fever. Generalized vasodilation may occur as a consequence of any significant fever, the vasodilation usually becoming more intense as the fever rises. Particularly intense vascular headaches may occur with pneumonia, tonsillitis, septicemia, typhoid fever, tularemia, influenza, measles, mumps, poliomyelitis, infectious mononucleosis, malaria and trichinosis. The vasodilation in these diseases is often intracranial as well as extracranial.

The most common nonmigrainous vascular headache is produced by fever.

Table 7-1. Causes of Toxic Vascular Headaches

Pathologic conditions		Total substances		Withdrawal from drugs
Febrile	**Other**	**Nonpharmacologic**	**Pharmacologic**	
Pneumonia	Alcohol hangover	Carbon monoxide	Nitrates	Ergot
Tonsillitis			Indomethacin	Caffeine
Septicemia	Hypoglycemia	Lead	Oral progestational medications	Amphetamines
Typhoid fever	Hypoxia	Benzene		Many phenothiazines
Tularemia		Carbon tetrachloride	tions	
Influenza			Oral vasodilators	
Measles		Insecticides		
Mumps		Nitrites		
Poliomyelitis				
Infectious mononucleosis				
Malaria				
Trichinosis				

Alcohol Headache

It is suggested that the hangover headache is due to vasodilation. It may be relieved by caffeine or ergotamine tartrate. The use of fructose, 30 gm, taken in the form of honey, can speed alcohol metabolism and thus reduce the frequency and intensity of hangover headache. The complaint is self-limited.

Hypoxic and Hypercapnic Headache

Any increase in carbon dioxide in the blood results in extreme dilation of cerebral vessels. Anoxia also produces throbbing headache. Thus, conditions such as high altitudes, carbon monoxide poisoning and anemias of sudden onset can cause headache. The subject complains of an intense, throbbing headache, a fullness in the head and a flushing of the face. Photophobia, injection of the conjunctiva and, rarely, cyanosis may also appear.

Nitrate and Nitrite Headache

Chronic exposure to nitrates or nitrites, either in industry (munitions) or in medications (for coronary heart disease), will cause vasodilation and cephalalgia. The headache is of a dull and aching quality and may be associated with a flushing of the face. Sometimes, tolerance to nitrates will occur with prolonged use. We have observed the recurrence of migraine-like symptoms in elderly patients who have previously suffered from migraine and were, for a long period, free of symptoms until they were given nitrates for their coronary insufficiency. Sodium nitrite, a preservative used in hot dogs, sausages and cured meats, can be a cause of vascular headaches; monosodium glutamate, found in soy sauce and other prepared foods, also can be a precipitator of vascular headache.

Caffeine Withdrawal Headache

Head pain after withdrawal of caffeine consequent upon a long history of ingestion can persist and be generalized for weeks. Eventually, it will disappear. This headache is quite common in heavy coffee drinkers who cease drinking coffee abruptly at their physician's request.

Withdrawal from caffeine and various drugs can produce headache.

Drugs and Poisons

Many poisons may evoke headache, including lead, benzene, carbon tetrachloride and insecticides. Treatment with monoamine oxidase inhibitors may cause a serious headache, especially when small amounts of catecholamines are ingested at the same time. The headache produced may be catastrophic and cerebrovascular accidents as well as deaths have been reported as a result of this combination.

Withdrawal from many pharmacologic agents may provoke headache. This is especially likely after prolonged therapy with ergot derivatives but may also follow the discontinuation of amphetamines and many of the phenothiazines. Treatment of arthritis with indomethacin may evoke headache, presumably by producing a chemical vasodilation.

Headache Associated With Arterial Hypertension and Toxemia of Pregnancy

Several categories of headache are associated with hypertension and deserve discussion. A sudden rise in blood pressure during violent exercise, anger, or sexual excitement, may be associated with bilateral pounding headache, usually short-lived or transient, which is rarely of diagnostic or therapeutic importance. Effort migraine occurring in athletes after a long race, or in mountain climbers experiencing anoxia, is a related phenomenon. Such episodes do not usually require specific therapy.

Sudden and extreme elevations of the blood pressure may occur with toxemia of pregnancy, in the malignant state of essential hypertension, and with end-stage renal disease. The syndrome termed hypertensive encephalopathy consists of severe headache, nausea, vomiting and convulsions, proceeding to confusion and coma. Papilledema is always present as a primary sign of increased intracranial pressure. The headache is more or less continuous, is generalized, pounding and difficult to relieve with simple analgesics. It is assumed that brain edema in some form produces the headache associated with hypertensive encephalopathy. The intravenous injection of osmotically active agents such as Mannitol will reduce its intensity. Oral glycerol is also effective. These agents produce relative dehydration of the brain, subsequent to which traction and displacement of pain-sensitive structures is reduced.

The neurologic signs of hypertensive encephalopathy occurring in toxemia are probably related to cerebral vasospasm, thereafter producing cerebral ischemia and cerebral edema. The primary therapeutic aim in hypertensive encephalopathy is to reduce the blood pressure, which is the only effective way to relieve the symptoms.

Vascular headache may also be associated with a paroxysmal rise of blood pressure as seen in a patient with a pheochromocytoma, but other physical findings should lead rapidly to that diagnosis.

What remains are those headaches associated with essential hypertension. With this common disease, the pain is vascular in nature and is best related to the contractile state of the extracranial and intracranial arteries. Should these arteries dilate, for whatever reason, hypertensive vascular headache will occur. Usually the pain is described as dull and aching with a pounding component, often present in the morning, and improving as the patient stirs, gets up and moves about. The pain is frequently increased by effort, stooping and by jolts to the head.

Hypertensive headache is rarely present unless the diastolic blood pressure exceeds 110 mm Hg.

Often the headache is relieved by rest in bed or by other methods of relaxation which reduce the blood pressure. A low salt diet may be helpful. Weight loss is often advised. The headache can be expected to respond to those medical measures which reduce the blood pressure to normal or near-normal levels. Though ergotamine tartrate may improve vascular headache related to hypertension, its routine use in this situation is not recommended.

Patients with minimal hypertension who complain of headache need careful evaluation. Often the tendency is to blame the headache on the hypertension when this may not be the case. As mentioned above, unless the diastolic blood pressure exceeds 110 mm Hg, another etiology should be sought in this situation.

Treatment of Acute Intermittent Migraine of Pregnancy

In ordinary circumstances, the cornerstone of medical therapy is ergotamine tartrate in one of its forms. In pregnancy, ergotamine tartrate is best avoided, for reasons of emotion and tradition, if not of science. The tendency of some of the natural ergot alkaloids is to increase the motor contractions of the uterus. Yet ergotamine tartrate, given by mouth, is without oxytocic effects on the human uterus. The problem is compounded by the important oxytocic properties of other ergot alkaloids. For example, ergonovine, sometimes used in migraine therapy, has prompt oxytocic activity when given orally. Hence the notion of avoiding all ergot drugs in therapy of pregnant migraine patients, since the clinician may become confused regarding which of the various forms of ergot are, in fact, oxytocic. (It may also be noted that, for the most part, ergot drugs are not effective abortifacients, particularly in the first two trimesters of pregnancy.)

Thus, treatment of acute intermittent migraine of pregnancy depends primarily on the use of analgesics and sedatives, much as any other self-limited pain syndrome. Chlorpromazine, by virtue of its analgesic and antiemetic effects, is particularly useful.

Treatment of Chronic Migraine of Pregnancy

This occurs only rarely in pregnancy. If simple analgesics and sedatives fail to relieve symptoms, cyproheptadine may be employed, beginning with 4 mg four times daily and increasing as necessary. Symptoms of anxiety and/or depression should be treated. Chlorpromazine 25 mg three times daily may be helpful. If depression is present, amitriptyline 25 mg three times daily is suggested.

Orgasmic Headache

Headaches may be related to sexual activity and particularly to orgasm. There appear to be two forms of headache associated with sex. The first which occurs with mounting excitement is related to muscle contraction in the head or neck. The second can be separated from that caused by muscle contraction or is superimposed on it. This headache, a more severe and explosive headache, usually appears immediately before the time of orgasm, and is thought to be vascular in nature. Some have termed this orgasmic headache.

The possibility of intracranial vascular or other lesions must always be borne in mind, particularly sudden rupture of a subarachnoid hemorrhage which is said to occur during orgasm. On the other hand, as noted above, headache syndromes do occur associated with sexual excitement in which no organic change can be demonstrated. Thus, there may be a benign orgasmic headache analogous to that associated with cough or with exertion which does not necessarily imply intracranial disease. If more serious intracranial disease occurs, the signs should be obvious to the clinician and further study would be warranted.

Exertional Headache

An exertional headache is defined as one that transiently interferes with complete comfort and follows exertional activities, such as coughing, sneezing, bending, running, lifting, or straining with a bowel movement. Of diagnostic importance is the fact that the onset is prompt and directly related to the activity, and the duration of the pain is short (from seconds to a few minutes).

In the past, these headaches were considered to have an ominous prognosis, and patients in whom they occurred were suspected to have brain or surrounding tissue disease. Rooke, in an excellent review on the subject, describes a large series of patients with benign exertional headaches he studied, some for as long as 10 years. Only about 10% of his patients eventually were found to have organic disease. Vigilance is a must, however, since exertional headache is more frequently found with a brain lesion.

The benign form is more prevalent in men and older patients and will usually improve or disappear after several years. Some authors have implicated dental disorders as a cause, but this has not been our experience. Care should be taken in all cases to rule out lesions such as Arnold-Chiari deformity and other foramen magnum conditions.

In older patients, a conservative approach is indicated and would omit invasive investigative procedures such as angiograms, pneumoventriculograms or myelograms in the absence of other neurologic signs. However, a computerized axial tomography study would be indicated. We have had some favorable response in treating benign exertional headaches with indomethacin, 25 mg three times a day, taken with meals.

Propranolol hydrochloride has also been of occasional help in doses of 20 to 40 mg four times daily.

Traumatic Dysautonomic Cephalalgia

N. Vijayan has described this post-traumatic syndrome. His patients did not suffer serious head injuries but had trauma of the soft tissues of the neck around the carotid vessels. Subsequently they developed recurrent episodes of unilateral vascular headaches associated with facial sweating and pupillary dilation ipsilateral to the site of the injury. Clinical and neuropharmacologic observations revealed evidence of partial oculosympathetic paralysis in between or immediately following the headache episodes. There were no premonitory neurologic manifestations as seen in classical migraine and the headaches did not respond to therapy with various ergot preparations.

Treatment with propranolol up to 80 mg a day in divided doses was effective in Vijayan's cases.

SELF-ASSESSMENT EXAMINATION

1 Visual field defects associated with migraine usually persist for 3 to 4 hours. True or False

2 In ophthalmoplegic migraine, permanent oculomotor palsy may ensue. True or False

3 In hemiplegic migraine prolonged vasoconstriction occurs with consequent cortical anoxia. True or False

4 Permanent paralyses are sometimes reported in hemiplegic migraine. True or False

5 Headache associated with hangover is most often due to muscular contraction. True or False

6 Withdrawal from chronic ergot therapy may be followed by a toxic vascular headache. True or False

7 Vascular headache appreciated at sea level is improved at high altitudes. True or False

8 In basilar artery migraine, usually occurring in young women, (a) vertigo and diplopia may occur; (b) fainting is reported; (c) elevated spinal fluid pressure appears frequently (d) bilateral incoordination is noted; (e) prolonged sensory complaints may be described

9 Hemiplegic migraine (a) often occurs in families; (b) is characterized by unilateral motor paralysis which may be persistent; (c) may produce residual neurologic damage; (d) all of the above; (e) none of the above

10 Ophthalmoplegic migraine is of importance because (a) it may be confused with an expanding berry aneurysm; (b) it is a common form of headache; (c) it occurs in childhood frequently (d) although troublesome, it never produces permanent ophthalmoplegia

11 Toxic vascular headache (a) is another name for cranial arteritis; (b) refers to classical migraine; (c) was the original term for cluster headache; (d) all of the above; (e) none of the above

12 Headache associated with overingestion of alcohol (hangover headache) (a) is vascular in nature; (b) should be treated by imbibing vodka; (c) may respond to vasoconstrictor agents; (d) may be improved by eating honey; (e) is usually self-limited

13 Alterations in the content of respiratory gases in the blood (a) rarely cause headache; (b) may be responsible for altitude headache; (c) may accompany carbon monoxide intoxication; (d) may accompany anemia; (e) are of little consequence

14 Industrial exposures of various types produce headache including (a) exposure to silica; (b) exposure to nitrites; (c) exposure to carbon monoxide fumes; (d) exposure to horse manure; (e) exposure to grass seed

15 Poisoning of various forms is associated with headache. Toxic materials include (a) lead; (b) benzene; (c) carbon tetrachloride; (d) insecticides; (e) all of the above; (f) none of the above

---

ANSWERS:

1—False; 2—True; 3—True; 4—True; 5—False; 6—True; 7—False; 8—a,b,d,e; 9—d; 10—a; 11—e; 12—a,c,d,e; 13—b,c,d; 14—b,c; 15—e

8

Traction and Inflammatory Headache and Cranial Neuralgias

Mass Lesions

Headache from intracranial sources is most often produced by inflammation, traction and displacement or distention of the pain-sensitive structures of the head, usually blood vessels. Most of the displacement is the result of traction; hence the term traction headache is used to identify this group. A traction headache can be elicited by hematomas of any sort, abscesses, nonspecific brain "edema" and lumbar puncture. It is, especially, a symptom of brain tumors (Fig 8-1).

A traction headache is a symptom of brain tumors.

Headache is certainly one of the cardinal signs of brain tumor, particularly a rapidly expanding lesion producing traction on the pain-sensitive structures of the head. This is especially the case if the ventricular system is compromised with obstruction of absorption or flow of cerebrospinal fluid, and hydrocephalus is produced. Headache is almost always a prominent finding with increased intracranial pressure. But with more slowly growing tumors, headache may be transitory, or mild, or easily relieved by common analgesics, and the patient's description of his head pain in this situation may be desultory. The worst head pains are not usually related to tumor, but to vascular headaches or the major neuralgias. Some generalizations concerning headache as an aid to localization in patients with brain tumor seem justified and these follow:

- Although the headache of brain tumor may be referred from a distant intracranial source, it approximately overlies the tumor in about one-third of all patients.

- If the tumor is above the tentorium, the pain is frequently at the vertex, or in the frontal regions.

- If the tumor is below the tentorium, the pain is occipital and cervical muscle spasm may be present (Fig 8-2).

- Headache is almost always present with posterior fossa tumor.

- If the tumor is midline it may be increased with cough or straining or sudden head movement. (This also occurs with migraine.)

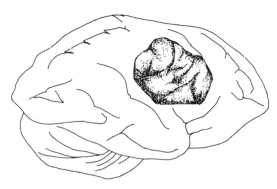

Fig 8-1. *Headache and brain tumor, neurologic signs: seizures, focal or general, progressive loss of neurologic function and mental symptoms. Headache pattern: onset usually intermittent, often dull and aching in character, increases in frequency and duration, sometimes altered by change in posture and tone.*

It has been possible to demonstrate localized skull tenderness at the site of meningiomas, or in the mastoid area, with a cerebellopontine angle tumor, presumably due to local involvement and extension into the skull or its structures by the tumor.

Treatment for this form of headache generally involves specific therapy for the associated underlying disease. Extensive investigation and consultation with other specialists may be required. Thus, the therapy for headache evoked by traction or inflammation of pain-sensitive cranial constituents is varied and may range from surgery to antibiotics. It is in this group that emergency treatment may be necessary. The headache is considered to be a secondary phenomenon which usually responds to alleviation of the primary disease.

Arteritis and Infections

Headaches can be caused by arteritis and infections. These headaches are related to inflammatory processes within or without the skull, in particular to meningitis, intracranial arteritis and phlebitis. The pain is evoked by an inflammatory response which includes those of the pain-sensitive structures of the head. The head pain is, in most instances, coincident with the course of the disease, usually abating as the disease is brought under control and is not recurrent or paroxysmal.

Much of headache pain relates to changes in blood vessels. In particular, arterial inflammation is considered to be painful, and angiitis occurs as a frequent complication of immunological disorders (Table 8-1). Headache is especially associated with periarteritis nodosa and giant cell arteritis. Headache is not commonly associated with systemic lupus erythematosus (SLE), unless there are other signs of involvement of the central nervous system.

In polyarteritis nodosa, there are multiple areas of arterial necrosis and inflammation affecting many organs. The arterial lesion appears to be identical to that found

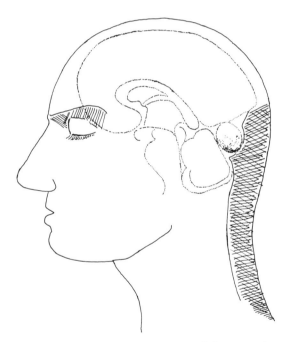

Fig 8-2. *Headache with tumors of the posterior fossa. Pain is referred to the occipital and neck areas.*

■ If the tumor is hemispheric, the pain is usually appreciated on the same side of the head.

■ If the tumor is chiasmal, at the sella, the pain may be referred to the vertex.

Table 8-1. Immunological Diseases and Angiitis

Periarteritis nodosa (polyarteritis nodosa)
Giant cell arteritis (temporal arteritis)
Connective tissue disease ("collagen disease") associated with
  Rheumatoid arthritis
  Scleroderma
  Poly- and dermatomyositis
  Rheumatic fever
  Erythema nodosum
  Sjögren's syndrome
Hypersensitivity angiitis:
  Drug reaction
  Henoch-Schönlein purpura
  Systemic lupus erythematosus (SLE)
  Mixed cryoglobulinemia
  Goodpasture's syndrome
  Hypergammaglobulinemic purpura
  C2 deficiency with vasculitis
  Australian antigenemia with vasculitis

in serum sickness. Gamma globulin may be identified in areas of fibrinoid necrosis. The role of this gamma globulin in the production of the arterial lesion is the subject of intensive investigation. Recently, 4 of 11 patients with biopsy-proven polyarteritis were found to have Australia antigenemia, suggesting that an immunologic reaction to a virus or virus-like particle had produced the systemic vasculitis. Circulating immune complexes were found in 3 of these patients and were composed of Australia antigen and immunoglobulin. Studies of tissue from 1 patient showed deposition of Australia antigen, IgM and β1C in blood vessel walls.

In temporal arteritis, a relatively similar pathologic picture occurs, except that the inflammatory reaction may be limited to the cranial arteries. The elastic tissues appear frayed or fragmented and giant cells within the vessel walls are almost a constant feature of the pathologic findings. The giant cells are most numerous in the region of the deranged internal elastic lamina.

Recent studies employing immunofluorescence have demonstrated that patients with temporal arteritis have anti-capillary antibodies in their sera, as well as deposits containing IgG which are localized to the arterial wall in temporal artery biopsies

procured for diagnosis. The capillary antibodies in sera of these patients are present in significant titer. Such antibodies are also found in certain rheumatic diseases, some of which, such as rheumatoid arthritis and SLE, are characterized by an arteritis. Capillary antibodies are discovered infrequently in normal controls or in blood donors.

Not all patients with "temporal arteritis" have headache, but when present, the headache is of high intensity, of a deep aching quality, throbbing in nature, and persistent, (Fig 8-3). In addition to the aching and throbbing, there is often a burning component, unlike most other vascular headaches. The headache is slightly worse when the patient lies flat in bed, and is diminished in intensity by the upright or half upright position. It is somewhat reduced in intensity by digital pressure on the common carotid artery on the affected side and is

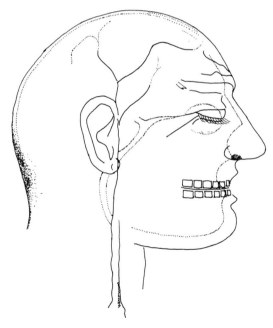

Fig 8-3. *Clinical features of cranial (temporal) arteritis: often unilateral headache, temporal artery is sometimes enlarged, rigid and tender, sudden or gradual loss of vision in one eye if the ophthalmic artery is involved. Early possible complaints include pain in the ear, pain with chewing, pain in the teeth or sometimes pain in the occiput.*

made worse by stooping over. There is hyperalgesia of the scalp, and the distended arteries are extremely tender, so that any pressure greatly increases the pain.

Some patients may suffer pain on mastication, and in some it may be the initial symptom. Facial swelling and redness of the skin overlying the temporal arteries, with the addition of the burning component of pain, are usually noted after the onset of headache. Immediate relief from burning pain and headache may follow biopsy of the inflamed temporal artery, and it is assumed that this follows the interruption of the afferents for pain about the vessel.

Prior to the onset of the full-blown picture of "temporal arteritis," there is often pain in the teeth, ear, jaw, zygoma and nuchal region and occiput. The distribution of these symptoms suggests primary involvement of other branches of the external carotid artery, notably the external and internal maxillary arteries.

Other arteries may also be involved, including the major vessels of the aorta, the coronaries, and the arteries of the limbs. Large- and medium-sized arteries are the principal sites of the inflammatory process. Aneurysm formation may occur in association with the arteritis.

The presenting complaint may be of ocular symptoms. It has become evident that more than a third of patients with temporal arteritis are threatened with partial or even complete loss of vision. Diplopia and photophobia have been noted, and ophthalmoscopic evidence of occlusion of the ophthalmic artery has been apparent in some cases.

Some patients have presented signs suggestive of cerebral damage and encephalitis during the acute stage of the illness. We have observed several patients with thrombotic strokes related to cranial arteries.

If loss of vision is the presenting complaint, then a medical emergency is in progress and the patient requires urgent treatment. This should not wait upon the specific method used to make the diagnosis, that of temporal artery biopsy. Prednisone or some other corticosteroid is the treatment of choice. As soon as the diagnosis is made, 40 to 60 mg should be given. The sedimentation rate should be followed as a guide to management with prednisone. It is generally necessary to continue therapy with prednisone at a low maintenance dose of approximately 10–20 mg for a prolonged period of time.

Postpuncture Headache

Postpuncture headache may be defined as the headache, mild or severe, that may appear a few hours to several days after lumbar puncture, lasting a variable period of days or, rarely, weeks. It is a sequel to lumbar puncture in approximately one out of every four patients. The pain is a dull, deep ache and may be throbbing. It is usually bifrontal and often also suboccipital. In the latter position it may be associated with moderate stiffness of the neck. Most characteristic are its occurrence when the subject is erect and its virtual elimination when he is horizontal. Shaking the head makes it more intense. It is usually resistant to all treatment except rest in bed in the horizontal position and the passage of time. Because of the frequency of its occurrence, the occasional severity of the discomfort, and the duration of the disability, headache of this type has been of clinical interest ever since the technic of lumbar puncture was introduced. Although theories concerning postpuncture headache have been clearly contradictory, the weight of the evidence supports the view that it is usually related to a loss of cerebrospinal fluid secondary to leakage through the dural hole.

Lasater has described a syndrome of primary intracranial hypotension, the symptomatology of which is identical to that of postpuncture headache. Headache is present in the upright position and is relieved by recumbency. Nausea, vomiting, vertigo, pallor and sweating may accompany the headache. The cerebrospinal fluid pressure is always very low. The symptoms last from 2 to 16 weeks and subside spontaneously. There is no specific therapy, and, to date, the cause is unknown. Lasater suggests that the syndrome may be the result of leakage of cerebrospinal fluid from a tear in the arachnoid or in the dural sheath of a spinal nerve root.

Disease of the Cranial or Neck Structures

Headache may be related to diseases of the eyes, nose, teeth or any of the other structures of the head. Noxious stimuli can be elicited by localized pressure phenomena, muscle contraction, trauma, tumor or inflammation. Generally, these headaches are confined to the affected area, although occasionally, due to central spread of excitation, their effects may be appreciated in more distant regions of the skull. Persistent painful stimuli may lower pain threshold and so evoke other forms of headache. For example, pain from ocular disease can be related to several different mechanisms and thus present a diagnostic challenge to the clinician. Eye pain may occur with increased ocular pressure, traction on ocular muscles, inflammation of the eye tissues, hyperopia or astigmatism, exposure to light, new growths or trauma (Fig 8-4). In pseudotumor of the orbit, severe pain is felt together with ophthalmoplegia, usually the result of an inflammatory lesion of the cavernous sinus or of the orbit itself.

Headache related to nasal disease is usually anterior and is often related to nasal vasomotor phenomena. The symptoms are accompanied by local pain and discomfort. Demonstration of a precise paranasal disease, such as sinusitis or allergic rhinitis, usually removes the headache from this category. This form of headache is frequently associated with vasomotor rhinitis and is assumed to represent a localized vascular reaction to stress.

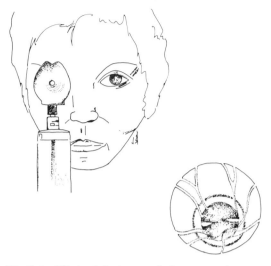

Fig 8-4. *Clinical features of glaucoma: intense headache involving the eye and supraorbital area, glaucomatous cupping of the optic disc, dilated pupil, pain in the eyeball, increased intraocular pressure.*

Cranial Neuritis and Neuralgias and Temporomandibular Joint (TMJ) Disease

Some forms of facial pain are considered to be related to the cranial nerves, *excluding* the trigeminal and glossopharyngeal neuralgias. They commonly include the atypical facial neuralgias, lower-half headache, vidian neuralgias, carotidynia and buccal neuralgia. Some of these syndromes are poorly developed and may not deserve a separate status. Some of them probably represent vascular pain or a form of migraine perceived in an unusual location. This is particularly true of lower-half headaches, which may respond to prophylaxis as with lysergic acid derivatives, such as methysergide.

Are there symptoms related to TMJ disease? The question is still being debated in the literature. A recent questionnaire on the subject finds that some 43% of physicians and 35% of dentists are in doubt or are uncertain that the syndrome even exists. We believe that facial pain can occur with TMJ disease, usually best appreciated locally, with radiation to the jaw, the neck and behind the ear, not neuritic in character. In our view, the syndrome consists of localized facial pain, limitation of motion of the jaw, muscle tenderness and joint crepitus. Usually the joint itself is normal in its radiologic appearance

The temporomandibular joint (TMJ) is the only moveable joint in the head, if one excludes the junction of the head with the atlas. It is our impression that disease of the temporomandibular joints is relatively rare. The most common complaint in TMJ disease is headache, of moderate intensity, located at the vertex, occiput or in the face overlying the joints. Diagnosis may sometimes be difficult. One should certainly palpate and auscultate the joints with significant pressure, with the patient opening and closing his mouth. If crepitus can be heard, osteoarthritis in the joint can be assumed. One may thereafter inject a local anesthetic such as 1 cc of a 2% solution of lidocaine into the joint to see whether or not there is alteration in facial pain. Here, again, consultation with a dentist who is knowledgeable in this field is essential. The point to be made is that patients with TMJ disease have pain primarily from muscular tension related to dental occlusive disease. Because of localized pain the patient begins to use the opposite side of the mouth on which to chew, attempting to splint the painful side but, in point of fact, this has exactly the opposite effect and makes the painful joint do all the work. For example, with right TMJ disease chewing on the left side moves the right temporomandibular joint excessively. There is no evidence that hearing loss, damage to cranial nerves, disturbances of equilibrium, development of Ménière's syndrome or difficulty with the eustachian tubes are in any way related to this syndrome. Current concepts of etiology are that occlusal disharmony and psychophysiologic factors play primary roles, with most of the dysfunction resident in the masticatory muscles rather than in the TMJ itself. Those pathologic changes which affect the joint, such as rheumatoid arthritis, may cause similar complaints, but are by definition different problems.

Attempts to relieve pain should be directed, then, at the relief of muscle spasm. Mouth reconstructions are not usually indicated in this situation and extensive surgery of the oral area should be undertaken with the greatest caution, since such procedures tend to reinforce the pain syndrome rather than relieve it. We suggest the use of simple sedatives and muscle relaxant agents such as chlorphenesin, if these prove to be helpful after a therapeutic trial. Placebo effects are very evident in this condition and have been reported. Physical methods of pain relief including heat, hot packs and massage should also be employed. The physician should work closely with a dentist in the therapy of this condition. Application of dental splints and similar maneuvers may prove helpful.

Attempts to alleviate pain should be directed toward relieving muscle spasm.

The syndromes delineated as trigeminal neuralgia (tic douloureux) and glossopharyngeal neuralgia are better characterized.

The Major Neuralgias

Trigeminal Neuralgia (Tic Douloureux)

The major neuralgias include trigeminal neuralgia and glossopharyngeal neuralgia. Trigeminal neuralgia (tic douloureux) is an episodic recurrent unilateral pain syndrome which occurs in the elderly. It almost never begins before the age of 30 years, unless the patient also has concomitant multiple sclerosis. The pain is of high intensity, and particularly occurs in association with trigger zones, which are areas of increased sensitivity on the face, particularly about the nares and mouth, which set off the attack when they are stimulated, often by trivial sensations (Fig 8-5). Thus, the behavioral characteristic of patients with trigeminal neuralgia is to avoid touching the face, or washing, or shaving, or biting or chewing, or any of the other maneuvers which stimulate the trigger zones and produce the pain. This avoidance technique is an invaluable clue to the diagnosis. In almost every

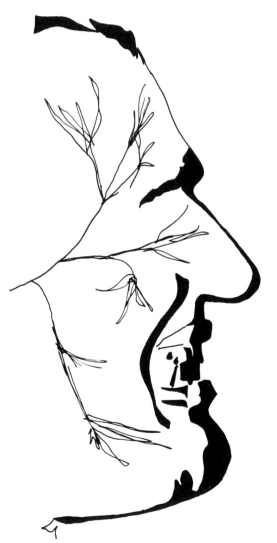

Fig 8-5. *Trigeminal neuralgia. Well localized lancinating pain in the distribution of one branch of the trigeminal nerve.*

other facial pain syndrome, patients will be found massaging the painful area, or abrading it, or applying heat or cold, but in trigeminal neuralgia exactly the opposite occurs, and the patient goes to great lengths to avoid any stimulation of the face or mouth whatever. The pain is usually a high intensity jab lasting less than 20 to 30 seconds, followed at times by a period of relief lasting a few seconds to a minute, again followed by another jab of pain. Repeated episodes of pain may occur, but the pain is not long-lived as is usually the case in other chronic facial pains.

Glossopharyngeal Neuralgia

Glossopharyngeal tic is a similar phenomenon, with the symptoms related to the anatomical base of the glossopharyngeal nerve. In this situation a pain similar to that described for trigeminal neuralgia is usually appreciated in the pharynx, the tonsils and the ear, and is often initiated by swallowing, yawning or eating. Syncope may occur during glossopharyngeal neuralgia, presumably related to asystole as a result of stimulation of the vagus system as well.

Treatment of Trigeminal and Glossopharyngeal Neuralgia

The treatment of trigeminal neuralgia is medical in most situations. Anticonvulsants reduce the sensitivity of the trigger zones, and relieve the pain, often dramatically within 4 to 24 hours. Generally one begins with carbamazepine 200 mg two or three times daily. If this dose is well tolerated and if the pain is rapidly relieved it may be continued for several weeks or months depending upon the course of the disease. One attempts to titrate the medication to the severity of the patient's pain. It may be necessary to continue the medication on a maintenance level such as 200 mg per day in order to keep the patient pain-free. If symptoms persist, diphenylhydantoin may be added to the regimen, and if there is no response to both drugs, then we commonly employ chlorphenesin 400 mg three to four times daily. By the time one reaches the three-drug treatment level, one should be considering referring the patient for appropriate surgery.

Our neurosurgical consultants commonly employ a percutaneous procedure whereby the Gasserian Ganglion is injured using thermal techniques. In elderly patients, this procedure can be done without craniotomy and is consistently effective.

The requirements for stereotaxic surgery include a controlled current, a patient who is awake or easily rousable, careful sensory testing, the preservation of touch, and the ability to relieve pain at the time the patient is on the operating table. In Dr. John Tew's 400 cases, 60% had right-sided pain, 39% had left-sided pain and only 1% had bilateral pain. Often more than one division was involved. In his procedure a stereotaxic surgical technique permitted precise localization of the various divisions of the trigeminal nerve as demonstrated by electrical stimulation. When the needle was in the proper position physiologically and radiographically, a radio frequency generator was turned on to a low voltage setting. The process was then repeated until the correct degree of sensory deficit had been created. Careful incremental lesions were necessary in order to prevent the creation of too much sensory deficit. Appropriate anesthesia was provided while the procedure was being done. Dr. Tew reported excellent results in pain control, but noted significant side effects in that 23% had masseter weakness, 11% had troubles of numbness of the face on the same side and 10% had an absent corneal reflex, with these problems lasting a variable length of time. Sometimes reoperation was necessary as well.

Dr. Peter Jannetta's clinical observations on the treatment of trigeminal neuralgia by suboccipital and trans-tentorial cranial operations are of great current interest. He found that 15 of 46 patients had mild sensory abnormalities in the region of the tic pain, and that abnormal sensory evoked potentials can be elicited in many patients with trigeminal neuralgia. In 100 operated patients he noted evidences of compression of the trigeminal nerve, in 88 by aberrant arteries, in 6 by tumors, 2 of whom had arterial venous malformations. The other 6 patients had multiple sclerosis. Dr. Jannetta's operative procedure is extensive, and requires an open craniotomy and the use of an operating microscope. His results as reported are excellent. In effect, he is suggesting that trigeminal neuralgia is, to put it simply, a compression neuropathy.

Headache Associated with Epidural Hematoma, Subdural Hematoma, Hypertensive Hemorrhage and Cerebellar Hemorrhage

Headache is a prominent symptom of all of the disorders mentioned above, but a complete discussion of these entities is beyond the scope of this monograph. Some clinical observations regarding headache in these conditions are:

1 Epidural hemorrhage is produced by rupture of meningeal vessels due to head trauma. Headache is sudden in onset and severe. There is rapid development of confusion, stupor or coma.

2 Headache in subdural hemorrhage is often nagging, but gradually increases in intensity, as other neurologic signs appear. The hematoma is almost always due to head injury, but may occur in an atraumatic fashion in anticoagulant therapy, blood dyscrasias, alcoholism and diabetes.

3 A high degree of suspicion is necessary on the part of the clinician making these diagnoses. They should be considered in all patients complaining of headache with associated clouding of consciousness, especially in the elderly and in the alcoholic. X-rays of the skull and a CAT scan must be done in this situation. The diagnosis may depend upon cerebral angiography.

Medina, Diamond and Rubino discussed the incidence of headaches in patients with transient ischemic attacks (TIA). They studied 25 patients with ischemic episodes who had been followed for 2–23 months. Episodic headaches occurred during or immediately after transient ischemic attacks but seldom preceded them. These headaches were present in 12 of the patients or 48%, and had a mean duration of 2 hours. The intensity was usually mild to moderate. Headaches involving the anterior circulation TIA were more often unilateral and tended more to appear in the frontal areas than those involving the posterior circulation.

Some Old Clinical Saws Which Should Be Discarded

Saws are defined as tools or devices for cutting. Medical saws, in addition to being useful to the orthopedist, can also be helpful as learning devices. Webster advises that, in addition to their utilitarian aspects, saws are further defined as sententious sayings, or maxims or proverbs. Proverbs are bits of information and knowledge which have persisted and which are often applicable to uncertain circumstances or to irksome situations. Much of folklore in human knowledge is transmitted through maxims and proverbs. Saws have the further advantage of being assimilated by rote learning, are easily understood, down-to-earth, and are proposed as common sensical. Proverbs or maxims may, however, also hinder learning, and they certainly dull the eye of the viewer to new experiences. Like the ritually repeated prayer, they roll off the tongue without thinking.

So it is with medical saws. Do they really save time? Do they enable the busy clinician to cut through the patient's verbiage, and to dazzle the house staff with vocal prestidigitation and footwork? Your observers believe that they may, with reservations. Like other bits of data they need constant revision and re-evaluation. The purpose of this section is to re-evaluate several medical saws concerning headache, and to comment more specifically upon them.

1 *When the headache is always on the same side, suspect an aneurysm* (Fig 8-6). Not so. This type of mischievous clinical advice has probably produced more unnecessary angiograms and furrows in the brows of attending physicians than any other piece of clinical memorabilia extant. Many patients with migraine *always* have their headache on the same side. There isn't any requirement which states that the headache should shift from side to side. In short, the persistence of unilateral head pain is a sign of migraine and not of aneurysm.

2 *Berry aneurysms are common in patients with migraine* (Fig 8-7). Not so. Migraine is a common disease and cerebral aneurysms also are common, so it is reasonable to assume that the two entities may occasionally appear in the same patient. But there is little evidence that the two syndromes are related. Asymptomatic aneurysms are asymptomatic. If an aneurysm begins to expand rapidly, it will produce a particularly severe localized pain which is not liable to be mistaken for recurrent vascular headache.

Headache is the most common symptom of subarachnoid hemorrhage and occurs in every conscious patient. It is usually of very

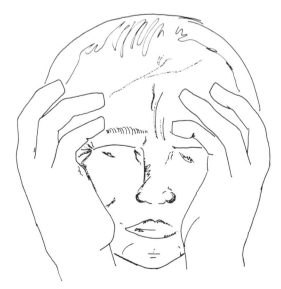

Fig 8-6. *Apoplexy with aneurysmal rupture. Headache is constant, severe, sudden in onset.*

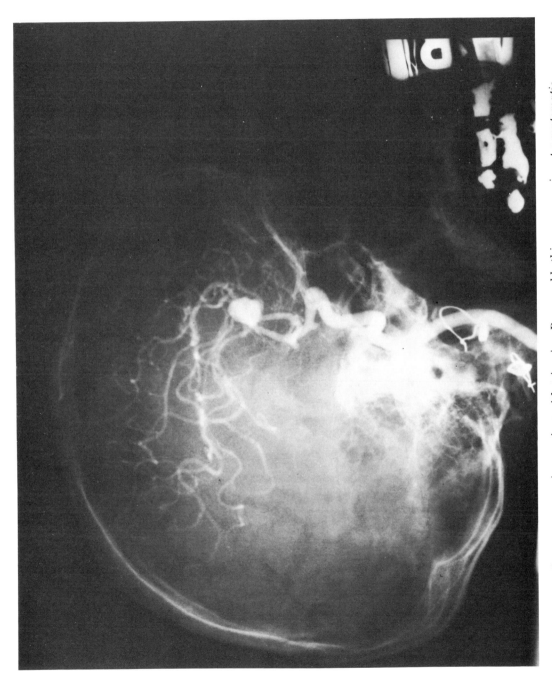

Fig 8-7. *Berry aneurysm in a patient with migraine. Presumably this aneurysm is not symptomatic. Such aneurysms are uncommon in patients with migraine.*

high intensity and of sudden onset. It is often described as "something snapping inside the head," followed by an intense throbbing ache. The ache at the start is commonly located in the occipital region, and then radiates down the neck and back. Less commonly it is first located in the frontal region, bilaterally or unilaterally, in the temporal region, at the vertex, or deep in the eye, but such headache soon radiates into the occipital region. When associated with neck rigidity the headache is made worse by flexure of the neck.

In over half the patients the attack of sudden intense pain is accompanied by vomiting and drowsiness, neck rigidity, and loss of consciousness. Convulsions occur after the onset of such a headache in approximately 10–15% of patients. In 10% of patients there are prodromes of a few hours to several days duration, such as low-intensity frontal or occipital headache, pain in the eye, pain in the back of the neck, backache, or pain in the hamstring muscles. Occasionally the severe headache is preceded by vertigo, photophobia, diplopia and rarely by vomiting.

The high-intensity headache following subarachnoid hemorrhage persists with but little modification for approximately 1 week from its onset, with subsequent complete elimination of pain within 2 months. Sustained, chronic or recurrent headache persisting longer than 2 months following rupture of intracranial aneurysm with subarachnoid hemorrhage is rare in patients who have not had headaches before the accident.

Headache may, on occasion, be a premonitory sign of cerebral embolism. The mechanism is not understood.

Headache of an intense degree also occurs with hypertensive intracerebral hemorrhage of a hemispheric nature. The catastrophic aspects of this disease should be obvious to the clinician, with headache appearing as only one manifestation of a profound neurologic disturbance. If the cerebellum is involved in a hypertensive hemorrhage, consideration should be given to

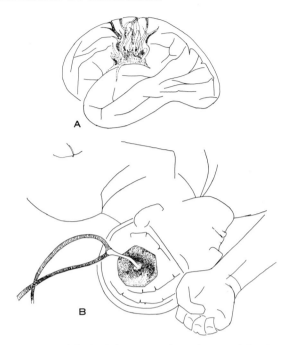

Fig 8-8. *Clinical features of angioma: 1) bruit over the site of angioma which may be calcified on x-ray (B); 2) persistent severe headache with meningeal signs, only if bleeding occurs; 3) disturbance of level of consciousness.*

a direct attack upon the involved hemisphere, which may be lifesaving.

3 *Migraine is a common feature of cerebral arteriovenous anastomoses.* Not so. This almost never occurs (Fig 8-8).

However, angiomas may leak briefly and repeatedly. Since the source of bleeding is usually from anomalous blood vessels, and is not arterial in type, the headache is often not so intense as in subarachnoid bleeding. If sufficient blood is liberated into the subarachnoid space, however, signs of meningeal irritation will also occur, indistinguishable from those which are associated with subarachnoid bleeding associated with rupture of a typical berry aneurysm.

4 *A specific migraine personality exists.* Not so. While some patients with vascular headache can be characterized as compulsive, obsessive and preoccupied with details (see below), occasionally they are dull, torpid and lethargic. It is unwise to assume that similar personality characteristics will always be found in a particular group of patients.

5 *Headache therapy is straightforward and easy, once the diagnosis is made.* Not so. The successful treatment of a patient with headache may not be easily accomplished. The physician will often find that his therapeutic suggestions have not brought forth the desired result. Patience and perseverance on the part of both physician and patient may be necessary. The art of medical practice may be more important here than scientific pharmacology. The physician must first remember to do no harm, since headache complications associated with analgesic abuse are almost always more dangerous than the headaches themselves. Nonetheless, with careful attention to the whole patient, some resolution of the problem can be achieved in the majority of patients who complain of headache.

6 *Migraine is caused by allergy.* Not so. It has not been possible to demonstrate that migraine results from an antigen-antibody reaction, whether the antigen be an inhalant pollen, an injected material or a food. There is no correlation between positive skin tests for various allergens and the appearance of migraine. Long trials of hyposensitization to presumed allergens are not indicated in the chronic treatment of migraine. Hives, allergic rhinitis, atopic eczema, bronchial asthma and other manifestations of true allergic reactions cannot be equated with the migraine episode.

Atypical Facial Neuralgias

The term atypical facial neuralgias is used for those pain syndromes which cannot be otherwise categorized, which are not associated with trigger zones, and in which a steady diffuse aching pain of hours' to days' duration occurs, which is not paroxysmal, and in which no consistent history can be obtained. It is our impression that multiple factors may be responsible for the production of this complaint. A careful search should be made for local pathology of the eyes, nose, teeth, sinuses and pharynx. Some patients with atypical facial pains may be suffering from a form of vascular or common migraine involving the face. This is particularly the case if the pain is throbbing in nature, when a trial on a vasoconstrictor agent of the ergot type may be helpful. If autonomic symptoms including cutaneous pallor, sweating, flushing, rhinitis and the like occur, attempts to alter responses to autonomic stimuli using beta adrenergic blockers such as Inderal can be employed. Many patients with chronic long-standing atypical facial pains require intensive inpatient evaluation. A pain center approach to the problem is indicated, to identify if possible the origins of the pain, medical or otherwise, to isolate factors contributing to the pain problem and to quantify or measure the severity of the pain the patient is experiencing. In this situation psychologic testing and pain measurements should be included in the evaluation. Treatment can include pain-relieving or analgesic medications, attitude influencing, or psychotropic medications, nerve blocks, electrical neurostimulation, biofeedback techniques for reduction of muscle spasm, activity management and family counseling.

Postinfectious Neuralgias

We speak here primarily of the pain of herpes zoster, particularly the postherpetic pain which occurs in the forehead and face of elderly individuals and which often dominates the waning years of their life. The pain is particularly intense, long-lasting, and associated with severe dysesthesias, frequently interrupting sleep at night, producing reliance on habituating drugs, depression and all of the problems of the patient with chronic pain, including a tendency toward consideration of suicide. Such patients are extremely difficult to manage. Medications which influence attitudes may be helpful, particularly the tricyclic antidepressants combined with a phenothiazine. When possible, electrical neurostimulation of the skin surface of the area involved by the herpes infection may be efficacious, but this is rarely possible when the face is involved. Local ablative surgical procedures are usually not helpful. Generally the patient requires patience, counseling, reassurance, and the understanding that he will need to live with the pain and that no treatment is liable to be curative.

SELF-ASSESSMENT EXAMINATION

1 Headache associated with brain tumor is due to extracranial vasodilation. True or False

2 Headache produced by traction of pain-sensitive structures is usually trivial. True or False

3 Traction headache is always severe and should be treated with narcotics. True or False

4 Cranial arteritis represents an inflammatory disease of arteries. True or False

5 Headache associated with lumbar puncture results from spasm of the back muscles. True or False

6 Sinus disease is responsible for many chronic headache syndromes. True or False

7 Drug therapy of the major neuralgias, such as trigeminal neuralgia, is rarely successful. True or False

8 The site of a brain tumor headache (a) always localizes the tumor; (b) is usually occipital, if the tumor is present in the posterior fossa; (c) is usually on the same side as the tumor; (d) is an unreliable sign, if increased intracranial pressure has appeared; (e) may be associated with local tenderness of the skull

9 Cranial arteritis (a) is another, more specific, name for temporal arteritis; (b) may occur in patients with polymyalgia rheumatica; (c) is a self-limited disease not requiring treatment; (d) is treated with aspirin and narcotics; (e) should be promptly treated with corticosteroids

10 Headache associated with a lumbar puncture (a) is self-limited; (b) is increased by sitting up; (c) is improved by recumbency; (d) is related to a spinal fluid leak; (e) is an occasion for emergency laminectomy

11 Headache associated with disease of the eye and eye pain (a) is always a sign of migraine; (b) rarely is serious; (c) occurs with cataracts; (d) all of the above; (e) none of the above

12 Chronic muscle contraction of head and neck muscles (a) often gives rise to nagging complaints of pain; (b) may be associated with tender nuchal nodules; (c) may respond to local injections of anesthetic agents; (d) may occur with cervical spondylosis; (e) is a specific indication for neck manipulations

13 Atypical facial neuralgia is a syndrome (a) easily diagnosed and treated; (b) related to disease of cranial nerve V; (c) improved with anticonvulsant therapy; (d) all of the above; (e) none of the above

14 Disease of the temporomandibular joint (TMJ) is (a) a concept well accepted by all physicians and dentists; (b) associated with localized facial pain and much muscle spasm; (c) always an indication for full mouth extractions; (d) sometimes produced by Ménière's syndrome; (e) often associated with ataxia and loss of equilibrium

15 In treating TMJ disease, the authors suggest (a) attempts to relieve muscle spasm; (b) treat the patient conservatively in association with a dentist; (c) radical mouth reconstructions; (d) extensive oral surgery; (e) use of simple sedatives and muscle relaxants

16 Trigeminal neuralgia is associated with (a) prolonged facial pain lasting hours; (b) spasm of facial muscles; (c) radiation of pain to the neck and occiput; (d) all of the above; (e) none of the above

17 Trigeminal neuralgia is best improved by (a) anticonvulsants; (b) narcotics; (c) aspirin and related compounds; (d) stilbamidine; (e) antidepressant medications

18 Glossopharyngeal neuralgia is (a) a nonspecific painful syndrome poorly characterized; (b) characterized by lancinating pain in the tonsillar area and ear; (c) a syndrome relieved by anticonvulsant agents; (d) initiated often by yawning, eating or swallowing; (e) sometimes associated with syncope

19 Headache which is always unilateral (a) usually implies aneurysmal dilation; (b) may be migrainous; (c) is never migrainous, since migraine should shift from side to side; (d) may be a sign of eye disease, if the orbit is involved; (e) never occurs in clinical practice

20 Migraine is related to allergy and (a) skin tests are indicated in its investigation; (b) if skin tests are positive, sensitization is indicated; (c) may be provoked by gastrointestinal allergic reaction to foods; (d) all of the above; (e) none of the above

---

ANSWERS:

1—False; 2—False; 3—False; 4—True; 5—False; 6—False; 7—False; 8—b,c,d,e; 9—a,b,e; 10—a,b,c,d; 11—e; 12—a,b,c,d; 13—e; 14—b; 15—a,b,e; 16—e; 17—a; 18—b,c,d,e; 19—b,d; 20—e

Muscle Contraction Headache

9

Definition

The terms "muscle contraction" and "tension" headache have been used synonymously for almost 40 years to describe chronic headaches of a nonspecific type which are not vascular and are not associated with traction and inflammation. It is our contention that the typical, occasional, episodic "tension headache," related to contraction of head and neck muscles, is relieved with over-the-counter medications, is associated with fatigue and temporary stress situations in life and is rarely seen in a physician's office. What the physician does see are patients with chronic muscle contraction headaches, a headache symptom complex in part due to psychologic problems, particularly present in those persons subject to depression.

Muscle Contraction Headache

The muscle contraction headache is a steady, nonpulsatile ache. Additional descriptive terms include "tightness" bitemporally or at the occiput; "bandlike" sensations about the head, which may become caplike in distribution; "viselike" ache; "weight," "pressure," "drawing" and "soreness." Distinct cramplike sensations and a "feeling as if the neck and upper back were in a cast" are also described (Fig 9-1).

These head pains and other sensations occur frequently in the forehead and temples or in the back of the head and neck as well as in other sites. They may be unilateral or bilateral, involving the temporal, occipital, parietal or frontal regions, or all, and any combination. Commonly, there is soreness on combing or brushing the hair or when putting on a hat. Although muscle contraction headache may be fleeting, with frequent changes in the site and intensity of recurrences, this is usually the type of headache which, localized in one region, may be sustained with varying intensity for weeks, months and even years. The intensity of the headache may diminish by assuming certain individually favored positions. The patient may limit the motion of the head, neck and jaws because it decreases his discomfort. There may be less discomfort when the head is supported by the hands.

Within the diffusely aching muscle tissues of the head, neck and upper back there may be found on palpation one or many tender areas, or "nodules," which are sharply localized.

Pressure on contracted, tender muscles may augment headache intensity and may elicit tinnitus, vertigo and lacrimation—features which also occur spontaneously. Such pressure on tender areas causes spread of the pain to adjacent portions of

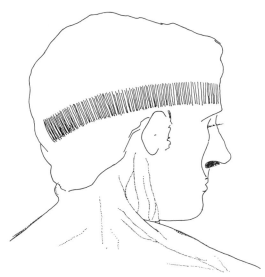

Fig 9-1. *Clinical features of muscle contraction headaches: the headache described as a tightness, with a hatband distribution of discomfort; tender areas over neck and scalp; limitation of motion; muscle spasm.*

the head. Muscle contraction headache is aggravated by shivering from exposure to cold.

Martin states that emotional factors are of prime significance in the causation of muscle contraction headache. He describes in detail psychiatric evaluations of a selected series of 25 patients with this complaint. There was no single psychologic determinant productive of muscle contraction headaches. Multiple conflicts were usually evident in patients suffering from such headaches. Poorly repressed hostility was often evident, but unresolved dependency needs and psychosexual conflicts were also frequently present. Martin suggests that psychophysiologic expression or somatization of anxiety in the form of increased skeletal muscle tension is uniformly present in cases of muscle contraction headache. The mother or other members of the family often play an unconscious role in fostering the headache. Secondary gain from muscle contraction headache is often present.

With muscle contraction headaches, the chronic headache may serve to obscure a serious emotional disorder, most often a depression. The patient's complaint is of specific and enduring headache for which no organic basis can be found. Anxiety and especially depressive symptoms are converted into acceptable (to the patient) physical symptoms. These patients are usually convinced of the somatic nature of their complaints. Other signs or symptoms of depression may be evident, including insomnia, loss of sparkle or spontaneity, lack of interest, early morning fatigue and irritability. Suicide may be contemplated.

Because of the central spread of the excitatory effect of noxious stimulation of the soft structures of the head, pain may be experienced at a distance from the site of noxious stimulation. Thus, orbital and frontal ache may be experienced when the condylar or basal region is stimulated by injecting hypertonic salt solution or by manual pressure in this region; occipital ache may follow such stimulation of the nuchal tissues. In contrast to the pain that results from sustained contraction of skeletal muscle, this type of remote pain comes on promptly with noxious stimulation and ends at once when the source of noxious stimulation is blocked by procaine.

Sex Distribution and Heredity

Both sexes are affected, but women predominate in most series.

These headaches tend to occur in families only because parents with these symptoms may leave the stigma with their children as an example of learned and inappropriate behavior.

Sleep History

There is almost always present an accompanying sleep disturbance in addition to the headache. Sleep disturbances, if they are related to anxiety, usually manifest themselves as difficulty in falling asleep; if the disturbance is associated with depression, there is frequent awakening during the night, early awakening and in some rare instances, hypersomnia (excessive sleep).

Psychogenic Determinants

As part of the headache history a careful and detailed psychiatric history should be obtained. An inventory should be made of the patient's

    marital relations

    occupation

    social relationships

    life stresses

    personality traits

    habits

    methods of handling tension situations

    sexual problems

This inventory must be reevaluated at each interview. It may take several appointments and a growth of confidence between patient and physician before the patient will ventilate the problems troubling him.

Chemical Determinants of Depression

In depression, a functional decrease in catecholamines occurs, particularly involving norepinephrine and dopamine. Medications which deplete the brain of catecholamines, including reserpine and alphamethyldopa, produce depression, although not invariably. Those medications which improve the symptoms of depression will increase the concentration of the brain catecholamines, although by different methods. The monoamine oxidase inhibitors decrease the rate of metabolism of the catecholamines, thereby preserving them. The tricyclic antidepressants inhibit the reuptake of the catecholamines into synaptic clefts and this preserves them in another manner.

Abnormalities in concentration of the indoleamine, serotonin, are also considered to play a role in the genesis of depression. Reserpine depletes the brain of serotonin

as well as the catecholamines. Metabolites of serotonin are altered in the depressed state. For example, the levels of 5-hydroxyindoleacetic acid in the cerebrospinal fluid are reduced in depression. Serotonin has been shown to be a neural transmitter in the pathways which mediate sleep in animals. Tryptophan, the amino acid precursor of serotonin, will cross the blood-brain barrier and can be used in the treatment of the depressed patient.

There is also evidence to suggest that adrenal and thyroid hormones may interact with catecholamines and serotonin. The corticosteroids potentiate the actions of the neurohormones. Addition of the thyroid hormone triiodothyronine (T_3) to tricyclic drug therapy has been reported to increase the effectiveness and rapidity of action of the antidepressant medications.

Depression may thus be considered as a heterogeneous illness involving multiple defects of neurotransmitters. The balance of these neurohormones seems crucial. One can postulate, for example, that some persons may be susceptible to alterations in the concentrations of the catecholamines, others to changes in serotonin and still others to changes in corticosteroids and/or thyroid hormones, or a combination of these.

Depression may be considered an illness involving multiple defects of neurotransmitters.

The regional distribution of the biogenic amines has been studied in detail. Norepinephrine is found in many areas of the brain, but the highest concentration is in the hypothalamus. Dopamine is found particularly in the basal ganglia. Serotonin is similar to norepinephrine in its distribution. Epinephrine is highly concentrated in the adrenal medulla; little is present in the brain itself.

The biogenic amines are found in considerable concentration in the limbic system, a part of the brain which is particularly concerned with the emotions. The limbic system is composed of the deeply placed amygdala, adjacent cortex and hippocampus (Fig 9-2). The functions of the limbic system are related to behavioral reactions, especially those of self-preservation, including fleeing, fighting, feeding and sexual activities.

Experiments in man and animals suggest that rage or attack behavior can be evoked by electric stimulation of either the medial amygdala, its hypothalamic projections or its tegmental projections. Chronic rage can also be produced by ablation of the lateral amygdala, ventromedial hypothalamus or septal nuclei. Conversely, rage can be suppressed by stimulation of portions of the limbic system. Rage provoked by stimulating one part of the limbic structures can also be suppressed by creating a lesion in its distal projections; this interrupts neuronal transmission.

Ascending pain pathways of the anterolateral pain system also involve the limbic nuclei, in addition to thalamic and reticular structures (Fig 9-3).

A classification of depression follows:

1. normal grief related to illness or death
2. reactive depression
   a. associated with physical illness
   b. associated with use of medications
   c. occurring in association with psychiatric illness
3. endogenous depression
   a. unipolar, recurrent or cyclic
   b. bipolar (manic-depression-manic)
   c. cyclic mania only.

In discussing these forms of depression it should be noted that no. 1, that is normal grief, is not truly a psychiatric disease and requires no further comment. Reactive depressions tend to be secondary to some problem, particularly physical illness, are usually less severe clinically than primary or endogenous depressions, often are self-limited or respond to support and nonspecific treatment and also respond to the tricyclic drugs.

A unipolar or endogenous depression may present with a history of previous episodes, a positive family history, and more obvious and prominent changes in so-called vegetative signs, that is sleep, appetite, sex, motor activity and the like.

Clinical Picture

The majority of patients with muscle contraction headache suffer from depression. The term tension headache is in part a misnomer. It is true that chronic muscle contraction occurs with these headaches. The question is—why are the muscles contracting? We suggest that most patients

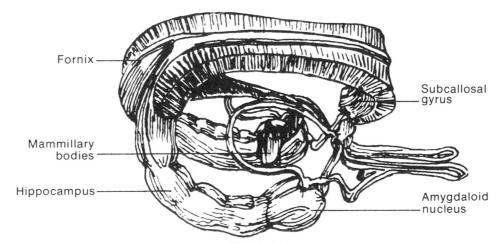

Fig 9-2. *The limbic system.*

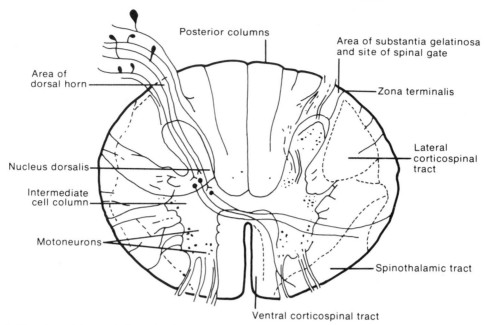

Fig 9-3. *The dorsal horn of the spinal cord and the area of substantia gelatinosa and site of spinal gate.*

with this form of headache are, in fact, suffering a depressive illness, with headache as one of their somatic complaints. Besides the constant generalized headache, one other prominent symptom that acts as a key to diagnosis is that of sleep disturbance, most often in the form of frequent and early awakening.

Most patients with muscle contraction headache suffer from depression.

Descriptions of this form of headache may be capricious and bizarre. They may involve the entire head or different parts of the head at different times. They are frequently increased on weekends, holidays and vacations. A depressed person will tell you he has had the headache for years or all of his life; the headache is more severe in the morning and the pain does not respond to the simple analgesics. It is for these reasons that he seeks medical help. The simple nervous or tension headache, described so often in literature and almost nonexistent in doctors' offices, is treated successfully by over-the-counter drugstore medications, usually aspirin or one of its derivatives, and does not have the long history of periodicity and/or chronicity so common to depressive headaches. Early morning awakening and frequent awakening during the night support the diagnosis. In addition to sleep disturbances, anorexia may be present. Rarely, some patients eat excessively with depressive illness. There may also be a history of decreased sexual activity, with men exhibiting impotence and females a decreased menstrual flow and frigidity. The depressed headache patient will evince, in addition, a multitude of associated physical, emotional and psychic complaints as shown in Table 9-1.

Occurrence

In the hours from 4:00 PM to 8:00 PM and from 4:00 AM to 8:00 AM, muscle contraction headaches most often occur. These are usually the periods of silent personal or family crises. Early in the morning the depressed patient awakens, with his fantasies of warfare with the members of his family, or his persistent work conflicts. Or, in contrast, in discussions with the depressed patient, we often find that his headaches begin when he leaves the quiet atmosphere of the office for a weekend at home. The headache may coincide with seemingly restful interpersonal situations in which the sufferer feels compelled to appear comfortable, relaxed, and agreeable although he is struggling to repress resentment toward someone whom he is expected to love and respect.

Depression and Bodily Symptoms

People with depressive illness may develop somatic symptoms and, conversely, people with painful organic diseases tend to become depressed. Even so, we suggest that too little attention is being paid to the depressive aspects of chronic pain and its treatment. The physical complaints often predominate to such an extent that the few simple questions necessary to uncover the underlying depression tend to be omitted.

Most patients come to consult the doctor with disturbances of body function. Often pain is the presenting complaint. We suggest a careful questioning of patients with chronic pain; the depressive symptoms may be instructive wherever the pain or its cause. Frequent complaints of fatigue, a heavy feeling, disturbances of sleep or appetite or sexual dysfunction are all clues to an underlying depression. The patients often report that the symptoms began after a specific experience which was judged to have started the sickness. Bodily injury or alteration is most frequently singled out. The patient complains, "I was never sick until I hit my head against the windshield of the car." A careful history will show that the patient was not knocked unconscious and that his x-rays were negative; but all his somatic symptoms started with the event. Depression is a common finding in compensation neurosis.

People with depressive illness may develop bodily symptoms, while people with painful organic diseases tend to become depressed.

Table 9-1. Patterns of Depression

Physical complaints	Incidence (percent)	Emotional complaints	Incidence (percent)
Sleep disturbances	97	Blue, low spirits, sadness	90
Early awakening	87	Crying	80
Headache	84	Feelings of guilt, hopelessness,	
Dyspnea	76	unworthiness, unreality	65
Constipation	76	Anxious or irritable	65
Loss of weight	74	Anxiety	60
Trouble getting to sleep	73	Fear of insanity, physical disease,	
Weakness and fatigue	70	death, rumination over the past,	
Urinary frequency	70	present, future	50
"Spells"—dizziness	70		
Appetite disturbances	70	**Psychic complaints**	
Decreased libido	63		
Cardiovascular disturbances	60	"Morning worst time of day"	95
Sexual disturbances	60	Poor concentration	91
Palpitations	59	No interest; no ambition	75
Paresthesias	53	Indecisiveness	75
Nausea	48	Poor memory	71
Menstrual changes	41	Suicidal thoughts; death wishes	35

Basic Questions

Two basic questions and their responses will give insight to a possible depression. First, ask about a family or personal history of previous depression. Ask if there have been similar symptoms in relatives or friends or if these symptoms have been experienced previously. Many will say that they felt like this 8 years ago, or they will give some obscure symptoms which are actually depressive equivalents. The second question in the history relates to the manner of onset. This may reveal that the depressive attack has followed upon a wide variety of events which the patient perceives as traumatic or feels as a personal loss, out of proportion to the severity of the resultant depression. The subject may say that he became sick after some form of bodily injury, some minor illness, getting an injection, an operation or even after a sigmoidoscopic examination—and that every one of his symptoms date from this event. The incident that precipitated the headache and other depressive equivalents is often trivial and seemingly not compatible with the subsequent incapacity of the patient. The patient may voice fears that he has been weakened or maimed by the event.

Patient's Emotional State

The emotional state of a depressed patient fluctuates widely. During the examination he may cry or look despondent or express the desire to cry; he is often markedly introverted, dwells on his illness and mistakes in a self-depreciatory manner. Prominent among his complaints are impairment of concentration, poor memory, loss of interest and difficulty in making decisions. The housewife who cannot follow a simple recipe and the practiced bridge player who consistently blunders badly are obvious examples.

Death of a loved one may produce depression and for a brief time this is considered normal. If depression persists beyond several months, however, the physician should be alerted, for chronic depression may then ensue. Headache often appears and may be persistent in this situation

Depression Associated with Drugs

Drugs can cause depression or increase a depressive state which may have been overlooked initially. A depressed patient may resemble an anxious patient at times, particularly if manic tendencies are present. Some of the sedatives and ataraxics, particularly the phenothiazine derivatives, barbiturates and rauwolfia alkaloids, may mobilize an incipient depression or exaggerate an existing one. This can be the first indication that the diagnosis of simple anxiety is wrong. The head pain caused by depression may be increased by sedative drugs. The primary duty of the physician is the recognition of the depressed patient. Once this is accomplished the patient can be adequately treated.

Treatment

Depression

Antidepressant drugs provide the most effective treatment for this condition. Amitriptyline hydrochloride (Elavil®), imipramine hydrochloride (Tofranil®), desipramine hydrochloride (Pertofrane® or Norpramin®), nortriptyline hydrochloride (Aventyl® HCl) and protriptyline hydrochloride (Vivactil®) are all effective. For example, amitriptyline hydrochloride may be used 50 mg at bedtime and may be adjusted upward as needed for control of the symptoms. The dosage of a tricyclic, such as amitriptyline hydrochloride, may be increased to 200–250 mg daily.

A number of antidepressant drugs are effective in treating psychogenic headaches.

The antidepressant class includes tricyclic antidepressants and monoamine oxidase (MAO) inhibitors. Tricyclics may have some primary analgesic effect, in addition to their mood-altering effect. Elavil and Doxipen are maximally sedating, and probably have about the same degree of anticholinergic side effects. Imipramine is less sedating than Elavil. Vivactil is the only nonsedating tricyclic, and consequently the majority of a day's dose should be given in the morning. The desmethyl derivatives (or secondary amines) have been represented as acting more rapidly, but this has not been borne out in clinical trials. Of the tricyclics, Elavil and imipramine are the most often used, since there is the most experience and literature with these two drugs. Choosing between the two largely hinges on the presence or magnitude of insomnia, or how much in the way of sedation appears desirable. The pamoate salt of imipramine, recently marketed, does not seem to offer major advantages over imipramine hydrochloride. Psychosis, marked agitation, or hostility in association with depression may warrant addition of a phenothiazine. Combinations such as Triavil and Etrafon are infrequently indicated, although frequently used. The dose of perphenazine is difficult to titrate using the combination, and many patients need not be exposed to the risks of phenothiazine administration, such as tardive dyskinesia.

In prescribing tricyclics, be sure to tell patients they will have some of the listed side effects as necessary evidence that an adequate dose is being given, and that onset of usefulness requires several weeks. A single daily h.s. dose is compatible with known pharmacokinetics, may help insomnia, lessens anticholinergic effects during the day, and may increase patient compliance. Too low a dose or too short a trial are primary causes of treatment failure. Tricyclics are far from being euphoriant drugs, and clinical lore has it that patients who do not need tricyclics do not tend to tolerate them. With the exception of Vivactil, the dosage range of tricyclics is generally between 50 and 300 mg per day. Blood level studies suggest that 80% of patients will have a therapeutic level at 150 mg per 24 hours.

Depending on the age and size of the patient, one may start out at 50 mg each evening, and increase the nightly dose by 25 mg each succeeding night or every other night until reaching the general therapeutic range or as limited by the side effects. The patient should be maintained at full doses for 3 or 4 weeks before deciding that the patient has not responded. A similar trial with a second tricyclic may then be in order, or one may proceed with an MAO inhibitor following a 10-day washout. If the depression is severe, and particularly if there is significant risk of suicide, consideration should be given to treatment with electroshock therapy.

MAO inhibitors are generally considered second line drugs for depression in terms of efficacy, and have more interaction problems than the tricyclics. The British school of psychiatry does not agree with this view, and there is increasing interest in the U.S. literature in using MAO inhibitors in "atypical depressions," especially those with major physical complaints as "depressive equivalents." Anthony et al. reported on the usefulness of MAO inhibitors in control of migraine, in 1970, and Lance has reported on this topic also. The MAO inhibitors appear to be useful in prophylaxis against vascular headache in some patients, but have not been widely accepted and may well be underutilized. If used, patients should be given written information as to necessary dietary restrictions and contraindicated drugs.

At one time it was considered poor practice to use the MAO inhibitors with the tricyclic compounds. However, M. Schuckit, E. Robins and J. Feighner (1971) have reviewed the case reports of assumed fatalities with combined therapy and have found that the concern regarding the severe side effects of the dual therapy was perhaps overstated. Our experience confirms theirs; on occasion combined therapy with tricyclics and MAO inhibitors is sometimes of value when no other therapy works, but the combined therapy should always be used *with caution*.

In rare instances, in which the patients are unresponsive to drugs, electroconvulsive therapy may be necessary to effect relief. If suicide is a serious threat, psychiatric consultation should be obtained.

Chronic Post-Traumatic Headache

Almost all persons who have had injury to their heads have local pain or tenderness at the site of impact for a few hours or even for a few days, after which many become symptom free.

Between one third and one half of all persons who injure their heads sufficiently to warrant hospitalization develop chronic post-traumatic headaches.

A small number of patients with headaches that persist after injury to the head have pain due to gross accumulations of blood in the epidural, subdural or subarachnoid spaces. The headache of subdural hematoma begins at the time of the blow or the regaining of consciousness and persists often for weeks or months until the hematoma is removed or, even more rarely, until spontaneous resolution occurs. Large amounts of blood in the subarachnoid space about the base of the brain induce headache because of traction, displacement, distention and rupture of pain-sensitive blood vessels and pia arachnoid. A still smaller group of patients have sustained headache after head injury due to adhesions involving pain-sensitive structures in the arachnoidea.

The vast majority of patients with post-traumatic headaches that persist or recur for long periods of time after head injury have no such intracranial abnormalities to explain their headaches.

Muscle Contraction Headaches, Cervical Arthritis (Spondylosis)

Many patients with cervical spondylosis have significant posterior headaches, particularly in the occipital region. Several pertinent points regarding this syndrome deserve repetition. The cervical spine films will show significant alteration in terms of osteoarthritic change, with associated muscle spasm and loss of the normal cervical lordotic curve. Treatment should invariably be medical. Examination of the patient with this form of headache will usually demonstrate one or more tender areas especially in the great posterior muscles of the neck as well as muscle contraction spasm of muscles, increase in tone and limitation of motion.

Anti-inflammatory and analgesic medications are effective in this situation, particularly the newer anti-inflammatory drugs such as ibuprofen (Motrin) and related analogues. We use these on a daily basis; a standard combination is ibuprofen 400 mg, three times daily with a muscle relaxant, for example, chlorphenesin 800 mg, at bedtime. Physical therapy with much laying on of hands and stimulation of the skin and subcutaneous tissue should be emphasized as the treatment of choice in this condition. Electrical neurostimulation and biofeedback training may be helpful. Local injection of tender areas with anesthetic agents and/or corticosteroids may be helpful as well. We suggest use of a cervical orthopedic pillow to retain the cervical lordotic curve during sleep. A posture program may be helpful.

One should consider operation for cervical spondylosis only if medical therapy fails and only when there is significant arm pain with an associated neurologic deficit which can be demonstrated on examination and which can also be recorded electromyographically. One does not operate for pain alone and particularly not for posterior occipital headaches. Operative section of the occipital nerve should be avoided. Extensive manipulation of the neck should be done with extreme care, especially in the elderly, if cervical spondylosis and early signs of cord compression are present.

SELF-ASSESSMENT EXAMINATION

1 The term muscle contraction headache is used to describe headache in wrestlers. True or False

2 Muscle contraction headache is a chronic headache symptom complex, with some elements of associated psychic disturbance. True or False

3 Muscle contraction headache is a particularly common complaint in an office practice. True or False

4 Muscle contraction headache may appear in families, as an example of learned and inappropriate behavior. True or False

5 Depression is a frequent finding in patients with muscle contraction headache. True or False

6 Pain in muscle contraction headache is most often unilateral and throbbing, with a pulsatile quality. True or False

7 Sleep disturbance is often associated with depression. True or False

8 Depression is a mental state characterized by (a) fatigue; (b) insomnia; (c) loss of interest; (d) loss of appetite; (e) absence of sparkle and spontaneity

9 Biochemical changes in the brain of a depressed patient may include (a) a decrease in norepinephrine and dopamine; (b) a decrease in serotonin; (c) an increase in epinephrine; (d) over-production of alpha ketoglutaric acid; (e) a reduction in hemispheric citrulline

10 The structure and functions of the limbic system include (a) the amygdala, the hippocampus, and the adjacent cortex; (b) behavioral reactions, including fear, anger and sexual activity; (c) the pontomedullary junctions; (d) profuse interconnections with the cerebellum; (e) ascending pain pathways from the anterolateral pain projection

11 Characteristics of headache in depressed patients include (a) capricious and bizarre complaints; (b) chronicity; (c) hat-band distribution; (d) poor response to analgesic agents; (e) pain improved by the recumbent position

12 Depression may be drug induced, and produced by (a) antibiotics, especially chloramphenicol; (b) reserpine and its derivatives; (c) phenothiazines; (d) barbiturates; (e) tricyclic drugs

13 Treatment of depressed patients may employ the following treatment modalities: (a) tricyclic antidepressants; (b) psychotherapy; (c) electroconvulsive treatment; (d) all of the above; (e) none of the above

14 Monamine oxidase inhibitors and tricyclic antidepressants are (a) never used simultaneously; (b) basically incompatible; (c) absolutely safe and frequently employed as the therapy of choice in chronic headache; (d) all of the above; (e) none of the above

ANSWERS:

1—False; 2—True; 3—True; 4—True; 5—True; 6—False; 7—True; 8—a,b,c,d,e; 9—a,b; 10—a,b,e; 11—a,b,c,d; 12—b,c,d; 13—a,b,c,d; 14—e

Headache in Children

Headache in children is a special subject and so deserves a special chapter. As with headache in adults, the large majority of children complaining of headache do not have organic disease as a basis for their complaints. Here again their headaches can be classified into three types: vascular, muscle contraction and traction and inflammatory.

Migraine

Vascular headaches in children may be classic in character, with premonitory symptoms, especially scotomata, followed by unilateral head pain. Severe nausea and hyperemesis are common in childhood migraine. Often the child appears pale, is obviously ill and "pasty," and usually retires to bed. Frequently also, the pain may be bilateral, rather than unilateral.

But migraine in children may not be so obvious as that described above. Some children note primarily periodic vomiting without headache ("abdominal migraine"). Only later in life does a recognizable migraine syndrome begin. Car sickness and other forms of motion sickness are frequent complaints, not necessarily associated with headache. In these situations, a family history of migraine is usually elicited.

Rarely, childhood migraine appears as an acute confusional state of self-limited duration, with significant associated electroencephalographic changes. The diagnosis is suspected if episodes recur, if there is a family history of migraine, and is confirmed when a more classic migraine pattern appears eventually.

Sillanpaa of Finland reported on the prevalence of headache in Finnish children starting school. In the two Finnish cities of Tampere and Turku, there were 4825 children, aged 7 years, who started their primary school in the autumn of 1974. At the first clinical examination performed by school doctors, 87.8% of the pupils and their mothers were interviewed to detect the occurrence of headache. The overall prevalence of headache proved to be 37.7%. Occasional headache, which was considered to be significant, was found in 32.7%. More frequent headache, occurring once a month or more, was found in 6.0% of cases. The prevalence of migraine was 3%. This contrasts with the study by Bille done in Upsala in 1962 on 9000 school children, where 39% were found to have headaches. On the other hand, the present study showed a two-fold higher frequency of migraine (3%) compared to Bille's series (1.4%).

It is important to realize that juvenile head trauma syndromes may be related to migraine and that migraine may occur after head trauma, particularly after trauma sustained in sporting activities such as football and baseball. Haas and his associates describe a clinical spectrum of juvenile head trauma in an analysis of 50 attacks in 25 patients. Attacks were grouped into four clinical types: (1) hemiparetic, (2) somnolent, (3) blindness and (4) brain stem signs. They suggest that these four types of juvenile head trauma syndromes are different manifestations of a common underlying process. All attacks followed mild head trauma after a latent interval, generally of 1 to 10 minutes. Forty of the 50 attacks occurred in patients under 14 years of age. Full recovery occurred after a variable period of time in all but one patient who demonstrated an occlusion of the branch of the middle cerebral artery on angiography. In their clinical and laboratory features these juvenile head trauma syndromes resemble classical migraine and presumably have a similar underlying mechanism.

In many of these children the migraine process probably involves the basilar artery. Symptoms include sudden onset of transient bilateral visual disturbances, gait ataxia, vertigo, pulsatile occipital headache with vomiting and dysarthrias of varying forms. In young women the attacks may be related to menstruation. As patients age, basilar artery migraine is often supplanted by more characteristic forms of vascular headache. Pediatric patients in whom there is a clinical picture of confusion related to basilar artery migraine and who have a family history of migraine and transient electroencephalographic changes may not require neurodiagnostic study, if the syndrome is recognized.

Cluster headaches have not been reported in children.

Muscle Contraction

Muscle contraction headache is common in children. The pain is described as diffuse, sometimes bandlike, and is not usually associated with nausea and vomiting. The pain may be relieved by simple analgesic agents. It is often associated with muscle spasm and complaints of neck tenderness. The headaches are almost always related to stress situations at school, or play, or to disturbed family relationships.

Muscle contraction headache is nearly always related to stress situations.

Traction and Inflammatory Headache

Headache associated with traction or inflammation of pain-sensitive structures of the head also appears in children. When associated with fever, meningitis or encephalitis should be suspected. Cranial arteritis does not occur in children, nor do the major neuralgias. If increased intracranial pressure occurs, the head pain is described as diffuse, often beginning in the occiput initially, but radiating thereafter to the frontal and temporal areas. Tumors involving the pituitary may produce a well-localized vertex head pain. With brain tumors, the same observations apply as described for adults. In addition, the pain is often present upon awakening and may be increased after exercise or head jolts. The pain becomes progressively more severe and is accompanied by obvious neurologic signs including increasing head size, ataxia and papilledema.

Planning the Work-up

Successful treatment of the child with headache depends upon the establishment of a specific diagnosis. A careful history and physical examination should be done. *Measurement of the head is essential.* Fontanelles and suture lines should be palpated. Fundoscopy should be performed as well as attempts to outline the visual fields. Skull films and an electroencephalogram are almost always ordered if the complaint is of significance or is chronic. If a tumor is suspected, a CAT scan should be done. Films of the cervical spine should be obtained if the pain is occipital in character. Children may be susceptible to occipital neuralgia, particularly after trauma to this region. If further neurologic work-up is indicated, the child should be hospitalized.

Treatment Suggestions

In general, we avoid using ergot and methysergide in childhood migraine in all but the most unusual circumstances (see Table 10-1). If the child responds to nothing else and ergot must be used, a rectal suppository can be employed, using half the adult dose if the child is aged 6 years or older. If the migraine episodes occur rarely, no specific therapy is indicated. If they occur frequently, perhaps weekly, we suggest therapy with anticonvulsant agents. Phenobarbital is frequently employed in a dose of 5 mg/kg, or in older children, 30 mg, t.i.d., providing somnolence is not severe. Occasionally diphenylhydantoin is added or used alone, if somnolence does become a problem. Cyproheptadine hydrochloride, 4 mg at bedtime, is helpful with migraine in children. If the electroencephalogram is dysrhythmic, the physician may feel more strongly about using anticonvulsant agents in the situation of recurrent headaches. If drug therapy is employed, careful and repeated examinations should be done.

Ludvigsson has described the use of propranolol in the prophylaxis of migraine in children. Thirty-two children between the ages of 7 and 16 years were included in a double-blind single cross-over study. Each child received propranolol and placebo for periods of 3 months, the preparations being allocated at random. It was demonstrated that propranolol has a very good prophylactic effect on migraine in school children. The drug did not seem to cause any noticeable side effects if certain categories of patients were excluded from treatment, particularly those with asthma, cardiac decompensation or cardiac arrhythmias. Begin with small doses, e.g., 10–20 mg/day.

Bille of Sweden has also described his experiences with prophylaxis of migraine in children. He advised that, initially, measures for maintaining sound biologic rhythms in terms of life, work and rest, meals and sleep should be followed, and sometimes prophylaxis with a mild sedative may be all that is required. If symptoms persist, it is important to try to counteract those trigger mechanisms which are suspected to provoke the migraine attacks, including dietary factors. Cyproheptadine and propranolol are both useful in the prophylaxis of migraine in children, as described above.

Muscle contraction headache of children rarely requires medication.

Table 10-1. Headache in Children

	Vascular (migraine)	Muscle contraction	Traction and inflammatory (Increased intracranial pressure)
Sex	Males 2:1	Females 3:1	No sex differential
Age of onset	4 to 10 years	6 to 12 years	At any time
Prodromata	Scotomata, pallor, abdominal complaints, malaise, irritability	None	None
Associated findings	Nausea, vomiting, hyperemesis, confusional state	Avoids school or other stress situations	Vomiting, lethargy, positive neurologic signs, progressive head pain
Family history	Positive for migraine	Disturbed relationships	None
Therapy	Phenobarbital, diphenylhydantoin, cyproheptadine, rarely ergot	Environmental manipulation, psychotherapy	As required by the lesion (surgery, radiotherapy, etc.)

Treatment of muscle contraction headache of children rarely requires the use of medications. Counseling should be provided. The patient and the parents should be interviewed separately and together. If there is no resolution of the problem, a psychiatric consultation should be obtained. Sometimes, simple behavioral and especially environmental manipulations will suffice to relieve the situation and formal psychotherapy will not be necessary. But if the headache is only one part of an obvious disorder of mood, thought or behavior, the patient should be referred quickly for formal psychotherapy. Depression can occur in children and these cases can be responsive to the tricyclic compounds such as amitriptaline (Elavil®).

In those unusual circumstances where muscle spasm and neck pain have produced chronic headache, use of simple measures of physical therapy and a Thomas' collar may prove helpful.

Sometimes, despite all efforts, attempts to diagnose and to treat the headaches which appear in childhood may be unsuccessful. In this situation, the wise physican resorts to periodic examinations and observation. Most frequently, the headache will be found to be a self-limited problem and will resolve spontaneously.

SELF-ASSESSMENT EXAMINATION

1 In general, headache in children can be classified into three types: vascular, muscle contraction and traction and inflammatory. True or False

2 Migraine in children may assume atypical forms. True or False

3 Migraine in children may appear as an acute confusional state. True or False

4 Cranial arteritis appears frequently in childhood and adolescence. True or False

5 Measurement of the head is an essential part of the neurologic examination of children. True or False

6 Muscle contraction headache is uncommon in children. True or False

7 Children may be particularly susceptible to occipital neuralgic pains, after trauma. True or False

8 Migraine in childhood (a) may be classical in character; (b) may be associated with severe nausea and vomiting without headache; (c) may appear initially as periodic vomiting; (d) occasionally presents as an acute confusional state; (e) often appears in the context of a positive family history of migraine

9 Variant forms of migraine in childhood include (a) progressive ophthalmoplegia; (b) carsickness and other forms of motion sickness; (c) intermittent abdominal complaints or vomiting; (d) a confusional state, short-lived and reversible; (d) progressive dementia

10 Muscle contraction headaches in children (a) are often related to difficult situations at home or school; (b) may respond to simple counseling and environmental manipulations; (c) are often poorly described and diffuse in character; (d) occur primarily in autistic children; (e) are familial

11 If a brain tumor is suspected in a child (a) a careful history and phsyical examination should be done; (b) measurement of the head is essential; (c) the fontanelles and sutures should be examined; (d) hospitalization may be required; (e) arteriography should always be done

12 Headache therapy in children (a) depends primarily on selecting exactly the right medication; (b) often requires the use of ergot preparations and methysergide; (c) never employs anticonvulsant agents; (d) all of the above; (e) none of the above

13 If occipital neuralgia of childhood is suspected, (a) cervical spine x-rays may be helpful; (b) a chiropractor should be consulted; (c) a Thomas' collar can be employed; (d) manipulations of the neck are indicated; (e) simple measures of physical therapy may relieve pain

14 If the clinician suspects a muscle contraction headache of childhood (a) counseling should be provided (b) formal psychiatric referral may be necessary (c) individual interviews of child and parents should be accomplished (d) medications are always indicated (e) on occasion, medications may be helpful

15 If despite all efforts, the source of a child's headache cannot be ascertained (a) admit the child to a hospital for ventriculography (b) follow the child carefully with periodic examinations and observation (c) send the child to the National Institutes of Health for consultation

ANSWERS:

1—True; 2—True; 3—True; 4—False; 5—True; 6—False; 7—True; 8—a,b,c,d,e; 9—b,c,d; 10—a,b,c; 11—a,b,c,d; 12—e; 13—a,c,e; 14—a,b,c,e; 15—b

11

Drug Abuse in Headache

Patients with headache may overuse or abuse their medications, although this is not invariably the case. The physician should at least suspect that the situation may occur in cephalalgic patients. If a proper history can be obtained, the diagnosis of analgesic abuse may be made. There are as yet no strict standards set down for establishing this diagnosis. The authors have devised their own list of criteria for this purpose, based upon personal experiences:

■ ingestion of more than 100 aspirin or associated compounds per month

■ consistent use of more than 10 mg of ergotamine tartrate or its derivatives per week

■ ingestion of more than 20 tablets of codeine (32 mg) per week

■ ingestion of more than 20 capsules of Darvon® (dextropropoxyphene) or Darvon® Compound per week

■ consistent use of habituating drugs including barbiturate compounds and other sedatives or tranquilizers, and narcotics

Sometimes the history of analgesic abuse is elicited easily; at other times the physician may find it imperative to question the patient and his family repeatedly about this problem, in hopes of obtaining the needed information. Patients may be secretive and secretly ashamed about ingesting medications and will put the physician off with inexact replies regarding medication use. This is particularly true in the case of over-the-counter drugs of a proprietary nature. It may be advisable to pursue the subject by asking your questions in an oblique manner. Here are some examples.

■ How long will 100 aspirin last?

■ Do you buy aspirin in large lots?

■ Do you always carry aspirin with you?

■ Do you place aspirin in strategic locations around the house or office or in your car?

■ Do you take aspirin or analgesics by the clock?

■ Do you always take several aspirin on awakening, or at bedtime?

No one of these questions, if answered affirmatively, is necessarily characteristic of patients with analgesic abuse. If several affirmative answers are obtained, however, then the physician's index of suspicion should be aroused and the diagnosis pursued further.

Different analgesics produce different clinical syndromes of analgesic abuse and these will be considered separately.

Aspirin and Aspirin Compounds

Aspirin is perhaps the least expensive and the most widely used medicine in the world. The consumption of aspirin in the United

States is about 50 million pounds per year. The aspirin industry is one main-stay of the advertising world, especially in public media including television and popular magazines. This massive consumption is not without its dangers. In pediatric practice, for example, between 25,000 and 100,000 cases of serious intoxication with aspirin occur yearly, sometimes resulting in death.

Since it is used so routinely by so many people, some effort should be made to establish the amount of aspirin taken by the individual patient over a period of time. Significant side effects of aspirin and aspirin compound ingestion are often seen in those who have taken more than 1 kg of these materials. Since 3 gm of aspirin is contained in the usual tablet, this would represent ingestion of about 3,500 tablets. In actual practice one finds that patients may have ingested considerably more than

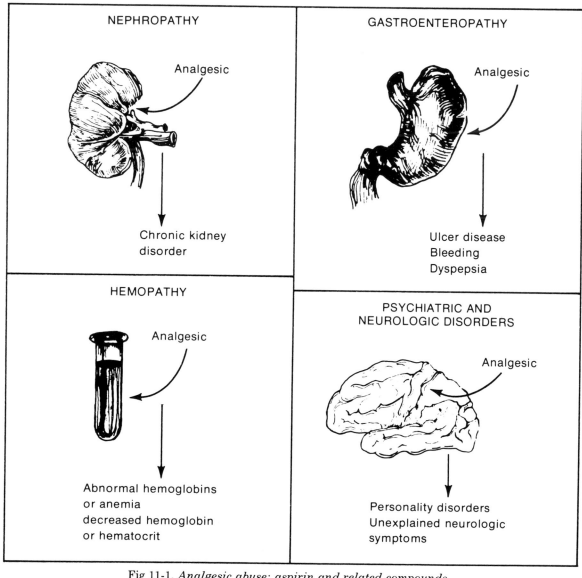

Fig 11-1. *Analgesic abuse; aspirin and related compounds.*

1 kg of aspirin or aspirin compounds, in the range of 2–70 kg of aspirin or its compounds. One study found an average ingestion, in patients with analgesic abuse, of 13 kg of phenacetin and 17 kg of aspirin.

Findings in Analgesic Abuse Compounds

Analgesic Nephropathy

The usual signs of renal abnormalities are present in this disorder (Fig 11-1). The blood urea nitrogen is raised in the majority of patients. Creatinine clearance is usually reduced. Bacteriuria or sterile pyuria may be demonstrated. The intravenous pyelogram is invariably abnormal, with reduction in renal size; calyceal deformities are also present. Calcifications of the kidneys, renal calculi, papillary necrosis and hydronephrosis are described. Isotope renography has been done in these patients, but the radioisotopic appearance of the kidneys is not striking.

There is uncertainty regarding which one of the major ingredients of common analgesics is most toxic to the kidney. Aspirin and phenacetin have been shown to be potentially nephrotoxic. Phenacetin is most commonly blamed for nephrotoxic effects, however. On the other hand, azotemic patients with analgesic abuse who have used only aspirin are described, and renal function has continued to deteriorate in some patients with presumed analgesic nephropathy who continue to use aspirin and not phenacetin.

Whichever of these substances is to blame, however, there is no doubt that the critical factor in treatment is withdrawal of the analgesic in question. Renal function will continue to deteriorate in patients who persist in analgesic abuse, whereas if the patient can be convinced that this pernicious habit must be terminated, renal function will usually stabilize and may indeed improve. In those who have abused analgesics, however, recurrent pyelonephritis remains a major hazard.

Phenacetin is particularly nephrotoxic.

Gastrointestinal Features

Dyspepsia is especially common in analgesic abuse, as is peptic ulcer (Fig 11-1). In a personal series of patients with peptic ulcer, 50% had overused analgesics or used them consistently. Approximately 20% of patients with analgesic abuse have demonstrable gastrointestinal bleeding, 30% have radiologic evidence of active or old peptic disease and 16% have had some form of gastric surgery. Given the magnitude of these figures, a search for a history of analgesic abuse should be made in all patients with chronic ulcer disease. It is foolhardy to treat the peptic aspects of analgesic abuse if the patient continues to use these drugs covertly.

Overuse of analgesics may be related to peptic ulcer, gastrointestinal bleeding and a reduction of red blood cell production.

Hematologic Features

Approximately 80% of patients with significant analgesic abuse have evidence of a reduction in red blood cell production, such as a fall in the hemoglobin to less than 12 gm/100 ml (Fig 11-1). While this may be related to decreased renal function, approximately 15% of these patients have hemolysis and in 7–10% sulfhemoglobinuria and/or methemoglobinuria can be demonstrated. Iron deficiency may also occur, associated with occult gastrointestinal bleeding.

Psychiatric and Neurologic Features

Rarely does one find analgesic abuse with aspirin and related compounds in patients with "organic pain syndromes." In one series, approximately one third of patients with analgesic abuse had required previous psychiatric therapy and another third were thought to be suffering from an unrecognized psychiatric disorder. Furthermore, unexplained neurologic symptoms occur in approximately one third of patients, including episodic unconsciousness, convulsions, tinnitus and deafness. A modest number of patients with analgesic abuse exhibit signs and symptoms of dementia.

Ergot Therapy and Ergotism

Ergot is a fungus which grows on grains, especially rye. The history of ergot intoxication dates from years before Christ. Ancient Greeks and Romans did not, however, employ rye extensively and it was not until the Middle Ages that written descriptions

of ergot poisoning appeared. The disease occurred then in epidemics and was characterized primarily by symptoms of ischemia, including tingling, burning, numbness and claudication, followed by gangrene of the hands, feet and legs (Fig 11-2). The illness had significant religious connotations. It was suggested that a type of Holy Fire was consuming the body. Subsequently, the name St. Anthony's Fire was also used, since a visitation to the Shrine of St. Anthony was sometimes curative. It is interesting that persons with ergotism were given a diet free of contaminated grain at the shrine and often recovered, further enhancing the belief in a divine cure. In addition to symptoms of peripheral ischemia, abortion was common with ergotism. Also, a form of ergotism associated with major motor seizures was described in those ancient epidemics of ischemia. In spite of this knowledge, outbreaks of ergot

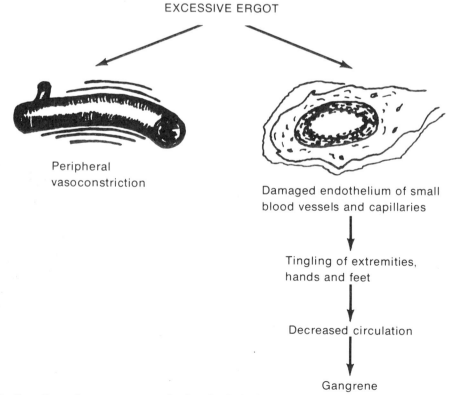

EXCESSIVE ERGOT

Peripheral
vasoconstriction

Damaged endothelium of small
blood vessels and capillaries

Tingling of extremities,
hands and feet

Decreased circulation

Gangrene

Fig 11-2. *Ergotism. Any artery may be involved, including peripheral arteries, coronaries and visceral arteries.*

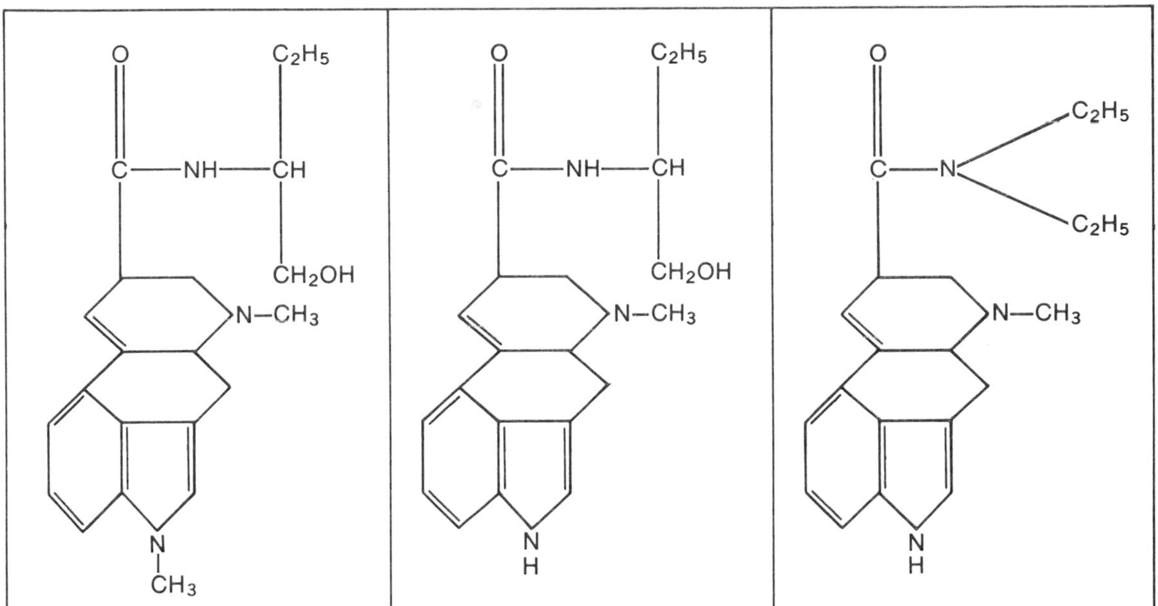

Fig 11-3. *Common ergot compounds.*

poisoning related to contamination of grain with the ergot fungus have continued to modern times.

The pharmacologic effects of the ergot compounds are complex, but for purposes of this discussion we will concentrate on their vascular effects. Ergotamine tartrate and related alkaloids produce peripheral vasoconstriction and also damage the endothelium of the capillaries and small blood vessels. Vascular stasis, thrombosis and gangrene may then ensue. The various ergot alkaloids differ significantly in these vasoconstrictor properties. Ergotamine is the most potent. Its effect in migraine is related largely to its vasoconstrictor properties.

Ergotamine tartrate is generally considered effective and safe in recommended doses, but can damage blood vessels.

Ergotamine tartrate is generally considered to be safe when used in its recom-

mended dose and migraine patients tolerate ergot well. If more than 10–12 mg per week are taken by mouth, however, or more than 1 ml per day parenterally, side effects may occur. These are usually not dangerous and include nausea, vomiting, severe thirst and other gastrointestinal discomforts. In chronic ergot poisoning, however, very striking and significant circulatory changes may occur. The distal extremities become cold, pale and numb, with slight sweating of the feet. Claudication becomes evident. The patient may complain of unusual susceptibility to the cold. Arterial pulses eventually disappear and gangrene may ensue. Since ergot is a nonspecific vasoconstrictor and may affect other arteries, including the coronary arteries, angina pectoris may appear and electrocardiographic changes have been documented. The visceral arteries may also be affected.

Unusual sensitivity to ergot therapy may appear in:

■ febrile states

■ liver disease

■   persons with compromised peripheral circulation

We therefore make it a rule never to employ ergot therapy in any patient with significant cardiovascular complaints and, in general, we avoid using the drug in persons over the age of 65 years.

Severe vasospasm may thus occur following ergot administration. On occasion this may occur related to overdose. On other occasions patients particularly susceptible to ergot may develop profound vasoconstriction as, for example, with Raynaud's disease.

Intravenous sodium nitroprusside may be helpful in this condition, where the signs and symptoms of peripheral ischemia are severe. The dose is 50 μg per minute, administered by a constant infusion pump, with careful monitoring of blood pressure in order to prevent hypotension. Chemical sympathectomy by lumbar and cervicothoracic sympathetic ganglion blockade may also be attempted in this situation and may prove to be therapeutic. Most often, watchful waiting, provision for symptomatic care, and withdrawal from ergot are the only treatment measures necessary.

Methysergide

Methysergide is, in fact, a methylated form of methylergonovine (Fig 11-3). It is of value in headache prophylaxis, by virtue of multiple sites of action (Fig 11-4).

■   When administered alone, methysergide may produce vasoconstriction.

■   When administered with catecholamines and some other vasoconstrictor agents, methysergide acts synergistically to increase peripheral vasoconstriction.

■   When administered either intravenously or by mouth, methysergide inhibits or alters the magnitude of central vasomotor reflexes.

Methysergide may also cause fibrosis of various areas of the body, which is relatively uncommon, but of sufficient intensity to cause great concern and to limit the usefulness of this drug in therapeutic situations. The most common fibrotic lesion produced has been retroperitoneal fibrosis, sometimes leading to the compromise of the kidneys and progressive renal failure. In addition, fibrosis has been observed in other areas, including the lungs and heart. The mechanisms by which fibrosis is produced is unknown. Although methysergide

Fig 11-4. *Structural formulas of methysergide and serotonin.*

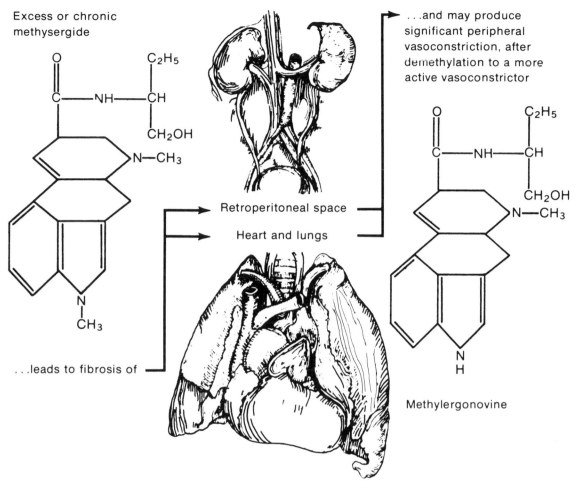

Excess or chronic methysergide

...leads to fibrosis of

Retroperitoneal space

Heart and lungs

...and may produce significant peripheral vasoconstriction, after demethylation to a more active vasoconstrictor

Methylergonovine

Fig 11-5. *Methysergide toxicity.*

is a powerful serotonin inhibitor, it has been suggested that it may, at times, act as a false serotonin transmitter (Fig 11-5). In diseases characterized by serotonin excess, such as the carcinoid syndrome, fibrosis does occur, particularly in the myocardium. But retroperitoneal fibrosis in the carcinoid syndrome is unusual.

Given the tendency of methysergide to produce fibrosis, it should be used sparingly and with care by the physician. We usually recommend that it not be used for longer than 90 days. If it is used for a longer period, the drug should be stopped for a full month every 6 months, at which time a careful reevaluation of the patient is mandatory. Renal function studies and a chest x-ray should probably be done at these times.

Other Drugs

Significant problems with analgesic abuse may appear with other medications and a thorough discussion of all of them is beyond the scope of this chapter. However, some general statements with respect to individual compounds can be made:

1 Compounds containing barbiturates have a significant capacity for addiciton.

2 Monoamine oxidase inhibitors may produce severe headache and hypertensive reactions if ingested with even small amounts of catecholamines. Patients taking these medications need careful guidance regarding diet and other therapy. Aged cheese contains tyramine which, if ingested while employing a monoamine oxidase inhibitor, may produce a severe hypertensive crisis. Even the small amounts of catecholamines present in proprietary cold pills and similar remedies should be avoided in this situation.

3 Phenothiazines are only occasionally abused in headache patients, but acute dystonic reactions may occur in some situations and must be recognized by the clinician.

4 Narcotics should not be given to patients with chronic headache. Addiction potential is especially significant where the pain is chronic and not acute, and where a tendency to overuse medication may already exist.

5 Cyproheptadine, if used for vascular headache prophylaxis, may produce undesireable weight gain.

6 Weight gain may also occur with prolonged use of tricyclic antidepressants. In addition, the tricyclic antidepressants have the potential of producing cardiac arrhythmias.

Summary

The syndrome of analgesic abuse occurs relatively frequently in patients with chronic headache. Unless the physician is aware of the syndrome and takes care in eliciting the history, the diagnosis may be missed. Abuse of proprietory headache nostrums may involve multiple therapeutic agents and may affect several organ systems. Abuse of compounds containing aspirin and phenacetin is common. This may lead to analgesic nephropathy, gastrointestinal symptoms and hematologic disorders. Overuse of ergot may produce undesirable vasoconstriction. Chronic use of methysergide is to be avoided; undesirable fibrosis of significance may appear, particularly in the retroperitoneal space. Recognition of the multiple components of the syndrome of analgesic abuse makes it imperative that the physician obtain a complete medication history from the patient.

SELF-ASSESSMENT EXAMINATION

1 Analgesic abuse should be considered in every patient complaining of chronic headache. True or False

2 A history of analgesic abuse is usually elicited easily from the patient. True or False

3 Analgesic abuse rarely involves proprietary headache remedies. True or False

4 Aspirin never produces signs or symptoms of analgesic abuse. True or False

5 Phenacetin ingestion in large amounts may lead to renal failure. True or False

6 Peptic ulcer is common in patients employing aspirin frequently. True or False

7 Ergotism refers to the hallucinogenic properties of LSD. True or False

8 Analgesic abuse can be suspected if the history reveals (a) ingestion of more than 100 aspirins or aspirin compounds each month; (b) consistent daily use of ergotamine tartrate; (c) patient consumes 2 aspirins weekly; (d) purchase of proprietary headache remedies in large doses; (e) employment of analgesics around the clock

9 Analgesic abuse which is symptomatic may (a) occur if more than 2 kg of aspirin or aspirin compounds have been ingested; (b) involve multiple organ systems; (c) commonly involve the kidneys; (d) be halted if the habit can be terminated; (e) be associated with abnormal hemoglobin compounds

10 Ergotism (a) has occurred throughout history in epidemics; (b) cannot occur with our present pure preparations; (c) is always reversible; (d) never leads to gangrene; (e) requires immediate surgical consultation and endarterectomy

11 The pharmacologic effects of ergotism include (a) vascular stasis and thrombosis; (b) endothelial capillary and arterial damage; (c) peripheral vasoconstriction; (d) all of the above; (e) none of the above

12 Chronic ergot poisoning (a) usually occurs in children; (b) rarely occurs in patients with reduced peripheral circulation; (c) is improved by fever; (d) all of the above; (e) none of the above

13 Methysergide, used for headache prophylaxis, is (a) unrelated to ergot in any form; (b) sometimes a vasoconstrictor agent; (c) used to reduce fibrosis caused by the carcinoid syndrome; (d) an inhibitor of serotonin; (e) an inhibitor of kinin effects

14 Monoamine oxidase inhibitors are (a) always contraindicated in the headache patient; (b) never contraindicated in the headache patient; (c) used with caution in the headache patient; (d) combined with small amounts of catecholamines; (e) served with cheese by a considerate hostess

15 Narcotics and barbiturates are (a) used with great caution in headache patients; (b) of specific aid in achieving headache analgesia; (c) the treatment of choice in chronic migraine; (d) of low addiction potential in the headache patient; (e) a frequent cause of dystonic reactions

ANSWERS:

1—True; 2—False; 3—False; 4—False; 5—True; 6—True; 7—False; 8—a,b,d,e; 9—a,b,c,d,e; 10—a; 11—d; 12—e; 13—b,d; 14—c; 15—a

Pain Mechanisms, The Pain Clinic, and Acupuncture

The nature of pain is a subject of continuous controversy in medicine. Pain is the primary symptom of most diseases, and as such is of concern to all physicians. Problems related to pain and its relief cut across narrow boundaries of specialties or categories of disease. The presence or absence of pain has been the impetus for some systems of philosophy, for aberrations of human behavior and for not a little of the world's literature. Many penal codes are based in part on pain or the threat of pain as punishment for wrongdoing.

Furthermore, there are at least two attributes of pain which tend to differentiate it from other subjective experiences associated with ordinary sensation and perception, such as touch, vision, hearing and the like. The first of these is related to the significant emotional experience which usually occurs with pain or threats of pain. This is to a considerable extent related to personality variables including fear, previous experience and previous conditioning. The second aspect is closely related to the first; this is the proposition that pain is a subjective sensation peculiar to the individual, which, at least in humans, requires an introspective report from the subject experiencing pain. This latter property of pain makes its precise measurement uncertain. Indeed, when dealing with clinical situations, it is often difficult to extract from the patient a reasonably accurate description of pain that can be correlated with descriptions of pain from others. Pain may not always be noxious, and some types of pain, especially those associated with sexual perversion, may in perverted individuals be experienced as pleasure.

Pain is a subjective sensation peculiar to the individual.

The Pain Problem

Pain is one of the few nearly universal human experiences and perhaps the greatest single cause of disability in the world.

Respecting no cultural, socioeconomic or racial boundaries, and afflicting people of all ages, pain exacts a heavy toll—figured in the billions of dollars annually in the United States alone. In terms of the human suffering it inflicts, pain is a health problem of even more monumental proportions.

People with severe, protracted pain often develop complications as significant as the original cause of their problem, and as the pain itself. Drug addiction or dependence, serious, even suicidal, depression, disability and invalidism are among the frequently encountered complications of long-term, intense pain. All can magnify the impact of the situation on the sufferer, his family, friends and lifestyle, as well as on the actual severity of the pain experienced.

For centuries, physicians and scientists have sought to understand and control this seemingly demonic force. As research produced more information about the human nervous system, and greater appreciation of its incredible complexity, pain phenomena became increasingly enigmatic.

Despite the magnitude of the problem, few physicians today receive formalized training in treatment of people with chronic pain and each medical specialty tries to deal with the problem in the framework of its own narrowly defined province. As a result, many practitioners, and most hospitals, are unable to cope with the special situation posed by pain patients.

Traditionally viewed as a symptom or "signal" of a disease or injury that will vanish when the disease is cured or the injury heals, pain—like many illnesses —can also become chronic. In such cases, *pain is a disease* and should be treated as one.

The Pain Clinic

In the past decade, significant strides have been made in pain *management*. There has been a surge of interest in research to uncover the biologic mechanisms underlying chronic pain and in development of new, better methods with which to evaluate and treat it.

Among the most outstanding developments of recent years has been the evolution of special centers in which efforts to solve the paradoxical and still mysterious puzzle of pain are being coordinated.

The significance accorded the emergence of such special facilities stems from the fact that, in this setting, *many* disciplines can be effectively integrated in a concerted and virtually simultaneous attack on each patient's pain problems.

While "cures" for pain are still in the future, notable and promising headway is being made in helping some to reduce or eliminate their pain and in teaching still others how to live useful, productive lives *despite it.*

Organization

The Pain Clinic may be operated by any interested physician. Our Pain Treatment Center (D. J. D.) is supervised by the Division of neurology, psychiatry and physchology, and is an amalgam of specialists in several different fields whose primary interest is chronic intractable pain.

Able to rely on our well-established diagnostic facilities to reveal underlying medical problems, a Pain Treatment Center concentrates on pain technologies—combinations of devices and equipment specifically intended for use in evaluation, treatment and management of chronic pain. Its staff includes a neurologist, psychologist, neurosurgeon and psychiatrists with a primary clinical or research interest in pain.

Although patients can be admitted to the hospital through the Pain Treatment Center when necessary or appropriate, most are cared for as outpatients. The emphasis on ambulatory treatment is a hallmark of our philosophy in treating the patient with chronic pain. It reflects the Center's orientation toward making life—outside the hospital—liveable for people with severe, chronic pain problems.

The Program

Headaches, neck and low back pains are the most common complaints for which people seek the help of a Pain Treatment Center. Other frequently encountered problems include injuries or diseases of the peripheral nerves, painful scars, thalamic pain following strokes, arthritic conditions and several types of neuralgias.

Although less common, phantom pain suffered by amputees and other kinds of paradoxical or esoteric pain syndromes are also evaluated at the Center.

The pain program includes three distinct components: evaluation, treatment and research.

Evaluation. Before a specific approach to a patient's pain problem is adopted, a thorough, comprehensive analysis and evaluation are completed to: (a) identify, if possible, the origins of the pain—medical or otherwise; (b) isolate factors contributing to the pain problem; and (c) quantify or measure the severity of the pain the patient is experiencing. The evaluation includes reviews of all available previous medical and surgical records (including tests, x-rays and special scans); the administration of psychologic tests; and, when indicated, other diagnostic medical procedures.

Most pain clinic patients have seen a number of different physicians and many have undergone several surgical operations for their problem. Medical history reviews help to define what has already been attempted and to eliminate *unnecessary* duplication of diagnostic tests. Coupled with the supplementary and comparative testing completed at the clinic, these records help to establish the cause underlying the patient's pain problem. In some cases, a correctible medical condition is uncovered. In others, where the cause cannot be "cured," efforts can then be focused on controlling or *managing* the pain itself.

Psychologic testing and pain measurements are routinely included in the Center's evaluations. These tests aid pain specialists in defining the nature and extent of psychic complications which are almost unavoidably created by a chronic pain problem.

Treatment. Except in cases where a medically or surgically correctible condition is uncovered in the preliminary evaluation, treatment at a pain clinic is usually focused on methods of controlling or reducing pain—of managing it—and permitting those it afflicts to lead near-normal lives.

Among the pain-management techniques employed at the Center, either singly or in combination, are:

Regulation of pain-relieving (analgesic) medications. Analgesics are often ineffective in chronic pain cases. Users develop a physical tolerance that inhibits the drug's ability to "kill" pain, and physical and psychologic addictions frequently occur after long-term use. However, carefully controlled administration of different analgesics can often produce substantial reduction of pain intensity and proper regulation of dosages—even with common aspirin—can successfully prevent episodes of severe pain.

Attitude-influencing (psychotropic) medications. Anxiety, depression or agitation—regardless of their origin—can increase pain markedly. Tranquilizers and particularly antidepressants can reduce pain and, at the same time, increase patients' ability to tolerate and function with their pain.

Nerve blocks. Anesthetics capable of temporarily deadening a nerve and eliminating, at least for a few hours, pain in the "deadened" area are sometimes used to interrupt cyclical pain syndromes—cases where pain activates complicating factors which, in turn, aggravate and intensify the pain, and so on in cyclical fashion. By interrupting the cycle, the nerve block can break the pain circuit and, in some cases, provide relief lasting weeks, or even months. Such blocks are frequently diagnostic as well.

Electrical neurostimulation. Sometimes referred to as "electronic acupuncture," electrical neurostimulation relieves pain by creating a mild electrical "shock" that replaces the sensation of pain with a gentle, even pleasant, tingling feeling. Although its effect is similar to that of a nerve block, electrical neurostimulation does not produce incapacitating numbness and its effect can be prolonged, amplified, or modulated directly by the patient.

Frequently affording significant relief for pain sufferers, neurostimulation employs a pocket-sized, battery-operated, transmitter/regulator and electrodes that are "worn" by the patient at regulated intervals. The electrodes are taped on the skin in the midst of the neurologic pathway which the pain signal follows to the brian. By overriding the pain impulse with its electrical stimulus, the device effectively "blocks" the sensation of pain.

Electrodes may also be surgically placed directly on a nerve fiber beneath the skin to reduce interference with the electrical stimulus created by surrounding tissue. This procedure, however, is rarely used at present.

Activity management. Incidence and severity of pain is often related to the types and levels of activity in which the patient engages. Increases in pain can result form too much, too little or just certain kinds of activity.

Proper analysis of the problem and the patient's living patterns can provide the pain clinic's staff with a basis for helping the patient adjust his lifestyle to minimize the pain—often by simply "pacing," rather than eliminating, various types of normal activity.

Family counseling. Especially in cases of intractable pain, the support provided by a pain patient's family is often a critical factor in his or her rehabilitation. Family members must learn how to *work with* the patient, reinforcing *normal*—not pain—*behavior.* Family counseling services offered through the pain clinic are intended to bring this important element into concert with other efforts to help patients cope with their problems.

Research. The puzzling, paradoxical nature of pain remains one of the most challenging *and important* areas in modern health research. An important dimension of any pain clinic's research should be the accumulation and analyses of day-to-day clinical data from which various therapeutic approaches can be evaluated. These studies help to isolate which methods either offer or promise long-term effectiveness, which therapeutic combinations are most successful, etc.

Our own research programs are focused on: development of new biofeedback systems, as well as evaluation of present approaches, the mechanisms of electrical analgesia (pain-reducing neurostimulation), more accurate objective measurement of pain and evaluation of new, nonnarcotic pain-controlling drugs.

Future research is anticipated to include studies of pain's underlying biologic and physiologic mechanisms.

The Gate Control Theory

It is generally agreed that patterning of input is essential to the production of pain. The excessive peripheral stimulation that occurs when one hits one's thumb with a hammer quite obviously evokes pain of an acute nature. In addition, there are specific neural mechanisms that account for the summation of stimuli in clinical situations of chronic pain, where the provoking stimulus may not be so apparent. Reverberating circuits in spinal internuncial pools may be set off by normally benign afferent input which could thereafter be interpreted centrally as painful. It is proposed that a specialized central system prevents this critical summation from occurring, in that it inhibits synaptic transmission of slowly conducting nerve fibers which ordinarily subserve pain. One must, therefore, evoke the dual concepts of central summation of pain and central inhibition of pain to explain pain as it occurs clinically. Malzack and Wall have modified this theory to propose that the substantia gelatinosa of the dorsal horn of the spinal cord functions as a gate control system which modulates the afferent stimuli before they are transmitted centrally.

Central to the concept of the gate control theory is the substantia gelatinosa, which runs throughout the length of the spinal cord. It is suggested that this area acts as a gate control system modulating the transmission of nerve impulses (Fig 12-1). Thus, the large, myelinated fibers inhibit pain signals, while the small, unmyelinated fibers facilitate their transmission. In each

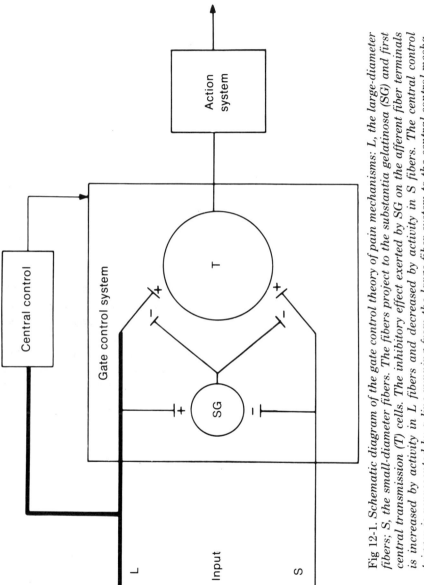

Fig 12-1. *Schematic diagram of the gate control theory of pain mechanisms: L, the large-diameter fibers; S, the small-diameter fibers. The fibers project to the substantia gelatinosa (SG) and first central transmission (T) cells. The inhibitory effect exerted by SG on the afferent fiber terminals is increased by activity in L fibers and decreased by activity in S fibers. The central control trigger is represented by a line running from the large-fiber system to the central control mechanisms; these mechanisms, in turn, project back to the gate control system. The T cells project to the entry cells of the action system. + = excitation, − = inhibitions. [From Melzack R, Wall PD: Pain mechanisms: A new theory. Science **150**:971, 1965. Copyright 1965 by the American Association for the Advancement of Science.]*

case, this is accomplished by the action of the substantia gelatinosa on the spinal cord cells that transmit afferent signals to the brain.

Effects of Analgesic Agents

Much information related to the study of pain has been obtained from the study of analgesic agents of varying types. It has been known for some time that receptors in the skin, termed nociceptors (responding to tissue-damaging stimuli), have both myelinated and nonmyelinated afferent fibers. Not all nonmyelinated fibers (C-fibers) are specific for nociceptive stimuli, since it has been shown that C-fibers will respond to temperature changes and to mechanical stimuli of only a few milligrams of skin pressure, which do not cause pain. It is important, therefore, to avoid the concept that C-fibers are specific in peripheral nerves for pain. Furthermore, it has been found that fluid obtained from areas where there has been tissue destruction, as in a blister which forms after burning, contains a pain-producing substance, which also has vasodilator and vasopermeability-increasing activity. This substance is a vasodilator polypeptide, related to the polypeptide bradykinin. This polypeptide may be a terminal portion of the gamma globulin molecule from which it can be liberated or separated by proteolytic enzymes. Injury to tissue activates the enzymes which lead to the formation of bradykinin. Prostaglandins are also liberated. Salicylates, such as aspirin and related compounds exert a peripheral analgesic effect by interfering with the actions of the kinins, and by inhibiting prostaglandin synthesis.

Wolff et al. have demonstrated that antidromic dorsal root activity plays some role in the liberation of vasodilator polypeptides of the bradykinin type. They suggest that neurogenically induced vasodilation may represent a direct contribution of the nervous system to the inflammatory reaction. Interactions within the spinal cord

may play a role in the central perception of pain. The flexor response in man is studied by recording electromyographically the response in the vastus medialis muscle when pain stimuli have been applied at different skin territories of the same limb. The flexor reflex consists of the contraction of the limb at the ankle, knee and hip, when noxious stimulation is applied, in order to withdraw the limb from the site of noxious stimulation. This is an integrated and organized reflex, which serves as a withdrawal response. Under hypnotic analgesia, inhibition is evoked and no excitatory activity follows. This illustrates that painful flexor reflexes in man are subject to modulation from higher centers.

Chapman et al. have demonstrated changes in tissue vulnerability induced during hypnotic suggestion. Following standard amounts of noxious stimulation of the forearm during hypnosis, decreased inflammatory reaction and tissue damage were observed when the suggestion was made that the arm was insensitive and numb, as compared to the reaction and tissue damage of the other arm which was suggested to be normally sensitive. When the suggestion was made that the forearm was tender, increased inflammatory reaction and tissue damage was observed, as compared with the normally sensitive arm. On the basis of these studies it is postulated that neural activity can alter inflammatory reactions in peripheral tissues.

Postulation: Neural activity can alter inflammatory reactions in peripheral tissue.

Narcotics exert a suppressive action on spinal reflexes, probably by augmenting supraspinal inhibition of cord reflexes. Reflex suppression by morphine is greater when the spinal cord is intact than when it is transected. Spinal cord reflexes can also be diminished using medications which are not analgesics in the usual sense, especially anticonvulsants. Studies on the use of the anticonvulsant carbamazepine in tic douloureux suggests that inhibition of spinal cord reflex activity may provide analgesia. Thus, tic douloureux, an extremely unpleasant pain syndrome, may be manifested by a state of abnormal reactivity of the spinal trigeminal nuclei, related to a decreased or defective central integrative system regulating sensory input. Tic douloureux has been proposed as a model for this type of syndrome, wherein the inability of the brain to suppress sensory input from normal or minimally damaged peripheral tissues evokes severe pain.

The Brain's Function

This latter proposition of pain related to abnormal spinal reflex activity leads naturally to considerations of central handling of pain in the brain. Here the dual functions in the somatosensory system of man should be emphasized. One component of this system is represented by the lemniscal system, which is a precise, topographic system of somatic sensation involving the peripheral nerves, the first order afferent fibers of the dorsal columns of the spinal cord, the neural elements of the medial lemniscus, the cells of the ventrobasal nuclear complex of the thalamus and of the post central region of the cerebral cortex (Fig 12-2). A second, phylogenetically older system, designated the anterolateral system, originates in the dorsal horn of the spinal cord.

In contrast, the anterolateral system is poorly defined and ascends in nonlinear tracts to multiple areas of the brain including the thalamus, midbrain, medulla, and especially to the reticular system and the limbic system. The anterolateral system is hard to illustrate in a precise neuroanatomic way, but is pictured schematically in Figure 12-3.

The neurons in this latter pathway have properties different from those in the lemniscal system. Their receptive fields are very large and not topographically organized, and often lack specificity. Medications such as narcotics exert their effects primarily on the anterolateral projection system, and thus produce diffuse pain-alleviating effects. There are other experimental studies in animals, which support this concept—that is, that the lemniscal and anterolateral systems differ in their pharmacologic reactivity. Melzack produced neural responses by stimulating the tooth pulp of cats; these neural responses appeared both in the lemniscal and in the anterolateral systems. It was shown in these experiments that nitrous oxide abolished selectively the response from the lemniscal system only. These pharmacologic differences may relate to differences in the size of the fiber tracts rather than to those in the number of associated synapses (Fig 12-4).

Antidepressants of the tricyclic type have been employed in the management of chronic pain syndromes, especially headache. These agents may decrease pain by altering central appreciation of the quality or intensity of pain as it occurs in the depressed patient. As a consequence of his depression, the depressed patient may misinterpret afferent stimuli at the cortical level and experience pain when, in fact, he should not. The structural relationship of the tricyclic antidepressants to anticonvulsants such as carbamazepine is striking. It is important to realize that the anterolateral system projects especially to those areas of the brain which have to do with basic behavioral mechanisms, with personality, with motivation and affect, and all of these aspects of central nervous activities strongly influence pain perception.

The depressed patient may misinterpret afferent stimuli and experience pain when, in fact, he should not.

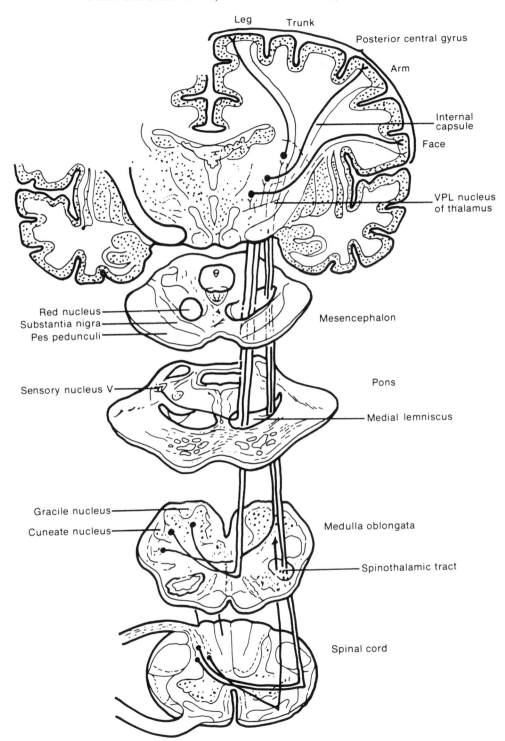

Fig 12-2. *A simplified diagram of the main features in the lemniscal somatosensory pathways. A surgeon's cut here is a cordotomy, used to relieve pain by blocking sensation.*

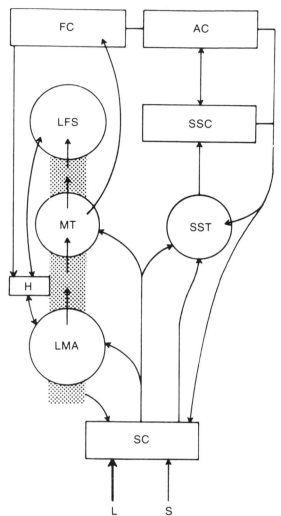

The brain itself exerts significant control over information it receives. Probably a portion of the brainstem reticular formation exerts a tonic inhibitory influence on information transmission. This may occur not only at the spinal gate, but at any other synaptic level where sensory information is projected rostrally. Thus, the gate control theory is also compatible with the clinical experience that pain can be intensified or decreased by psychologic factors. Just as in biofeedback experiments, where there is brain control over sensory input, so methods of conditioning may be employed in situations of chronic pain. In cases of chronic headache, for example, where a chronic pain cycle has been produced, it should be possible, using methods of relaxation, suggestion, biofeedback control, and, possibly, hypnosis, to reduce pain perception through cortical activity, which acts to increase inhibition at the spinal gate and other synaptic levels.

Thus, what we are saying in so many words is that the brain itself can modify and change painful stimuli, and it can do this is at least two ways (Fig 12-5):

1 peripherally, by closing the spinal gate and not letting the stimulus into the spinal cord and

2 centrally, by modifying ongoing central nervous activity.

Thus it may be seen that pain is an integrated experience which is dependent upon an intact and functioning central nervous system involving the peripheral nerves, the spinal cord and the brain. Psychologic factors such as past experience, attention and emotion may influence pain response and perception greatly. It is to be emphasized that the quantitative measurement of pain is hazardous, that pain is an individual perception which the perceiver

Fig 12-3. *Schematic diagram of the anatomic foundation of the proposed pain model. On the right: thalamic and neocortical structures subserving discriminative capacity. On the left: reticular and limbic systems subserving motivational-affective functions. Ascending pathways from the spinal cord (SC) are: (1) the dorsal column-lemniscal and dorsolateral tracts (right ascending arrow) projecting to the somatosensory thalamus (SST) and cortex (SSC), and (2) the anterolateral pathways (left ascending arrow) to the somatosensory thalamus via the neospinothalamic tract and to the reticular formation (stripped area), the limbic midbrain area (LMA) and medial thalamus (MT) via the paramedial ascending system. Descending pathways to spinal cord originate in somatosensory and associated cortical areas (AC) and in the reticular formation. Polysynaptic and reciprocal relationships in limbic and*

ations: FC-frontal cortex; LFS-limbic forebrain structures (hippocampus, septum, amygdala, and associated cortex): H-hypothalamus. [From Casey K: Toward a neurophysiology of pain. Headache 8:141, 1969.]

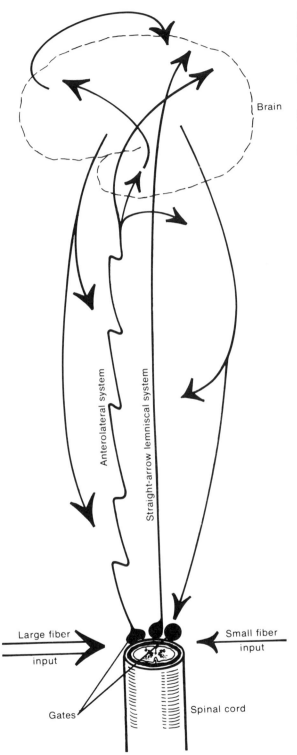

Fig 12-4. *Another view of the gate control system.*

may communicate only poorly, and that laboratory models of experimental pain may be difficult to interpret, especially in terms of clinical situations wherein analgesia is sought.

Measuring Pain Severity

Sternbach has shown that it is possible to relate the patient's pain estimate to a tourniquet pain ratio in an attempt to more adequately measure the amount of suffering the patient is experiencing. This is important, not only for its help in making a correct diagnosis, but also to decide to what extent medical and/or surgical procedures may be necessary to relieve the pain. If one relies solely on the patient's description of the intensity of the pain, one invites error from other factors, particularly personality variables and cultural differences in pain appreciation.

The pain estimate is obtained by asking the patients to rate the intensity of their pain on a scale of 0–100. Zero represents no pain at all, and 100 is pain so severe that one would commit suicide if it had to be endured. The patients frequently estimate the pain daily at the same time that activity management in terms of hours up and out of bed are calculated. In addition, the tourniquet pain ratio can be obtained using an ischemic test developed by Smith, which makes use of partial ischemia of the arm associated with exercise. (See Tourniquet Pain Test Procedures.) Neither the pain estimate nor the tourniquet pain ratio appear to be correlated with any clinical personality variable on the Minnesota Multiphasic Personality Inventory (MMPI) or on a Health Index, but the pain estimate is usually higher than the tourniquet pain ratio, presumably due to a mixture of pain perception and communication needs.

Tourniquet Pain Test

Procedures

1. Have patient lie down.
2. Identify which is nondominant arm (opposite from one used for writing). Ask patient if there is anything wrong with that arm. If the nondominant arm is o.k., it will be used for the test on each occasion. Otherwise, the dominant arm should be used.
3. Have patient remove any jewelry (watch, rings, etc.) from arm to be used.
4. Explain the basic procedure to the patient in a brief fashion and mention that he may ask questions if he wishes.
5. Raise the arm to be used, and then begin wrapping arm with rubber Esmarch bandage. Wrap the arm very tightly, starting with the top of the finger tips to just slightly beyond the elbow. Tuck any extra bandage roll into the wrappings.
6. Inflate blood pressure cuff to 250, with the cuff placed in the normal position, and just at the end of the Esmarch bandage.
7. Remove Esmarch bandage.
8. Lower arm and begin stop watch for a 60-second pause. During this period, make sure the cuff stays at 250.
9. Give patient hand exerciser and tell him to squeeze-release, every 2 seconds for 20 squeezes. When second hand passes 1 minute 20 seconds, he will have completed 20 squeezes.
10. *Restart* stop watch by pressing side button. Timing begins when last squeeze completed.
11. Ask patient to tell when what he feels in his arm feels similar to: (a) the average pain he has had for the past week; and (b) the "un-bearable" level (the most he can take).
12. When patient says the pain in his arm is unbearable, stop the watch by pressing the large center knob and release the cuff. That is the end of the test.

NOTE: Be sure patient compares arm feeling to pain he has had. Question him if he says it is "unbearable" and has not mentioned clinical pain.

If patient does not reach "clinical" level in 15 minutes, stop the test and remove cuff.

Compute ratio: $\dfrac{\text{Clinical pain level}}{\text{Maximum tolerance}}$ $\times 100$;

Example: $\dfrac{3 \text{ min, } 10 \text{ sec}}{5 \text{ min, } 40 \text{ sec}} = \dfrac{190}{340} = 56\%$

Instructions to Patients

(Read or repeat to patients on their first testing.)

We're going to do an experiment to test your pain thresholds, to help the doctors understand the level of pain you feel.

I will first wrap your arm tightly with this rubber bandage. Then, I'll inflate a blood pressure cuff on your arm, and then have you squeeze a hand exerciser 20 times. This is in order to drain the blood from the veins in your arm as much as possible.

Then you will just lay your arm down, and then I want you to tell me when what you feel in your arm equals the pain which you have had for the past week. It may be a different kind of pain, but when the severity is the same, or it hurts as much, let me know.

Then, I want you to tell me when what you feel in your arm is unbearable. When you tell me it is unbearable, that you cannot take any more, I will take the cuff off and the test will be over.

Remember, I want you to tell me when the level of pain in your arm equals your clinical pain.

Please don't move or talk during the test. Do you have any questions?

Morphine, Opiate Receptors, Enkephalins and Pituitary Endorphins

Morphine and its derivatives exert their effects by binding to specific receptor sites on cells in the brain and spinal cord. Morphine-like substances which occur naturally in the body may also act at those sites. Opiate receptors in the brain have been identified by measuring the specific binding of radioactively labeled opiate drugs to cell fragments from different brain areas. Much the largest amount of binding was found in cells of the limbic system. This suggests that the opiates exert their analgesic and euphoria-producing effects by binding to receptors in the limbic system.

Optical isomers of the opiate analgesics have different pharmacologic activities. Only the levorotatory isomer produces the characteristic analgesic effects of the drug. The dextrorotatory isomer is totally inactive. This stereospecificity of opiate actions supports the model of a highly specific receptor which can recognize the mirror image form of the opiate molecule.

Opiate antagonists are substances that specifically block the analgesic and euphoric actions of opiates without eliciting any such effects themselves. These antagonists turn out to be opiates which are transformed by only very slight molecular modifications into antagonists. It seems likely that opiate antagonists will occupy opiate receptor sites, are inert themselves, but prevent the opiates from reaching the receptor sites and in this manner inhibit analgesia and euphoria.

The opiates are also of interest with respect to the two major brain pathways im-plicated in the perception of pain. Opiates are considerably more effective in interfering with dull, chronic and less localized pain which is transmitted to the central nervous system through the paleospinothalamic pathway. Sharp and well-localized pain, transmitted through the lemniscal system, responds more poorly to opiates. If one maps the distribution of opiate receptors in the brain, one finds that they parallel in a striking fashion the paleospinothalamic pathway. Similarly, spinal cord opiate receptors can be localized in the area about the substantia gelatinosa, which, as discussed before, is a way station for the brainward conduction of sensory information associated with pain.

Since specific opiate receptors are a characteristic of most animals and man, the speculation arose that a natural neurotransmitter, morphine-like, would be found in the brain, acting at opiate receptors. In a series of brilliant studies, Hughes, Kosterlitz, Pasternak and Snyder were able to isolate a morphine-like factor from the brains of animals, particularly pigs, and found that it consisted of two closely related peptides made up of five amino acid units. The term enkephalin was given to these peptides. Evidence has now accumulated to suggest that the enkephalins are neurotransmitters of specific neuronal systems in the brain which mediate information having to do with pain and emotional behavior. Furthermore, enkephalin brain levels tend to parallel the distribution of opiate receptors.

The enkephalins work by inhibiting the polarization of brain cells by excitatory transmitters. In effect, enkephalin will mimic morphine, to the extent that the inhibition of enkephalin, like that of morphine, is blocked by the opiate antagonist naloxone. This suggests that both morphine and enkephalin act at the same receptor. The relationship between enkephalins and morphine has led to suggestions that the naturally occurring enkephalins may be important in the production of physical addiction.

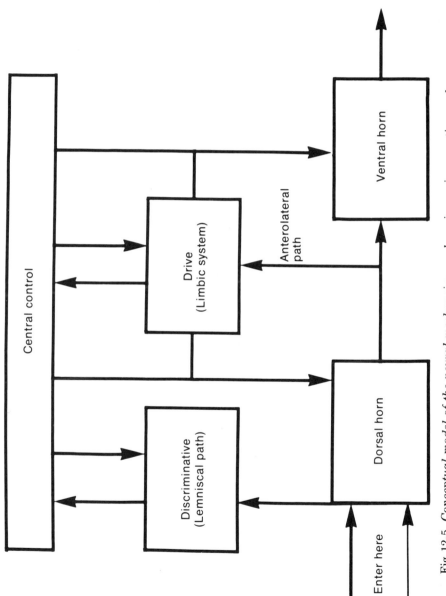

Fig 12-5. *Conceptual model of the neural mechansisms subserving pain sensation and response. Small and large diameter afferent fibers enter at the spinal cord dorsal horn. Large fibers activate the discriminative system. Both fiber types interact at the dorsal horn to produce a dorsal horn output which activates spinal reflexes (ventral horn) and, via a paramedial ascending system, drive mechanisms in the limbic system. All stages of the system are reciprocally connected with the central control system. [From Casey K: Toward a neurophysiology of pain. Headache 8:141, 1969.]*

Even more recently, Goldstein and Li have discovered that natural opiate-like peptides are contained in the pituitary gland. Li has named these peptides endorphins for endogenous morphine. These have a high degree of analgesic activity and again are directly blocked by naloxone, a specific opiate antagonist. Guillemin of the Salk Institute has isolated several other peptides from a mixture of hypothalamus and pituitary tissue of pigs. The function of the pituitary endorphins is uncertain, but they may regulate pituitary functions which are known to be altered by opiates, such as the release of the antidiuretic hormone from the posterior pituitary by morphine.

Some of the naturally occurring "internal opiates" have also been demonstrated to produce catatonia and other signs of psychiatric disturbance, leading to the further supposition that they may be implicated in various forms of mental illness. Clearly, the discovery of the opiate receptors, and their internal opiates, is one of the most exciting developments in neurochemistry in recent years. Their relationship to chronic pain states, to addiction, and possibly to basic forms of mental disease will be of concern to all physicians for the foreseeable future.

Everything You Always Wanted to Know About Acupuncture

Question: Just exactly what is acupuncture?

Answer: Acupuncture is a method of treatment several thousand years old, which has been used by the Chinese in curing disease and protecting health. In primitive society, acupuncture was administered with a piece of sharp stone called a pien. A cure was effected by pressing or pricking a certain section of the body. Later the pien was replaced by needles made of stone, bone or bamboo. After metals were discovered, copper, iron and silver needles were used. Modern acupuncture is performed with fine needles of stainless steel.

Q: What is the basis of classical acupuncture?

A: This is related to the ancient Chinese theory that a balance of two forces, the yin and the yang, exists in the universe—and in the human body. The yin represents negative forces including darkness, femaleness, cold and passivity, while yang represents the positives of light, maleness, heat and activity. A disease may result when there is an imbalance of the yin and the yang, which disrupts the orderly flow of life energy through the body. According to this theory, the major body organs, 12 in all, are divided between the yin and the yang. The yin organs include the liver, the spleen and the heart, while the gallbladder, large intestine and stomach are yang organs. Life energy is said to flow from organ to organ through a network of channels beneath the skin, termed meridians. There are 12 meridians, representing the organs, running on either side of the body with two extra meridians, one along the center, in front of the body, and one in the back. In addition, the network of meridians contains 500 to 800 points which the acupuncturist must learn in order to correctly place his needles and "correct the energy and balances." These points are quite specific. One point on the hand, for example, is for toothaches, sore throat and anesthesia. One point on the leg is for stomachache and appendicitis. Another point on the foot is used for treating ulcers, fever, coughing and so on. Manual manipulation of the acupuncture needle or heating may be incorporated into this treatment.

Q: What is acupuncture anesthesia?

A: In acupuncture anesthesia one or more needles are inserted at certain points on the patient's limbs, ears, nose or face. Anesthesia follows after a period of inducement or stimulation, often one half hour, and then the operation is performed. Patients are fully conscious during operations when this kind of anesthesia is used. They may receive some preanesthetic medications, but the amount and type of preanesthetic medication is not usually emphasized in Chinese publications on the subject. Evidently there are many patients who receive no preanesthetic medication. In some situations during acupuncture anesthesia, electrical stimulation of the needles is necessary to achieve pain relief.

Q: How many patients have received this type of acupuncture anesthesia?

A: The Chinese claim that more than 400,000 patients have received acupuncture anesthesia for surgical operations, including children and people in their 80s. They claim a success rate of 90%. Operations have included procedures on the brain, removal of the lung and even correction of congenital cardiac defects. Acupuncture anesthesia does not need complicated apparatus and is applicable regardless of equipment, climate and geographical conditions. It can therefore be widely used in the cities and is particularly suitable to mountainous and rural areas and under conditions of war.

Q: What sort of knowledge is required to use acupuncture anesthesia?

A: So far as can be determined, acupuncture anesthesia can be learned quickly and does not require elaborate professional instruction. Chinese publications show medical workers experimenting on each other, placing needles in order to locate the most effective points for producing anesthesia.

The Chinese use acupuncture for a whole series of medical problems related to pain.

Q: Is acupuncture helpful in medical conditions?

A: The Chinese use acupuncture for a whole series of medical problems related to pain. These include especially arthritis, headache (including migraine) and hypertension. The Chinese make great claims for treatment of eye diseases with acupuncture, including glaucoma and even blindness. It should be recognized that Chinese physicians do not believe in rigidly controlled studies, and some of the claims for treatment of medical diseases particularly should be viewed with great scepticism. There is no question, however, that in some situations acupuncture works.

Q: Is acupuncture anesthesia a new concept?

A: According to Chinese publications, this form of anesthesia is a direct result of the teachings of Chairman Mao who pointed out that "Chinese medicine and pharmacology are a great treasure-house; efforts should be made to explore them and raise them to a higher level." In responding to this call in the 1950s, Chinese medical workers developed a "revolutionary spirit" and applied modern scientific knowledge and methods to acupuncture. It is of interest that the entire story of acupuncture anesthesia as described by the Chinese is full of political implications. Thus, for example, it is stated in a book on acupuncture anesthesia produced by the Foreign Languages Press of Peking, in 1972, that "no sooner had acupuncture anesthesia appeared than it was repressed by Liu Shao Chi's counterrevolutionary revisionist line and attacked by bourgeois experts. In a vain attempt to nip it in the bud, they raved that it was not scientific, without any practical value, and a retrogression in the history of anesthesia."

It is further stated that "the great proletarian cultural revolution swept away the bourgeois trash, and revolutionary medical workers relentlessly criticized Liu Shao Chi's counterrevolutionary revisionist line and work in scientific research. This facilitated great development in improvement in acupuncture anesthesia." Political diatribes such as this, which appear in the discussion of a scientific method of anesthesia, make Western observers critical of acupuncture, and of Chinese studies of its efficacy.

Q: Is acupuncture anesthesia invariably effective?

A: Even the Chinese admit that it may still have "some imperfections." They admit that at certain stages in some operations patients still "feel some pain" and "some feel uncomfortable when the internal organs are pulled." They further state that "Chinese medical and scientific workers are making still greater efforts in studying Marxism-Leninism-Mao Tse Tung thought and are using dialectical materialism to guide their medical work in scientific research. Daring in practice and in breaking new ground, they are bending their efforts to perfect acupuncture anesthesia."

Q: How might acupuncture anesthesia work?

A: Surprisingly, there are few suggestions in Chinese writings which indicate the mechanism by which acupuncture anesthesia works, and there is apparently little interest in this subject. The explanation for acupuncture, on a scientific basis, has come by and large from Western medicine. It has been known for years that stimulation of the skin tends to reduce pain, related primarily to the speed of conduction of pain sensations as related to those of touch. Sensations of touch are conducted along the nerves at a much more rapid rate than are those of pain. It is theoretically possible therefore to block out sensations of pain by producing simultaneous stimulation of the skin. We all know this well. For example, when a child falls down, his mother advises him to rub the uninjured area around the skin abrasion and, frequently, this reduces the pain. Grandmother produced the same effect with her mustard plasters and, even now, irritating rubs are sold to reduce muscle pain. Presumably these act by producing counterirritation and stimulation of the skin and thereby block out the pain from the aching muscles. This concept—of a gate control mechanism regulating pain—was first formulated by Drs. Melzack and Wall, who proposed that a specific area of the spinal cord functions

as a gate modulating the amount of stimuli that are allowed to flow into the spinal cord and eventually to the conscious waking brain.

It is suggested that the scientific basis of acupuncture can be explained in part by its counterirritative or gating effect.

Q: Can acupuncture anesthesia be considered a form of hypnosis?

A: There is no question that some aspects of hypnosis may play a role in acupuncture anesthesia. But it is unlikely that the entire explanation for acupuncture anesthesia can be related to hypnotic effects. Operations under hypnosis are effective in perhaps 10 to 20% of patients. Operations under acupuncture have a considerably higher success rate, approaching 90% effectiveness in some body areas, such as surgery of the thyroid. Although conditions in China may lead to a greater acceptance and confidence in the mystique of acupuncture, as representing a method of anesthesia officially approved by the government, it seems unwise to us to assume that the beneficial effects of acupuncture anesthesia are entirely related to a hypnotic trance effective in a particular cultural milieu.

Q: In other words, acupuncture anesthesia probably has a neurophysiologic basis?

A: Correct. Whether it is related to the gating effect mentioned above, to an increase in cortical inhibition of afferent input, to alteration in postsynaptic inhibition of impulses or to spreading depression of the sensory cortex itself, all of which have been suggested as possible explanations, is currently moot. Obviously this is a method of anesthesia that requires further study.

Q: Would acupuncture anesthesia be an improvement over modern anesthetic techniques?

A: Although it is obvious that modern anesthetic techniques should not be abandoned, there are certain aspects of acupuncture anesthesia which deserve serious thought and consideration. Anesthesia by acupuncture helps to prevent disorders of the patient's physiologic functions during operations, and avoids the harmful side effects of the use of anesthesia after its completion. The patient's blood pressure, pulse and breathing in general remain normal. Incisions tend to heal more quickly and functions of the internal organs are restored quickly and more satisfactorily after the operation, as a consequence of which the patient can move about and take food early. Acupuncture may have its particular application in patients who are poor operative risks because of poor functioning of the liver, kidneys or lungs, in which administration of anesthesia by drugs is not advisable. Certainly it promotes early ambulation, a goal of Western anesthetic practices as well.

SELF-ASSESSMENT EXAMINATION

1 Pain is (a) conducted over large myelinated fibers of peripheral nerves; (b) conducted only by small unmyelinated fibers of peripheral nerves; (c) conducted over thinly myelinated and unmyelinated fibers

2 (a) All small unmyelinated fibers of peripheral nerves conduct pain; (b) Some small unmyelinated fibers of peripheral nerves conduct pain, and some conduct other forms of sensation, such as temperature; (c) All small unmyelinated fibers of peripheral nerves are larger than 14 in diameter. Which statement is true?

3 Pain is conducted (a) centrally over two major pathways, the lemniscal system and the anterolateral system; (b) only over the anterolateral system; (c) only over the lemniscal system

4 (a) Pain is a specific sensation which has its own neurologic apparatus, the pain fiber; (b) Pain is a nonspecific sensation involving the entire spinal cord; (c) Joe Namath is a quarterback with painful knees. Which statement is true?

5 The lemniscal system is designed to transmit sensation rapidly and discretely to the thalamus and cortex. True or False

6 The lemniscal system is designed for slow, nonspecific conduction of sensation and sometimes reaches the conscious level. True or False

7 The lemniscal system is a figment of the anatomist's imagination. True or False

8 The anterolateral system of sensory conduction (a) is not organized to provide discrete information regarding sensation; (b) provides direct and rapid ascent to the cortex; (c) is not related to the limbic system

9 Central control of sensation and pain (a) almost never occurs; (b) is of considerable importance; (c) refers to a computer in Washington which programs the activities of the FBI

10 The gate control system (a) functions at the spinal level to modulate sensory information passed on to conscious levels; (b) is located in the thalamus; (c) acts to speed sensory messages to the brain

11 The gate control system position (open or closed) is (a) determined by a balance between peripheral sensory and central inputs; (b) opened by increasing central control or tone; (c) closed by increasing small fiber input to the gate

12 If small fiber input to the gate control system is reduced, (a) pain will increase; (b) pain will decrease; (c) not a thing will happen

13 In cordotomy, the (a) nerves are sectioned; (b) nerve tracts in the spinal cord are sectioned; (c) the sensory portion of the cortex is destroyed

14 Pain is (a) always noxious; (b) not always noxious, sometimes ignored, and sometimes, in perverse states, described as pleasurable; (c) a philosophical concept signifying the absence of pleasure

---

ANSWERS:

1—c; 2—b; 3—a; 4—c; 5—True; 6—False; 7—False; 8—a; 9—b; 10—a; 11—a; 12—b; 13—b; 14—b

13

Biofeedback and Operant Conditioning

Introduction

Over the past two decades, medical researchers have devised a new technique which has proven to be very useful in the treatment of certain forms of headache. This technique, known as biofeedback, combines modern electrical technology with ancient Eastern practices and modern psychology. Complex electrical devices are employed which carefully monitor various bodily functions such as heart rate, blood pressure, temperature, muscle tension and brainwave activity, the functions of which we are generally unaware. By relating the status of these various functions back to the individual, a person can learn to control a previously unused or involuntarily controlled function of his body.

Such control of bodily functions can be related to psychologic self-discipline practiced in Eastern cultures by yogis and Zen masters. As we shall see, such control has proven to be quite useful in treatment of headaches.

Background

The basic principle behind biofeedback technique or instrument learning goes back to the Russian scientist, Ivan Pavlov, and his conditioned reflex theory (Fig 13-1). From this emerged the theory of operant conditioning (Fig. 13-2), the basis for biofeedback technique, which provides the conditioned stimulus along with an opportunity to respond in various ways. The desired response is then reinforced or rewarded. After several reinforcements, the stimulus serves as a signal for the subject to perform the learned response.

Working at almost the same time as Pavlov, Johannes Schultz, in Germany, developed a mind-body training system called autogenic training. In Schultz's system, the patient directed himself, repeating a series of phrases to help him relax. This technique came into the realm of self-regulation, as the role of the physician was purely as a teacher. These procedures are remarkably like yoga, where the disciple chants a series of mantras to help him achieve inner discipline. And in yoga, too, the master is simply a teacher, showing the disciple the way, but never intruding.

The idea of using a combination of biofeedback and autogenic training to alleviate the problems of migraine headache patients was first suggested by Dr. Elmer Green of the Menninger Foundation. A volunteer in a training program to learn control of brainwaves and to reduce electromyographic (EMG) potential in the forearm muscle structure and increase blood flow in the hand was fortuitously discovered to be able to abort a migraine headache by raising the temperature of her hand. Further tests

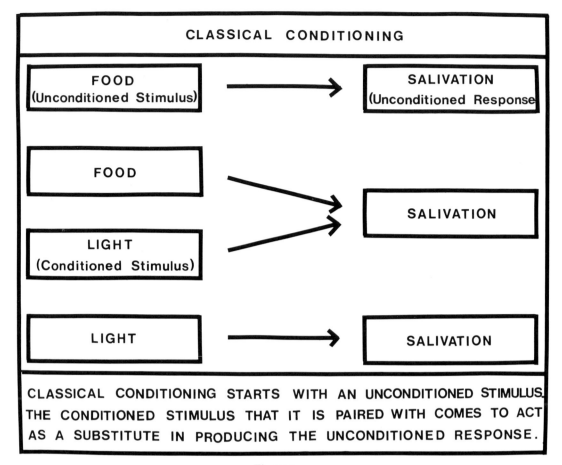

Fig 13-1.

led to the development by Sargent, Green and Walters of the so-called "hot-hand theory" for treatment of migraine headaches.

Work by Green and his staff had shown that local peripheral temperature is directly related to the blood flow in that area, as measured by a photoplethysmograph. In the case cited above, it was noted that the increase of blood flow to the hand was accompanied by a spontaneous remission of the migraine headache. This provided the initial stimulus for further research in the area.

As an aid in training patients to raise the temperature in their hand, Sargent used the autogenic training phrases of Johannes Schultz (Fig 13-3). The idea stemmed from previous reports by Schultz which had shown that, in some cases, subjects were able to alleviate migraine attacks while per-forming the autogenic training exercises. The combination of biofeedback training and autogenic training has proven to be quite useful in our own clinical work.

At approximately the same time a similar breakthrough was made for muscle contraction headaches. Thomas Budzynski, Johann Stoyva and Charles Adler, working at the University of Colorado Medical Center, described a technique for producing deep muscle relaxation by means of an informational feedback system in which the subject hears a tone with a frequency proportional to the electromyographic level of the muscle being monitored. With this biofeedback training and relaxation method, patients with muscle contraction headaches not only learned to produce low frontalis muscle EMG levels, but also showed substantial reduction of headache frequency.

This combination of techniques known as autogenic-biofeedback training, solicits the patient's direct involvement in his own treatment and, therefore, delegates much of the responsibility for the control of headaches to the patient himself. This is a breakaway from the traditional doctor-patient relationship in which the physician has total control of the therapy. It is a return to a holistic form of medicine in which the patient plays an integral role in his own treatment. Through biofeedback training the patient first develops a new internal awareness to the manner in which he responds subjectively to situational or external stimuli. This expanded awareness includes a concrete sense of physiologic responses to such stimuli. It is, thus, our goal, using biofeedback training, to help patients reach this individual realization and to apply it to the next stage of the learning process, that is, acquisition of voluntary control over physiologic functions which have demonstrable effects upon headache problems.

Autogenic-Biofeedback Training

In this section the techniques employed in the different forms of biofeedback training will be reviewed. The conventions which will be discussed here have emerged from our extensive experience with a great many headache patients. They are basically designed to teach the patient to develop new voluntary physiologic control skills which have proven to be effective in reducing both the severity and the frequency of headaches. It must be emphasized that the proper training in these techniques is essential if the full potential benefits of biofeedback therapy are to be realized.

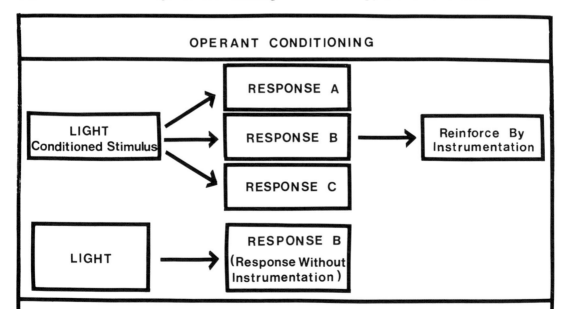

Fig 13-2.

TEMPERATURE TRAINING PHRASES

I FEEL QUITE QUIET....I AM BEGINNING TO FEEL QUITE RELAXED....

MY FEET FEEL HEAVY AND RELAXED....MY ANKLES, MY KNEES,

AND MY HIPS, FEEL HEAVY, RELAXED, AND COMFORTABLE....

MY SOLAR PLEXUS, AND THE WHOLE CENTRAL PORTION OF MY

BODY, FEEL RELAXED AND QUIET....MY HANDS, MY ARMS, AND

MY SHOULDERS, FEEL HEAVY, RELAXED, AND COMFORTABLE....

MY NECK, MY JAWS, AND MY FOREHEAD FEEL RELAXED....THEY

FEEL COMFORTABLE AND SMOOTH....MY WHOLE BODY FEELS

QUIET, HEAVY, COMFORTABLE AND RELAXED.

I AM QUITE RELAXED....MY ARMS AND HANDS ARE HEAVY AND

WARM....I FEEL QUITE QUIET....MY WHOLE BODY IS RELAXED

AND MY HANDS ARE WARM, RELAXED AND WARM....MY HANDS

ARE WARM....WARMTH IS FLOWING INTO MY HANDS, THEY ARE

WARM....WARM.

Fig 13-3.

In order to ensure an appropriate response from the patient, it is necessary to use the correct choice of biofeedback modality. In the treatment of patients with vascular headaches there are two methods of choice. In cases where the patient exhibits the "classical" migraine symptoms, we have found that temperature training is the preferred method. These people first get a warning preheadache and can, therefore, best utilize the vascular control skills learned through temperature training, at the first warning signs. This will frequently abort or at least diminish the severity of the subsequent attack. However, since stress can provoke migraine, we have found that patients do better when they receive EMG feedback in addition to temperature feedback.

On the other hand, patients who exhibit nonclassical migraines or a mixed diagnosis of vascular and muscle contraction headache, are best treated with a combination of temperature training and EMG feedback training. In those patients with exclusively muscle contraction headache, EMG training is the preferred choice of treatment. Since many migraine headaches appear to have a psychogenic component and vice versa, most patients receive both the temperature and EMG feedback training.

Temperature Training

The general procedures employed in temperature control training focus on the patient's capacity to increase finger and hand temperature (Fig 13-4). The training period generally consists of 4 to 5 weeks of intensive biofeedback training with follow-up biofeedback practice at gradually decreasing intervals as well as regular practice without biofeedback. Local patients are seen twice weekly for biofeedback treatments in the first month. If the patient is from out of town, twice daily sessions for the first 2 weeks are arranged.

During office visits, the patient sits in a quiet, dimly lighted room in a reclining chair. The decor of the room is comfortable and relaxing, quite different from the traditional office setting. External distractions are kept to a minimum. This has proven to be important particularly at early stages of the learning process where patient relaxation and concentration are both essential.

The initial training consists of three elements: (1) A temperature biofeedback signal supplied by the monitor; (2) Patient exercises, which are first done while receiving biofeedback, and (3) Careful record-keeping to identify problem areas and chart progress. At the start of each session the patient's hand temperature is determined and recorded. At the conclusion of the session, similar data are noted with special attention to any change, as well as the patient's subjective assessment of mood change and relaxation achieved during the session.

As the training period progresses the patient is slowly weaned from the biofeedback monitor. This is accomplished by alteration of his home exercise sequence. The patient is instructed to practice twice daily with the temperature trainer and twice a day without it. This is essential, since the ultimate goal of the training program is to develop new patient control skills which do not depend upon biofeedback machines.

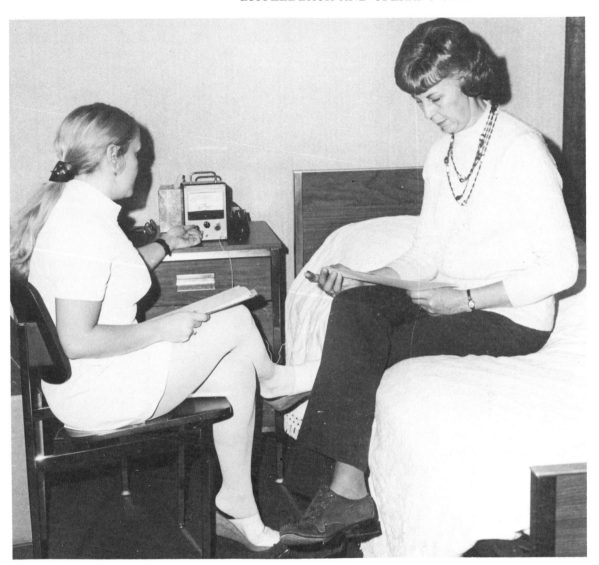

Fig 13-4. *Autogenic trainer teaches patient to raise temperature in the hands.*

Thus, biofeedback is only a temporary facilitating mechanism, a therapeutic tool, which, when the task is completed, should be laid aside. This concept should be made clear to the patient.

After the training period is concluded, follow-up visits are indicated. These will generally decrease as most patients require only a few reinforcement sessions. Out-of-town patients are generally seen monthly for 3 to 6 months. If, for whatever reason, the patient's condition regresses, an increase of follow-up visits and additional

months of home use biofeedback trainers may be considered necessary.

As previously mentioned, autogenic training is used in addition to the biofeedback. An inventory of autogenic phrases adopted from the work of Johannes Schultz is given to the patient (Fig 13-3). The phrases are autosuggestive in nature, focusing on feelings of warmth and relaxation. In addition to these phrases the patients are advised to focus on warm images. (The word "focus" is stressed rather than "concentrate" as the patient may work too hard at the exercises.) They may imagine putting their hands in a hot tub of water, sitting on a hot beach or by a fire. They are also told to focus on a relaxing image, like being on a rubber mattress in a pool with the sunlight streaming down on their hands. We have also found that it is very helpful to listen to a tape of the autogenic phrases while on the monitor. Success at training has been particularly demonstrated when the patient listens to his own voice reading the phrases since they sometimes tend to resist training when listening to a tape in the clinician's voice.

Home Practice. As mentioned, the techniques just described are sufficiently learned only with diligent home practice by the patient. All patients are given detailed instructions to accomplish this. A temperature biofeedback monitor is provided on a rental basis for at least the first 4 weeks of therapy, as an integral part of the home training program. In addition to the monitor, the patient is also provided with either a list or a tape of autogenic phrases to be used in conjunction with the biofeedback as is done in the Clinic.

Patients are instructed to use their home trainer twice daily, for 10 to 15 minutes in each session. They are also encouraged to employ it with their emerging control skills whenever preheadache warnings occur, or at the time of headache onset. The importance of twice daily practice must be stressed at this point. The patient is told repeatedly, that in this way he builds the very self-control skills which decrease the chance of his experiencing a headache. Since many patients experience early awakening due to headaches, or wake up in the morning with a headache already present, they are also instructed to practice immediately before bedtime.

Each patient with a temperature feedback monitor at home is encouraged to keep a daily diary and record what occurs during all practice sessions. The patient should first record the degree of warmth, pretraining session. If he is aware of his hands being quite warm before he starts to

practice, he should not be discouraged by a small increase in temperature during the session, as he began in a state of substantial vasodilation. At the end of each session, patients should record their degree of relaxation as well as possible change of mood during the session. If patients concentrate too hard they may experience post session tension. This should all be recorded, as well as the exact amount of change in the hand temperature during the session, in degrees.

After the first week of training the patients should begin to record the speed at which they achieve warmth. This is important as the patient may need only a 2- or 3-degree change in temperature to successfully abort a migraine. If this can be accomplished in 1 or 2 minutes, the patient may be able to use his new skill effectively at the first signs of a headache. The patient should try to elevate his hand temperature 1 degree in 1 minute. When this goal is achieved it should be increased to 1½ degrees and increased thereafter, assuming, of course, that the first goal has been achieved.

EMG Feedback Training

Following each in-clinic temperature training session, an electromyographic session is administered (Fig 13-5). The EMG trainer is used exclusively in the office. Patients make two or three Clinic visits per week during the first month, with the visits gradually decreasing from then on. Out-of-town patients receive more intensive training and are seen twice daily for 2 weeks. To record the patient's progress, a daily chart is kept (Fig 13-6) noting frequency, severity and duration of headaches.

The sessions generally last 20 minutes and are conducted in a dark, quiet room, immediately following the temperature session. The patient remains in a reclining position and is told that we are monitoring frontalis muscle activity, and that if facial, shoulder and/or neck muscles are tense, a high pitched tone is produced. It is suggested that he focus on relaxation of the entire body while receiving biofeedback. As

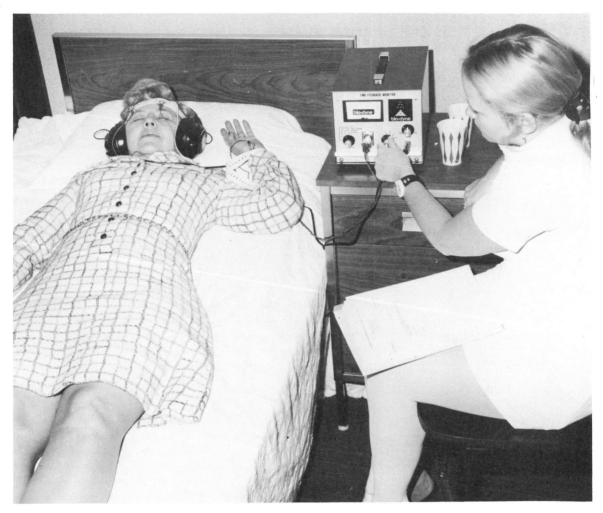

Fig 13-5. *Patient learns to relax by means of electromyographic biofeedback.*

relaxation is achieved, the pitch of the tone will decrease. The patient is advised to experiment with positions, moving around in the chair until maximum relaxation is achieved.

Electrodes are placed on each temple and a set of stereo headphones is used to minimize external distractions. The EMG monitor is equipped with variable sensitivities so that, as the patient reduces tension at one level, the monitor can be reset to the next higher sensitivity. With each level, decreasing the tone becomes more challenging.

As with temperature training, instructions are used to assist the patient in discovering how to relax the frontalis muscles

and the other target muscles just described. The patient must learn to identify certain tensor points in his facial, neck and shoulder areas, while using the biofeedback monitor. In order to aid the patient in this task, certain progressive relaxation exercises adapted from the work of Joseph Wolpe are given to the patient (Fig 13-7). These exercises should be practiced at home twice daily, without biofeedback instrumentation. If the patient is also using the temperature trainer, then the EMG exercises should be done second. There is a tendency for the hands to become warmer during progressive relaxation exercises, thereby diminishing the effect of the hand-warming procedures. As with temperature control,

HEADACHE CALENDAR

PATIENT'S NAME: _____

DATE STARTED: _____

DATE	TIME	SEVERITY OF HEADACHE	MEDICATION FOR PAIN	DOSE	RELIEF

1. Record all headaches:
    SEVERE   -- Incapacitating, unable to carry on with every day duties
    MODERATE -- Annoying but not incapacitating
    MILD   -- Able to carry on with normal duties
    NONE   -- Free from headache

2. Record any medication taken for headache and the amount taken

3. Record relief from headache pain:
    COMPLETE   -- Free from pain
    ALMOST COMPLETE - Pain present but not disturbing patient
    MODERATE   -- Has discomfort but not as severe as prior to taking medication
    SLIGHT   -- Minimal improvement of questionable significance
    NONE   -- No relief

4. Time: A.M., P.M., OR NITE

Fig 13-6.

E M G   FEEDBACK EXERCISE

RELAXATION OF FACIAL AREA WITH NECK, SHOULDERS AND UPPER BACK

TIME: 4 – 5 MINUTES

LET ALL YOUR MUSCLES GO LOOSE AND HEAVY. JUST SETTLE BACK
QUIETLY AND COMFORTABLE. WRINKLE UP YOUR FOREHEAD NOW;
WRINKLE AND SMOOTH IT OUT. PICTURE THE ENTIRE FOREHEAD AND
SCALP BECOMING SMOOTHER AS THE RELAXATION INCREASES....NOW
FROWN AND CREASE YOUR BROWS AND STUDY THE TENSION....LET
GO OF THE TENSION AGAIN. SMOOTH OUT THE FOREHEAD ONCE MORE....
NOW, CLOSE YOUR EYES TIGHTER AND TIGHTER. FEEL THE TENSION....
AND RELAX YOUR EYES. KEEP YOUR EYES CLOSED, GENTLY, COMFORTABLY,
AND NOTICE THE RELAXATION....NOW CLENCH YOUR JAWS, BITE YOUR
TEETH TOGETHER; STUDY THE TENSION THROUGHOUT THE JAWS....
RELAX YOUR JAWS NOW. LET YOUR LIPS PART SLIGHTLY....APPRECIATE
THE RELAXATION....NOW PRESS YOUR TONGUE HARD AGAINST THE ROOF
OF YOUR MOUTH. LOOK FOR THE TENSION....ALL RIGHT, LET YOUR
TONGUE RETURN TO A COMFORTABLE AND RELAXED POSITION....NOW
PURSE YOUR LIPS, PRESS YOUR LIPS TOGETHER TIGHTER AND TIGHTER....
RELAX THE LIPS. NOTE THE CONTRAST BETWEEN TENSION AND RELAXATION.
FEEL THE RELAXATION ALL OVER YOUR FACE, ALL OVER YOUR FOREHEAD
AND SCALP, EYES, JAWS, LIPS,TONGUE, AND YOUR NECK MUSCLES. PRESS
YOUR HEAD BACK AS FAR AS IT CAN GO AND FEEL THE TENSION IN THE
NECK; ROLL IT TO THE RIGHT AND FEEL THE TENSION SHIFT; NOW ROLL
IT TO THE LEFT. STRAIGHTEN YOUR HEAD AND BRING IT FORWARD AND
PRESS YOUR CHIN AGAINST YOUR CHEST. LET YOUR HEAD RETURN TO A
COMFORTABLE POSITION, AND STUDY THE RELAXATION. LET THE
RELAXATION DEVELOP....SHRUG YOUR SHOULDERS RIGHT UP. HOLD THE
TENSION....DROP YOUR SHOULDERS AND FEEL THE RELAXATION. NECK
AND SHOULDERS RELAXED....SHRUG YOUR SHOULDERS AGAIN AND MOVE
THEM AROUND. BRING YOUR SHOULDERS UP AND FORWARD AND BACK.
FEEL THE TENSION IN YOUR SHOULDERS AND IN YOUR UPPER BACK....
DROP YOUR SHOULDERS ONCE MORE AND RELAX. LET THE RELAXATION
SPREAD DEEP INTO THE SHOULDERS, RIGHT INTO YOUR BACK MUSCLES;
RELAX YOUR NECK AND THROAT, AND YOUR JAWS AND OTHER FACIAL
AREAS AS THE PURE RELAXATION TAKES OVER AND GROWS DEEPER....
DEEPER....EVER DEEPER.

Fig 13-7.

many patients have noted a decrease in the
severity of their headaches when they practice the progressive relaxation exercises at
the first symptoms of a headache.

Home use of these exercises and clinical
sessions on the EMG monitor assist the
patient in recognizing stress points. Common stress points often identified by patients include: teeth grinding, jaw clench-
ing, tightening of the forehead, wrinkling
of the brow, obvious tension in the neck
and tightening of the shoulders. By learning

to relax these points under times of stress, the first symptoms of headaches, and at bedtime, patients have noticed a reduction in the severity of their headaches. Patients who are diligent in practicing the temperature and EMG exercises will usually experience a decrease in the frequency of their headaches as well. A common occurrence is the patient who experiences a decrease in the frequency of migraine headaches and an increase in the milder muscle contraction headache. What seems to be happening, in reality, is that the more severe migraine has masked the muscle contraction headache, and when this disappears, the milder form draws more attention. These too will eventually disappear with continued practice of the temperature and EMG exercises.

The Therapist

In the biofeedback training program the role of the therapist, or the technician, is a focal one and it must be emphasized. On the first visit the therapist explains the goals of biofeedback training. Current articles about biofeedback are also furnished for the patient to read. A clear understanding of biofeedback is very important for establishing the correct cognitive orientation of the patient. The therapist also instructs the patient in the use of the temperature or the EMG trainer. At this visit, a one-to-one relationship is established between therapist and patient.

On follow-up visits, the therapist should report any problems to the physician. This is important to keep in close touch with the patient's progress. The therapist also plays a key role by encouraging the patient, emphasizing and praising all progress and helping to stimulate motivation. This is a key part in any effective therapy program.

Goals are not generalized, with the training continued on an individual basis. External factors affecting training are identified. For example, patients may be told that warm hands before the session may result in a small increase on the temperature monitor. The patients are assisted in recognizing stress points, any patterns in headaches and in reviewing and redesigning biofeedback techniques. All those functions require careful diligent attention from the therapist. Obviously, the attitude of the therapist can affect the patient's success. A relaxed manner is necessary, along with confidence in the use of various instruments. Flexibility in the various techniques will help in each patient's therapy. Firmness is also required with the patients in stressing home practice and in maintaining high motivational levels.

Outcome Audit of Biofeedback

The results of a survey of patients treated at the Diamond Headache Clinic are reported below. A questionnaire was mailed to the 556 patients instructed in both electromyographic and temperature feedback over the past 5 years asking their opinion about the effectiveness of the therapy. Of these patients, 413 answered the questionnaire. Their ages ranged between 9 and 71 with an average age of 36 years. The distribution of types of headache was: 115 patients had migraine, 15 muscle contraction headache and 283 mixed muscle contraction and migraine headache. They terminated their training period between 3 and 62 months ago. Of 413 patients, 120 (29%) thought that biofeedback did not help their headaches, 133 (32%) noted transitory improvement, and 160 (39%) permanent relief. The patients with transitory improvement did benefit from 1 to 36 months with an average of 9.5 months. The patients permanently improved have done well from 4 to 52 months with an average of 25 months. Seventy-one percent of the patients believed that the technique was helpful for headaches.

Operant Conditioning

Further support for the effectiveness of autogenic-biofeedback training comes indirectly from the recent work of Wilbert Fordyce concerning chronic pain. Fordyce has shown that there are two sets of factors influencing chronic pain: (a) the organic factors and (b) the learning or conditioning factors. The former considers the traditional Disease Model perspectives whereas the latter is much more complex and in many ways more difficult to recognize and to treat. These learning factors can promote and maintain a pain habit. Pain of this nature is referred to as operant pain.

The basic idea here is that, if the environmental consequences which occur either before, during or after the onset of pain are consistent enough to constitute a pattern, then the occurrence of those consequences may be sufficient to bring about pain even after the organic factors have been eliminated.

Probably the most significant learning factor is the way people who are important to the patient react to his behavior while he is experiencing pain. If excessive family attention or extra physician concern are shown toward him when he hurts, then these elements of their behavior become contingent on his being in pain. For example, a spouse may be extra-loving, or the physician may give the patient extra time and attention, and prescribe rest and medication. These reactions become the environmental consequences of his being in pain. They happen when he hurts and do not happen when he is well. This systematic set of environmental consequences to pain behavior may prove sufficient to maintain pain (or, as in our case, headaches) even after the original organic factor is gone.

Almost all chronic headache patients will display some degree of operant or learned pain. Since learned pain exists because of the automatic effects of learning, it can be reduced only by following a systematic learning or "unlearning" process. We attempt to explain to the patient and his family about learned or operant pain. This is done by carrying out the followg objectives: (a) We reduce pain behavior by withdrawing any positive reinforcement form of behavior; (b) We give positive reinforcement for increased activity and when the patient is feeling well; (c) We attempt to retrain the family unit to reinforce well behavior and to avoid reinforcement of pain behavior; and (d) if the patient has a pain or headache syndrome which has a basis for treatment, the organic or treatable factors should be corrected so that the operant behavior therapy can also be effective.

SELF-ASSESSMENT EXAMINATION

1 Temperature training is used for muscle contraction headache. True or False

2 Pavlovian conditioning, or classical conditioning, is the theory behind biofeedback. True or False

3 Johannes Schultz developed the system of autogenic phrases used with temperature biofeedback treatment. True or False

4 Anyone can learn how to use biofeedback. True or False

5 Operant conditioning is the theoretical basis for the effectiveness of biofeedback. True or False

6 The frontalis muscle is used to measure electromyographic feedback in muscle contraction headache. True or False

7 Pain is a learned behavior. True or False

8 The machines used in biofeedback teach one how to control his body without practice. True or False

9 Autogenic phrases are used in electromyographic feedback. True or False

10 The family of a patient with chronic headaches should sympathize with his illness. True or False

11 Biofeedback teaches a person to control his own body mechanisms. True or False

ANSWERS:

1—False; 2—False; 3—True; 4—False; 5—True; 6—True; 7—True; 8—False; 9—False; 10—False; 11—True

SELECTED REFERENCES

Adams F: Extant Works of Aretaeus the Cappadocian. London, The Sydenham Society, 1856

Ad Hoc Committee: Classification of headache. JAMA 6:717, 1962

Alestig K, Barr J: Giant-cell arteritis. Lancet 1:1228, 1963

Anthony M, Lance JW: Histamine and serotonin in cluster headache. Arch Neurol 25:225, 1971

Anthony M, Hinterberger H, Lance JW: Plasma serotonin in migraine and stress. Arch Neurol 16:544, 1967

Aurelianus C: Liber 1. De Capitis Passione, quam Graeci Cephalaean Nominant: Medici Antiqui Omnes Qui Latinis, etc., Venetiis. 4:249, 1547

Background to Migraine: Proceedings. 1st Symposium on Migraine. London, 1966. R Smith, ed. New York, Springer-Verlag, 1967

Background to Migraine: Proceedings. 2nd Symposium on Migraine. London, 1967. R Smith, ed. New York, Springer-Verlag, 1969

Background to Migraine: Proceedings. 3rd Symposium on Migraine. London, 1969. AL Cochrane, ed. New York, Springer-Verlag, 1970

Bickerstaff ER: Basilar artery migraine. Lancet 1:15, 1961

Blom S: Tic douloureux treated with a new anticonvulsant. Arch Neurol 9:285, 1963

Bradshaw P, Parsons M: Hemiplegic migraine: A clinical study. Q J Med 34:65, 1965

Brodie BB, Shore PA: A concept for the role of serotonin and norepinephrine as chemical mediators in the brain. Ann NY Acad Sci 66:631, 1957

Budzynski T, Stoyva J, Adler C: Feedback-induced muscle relaxation: Application to tension headache. Behav Ther Exp Psych 1:205, 1970

Carliner NH, Denune DL, Finch CS, Goldberg LI: Sodium nitroprusside treatment of ergotamine-induced peripheral ischemia. JAMA 227:308, 1974

Catino D: Ten migraine equivalents. Headache 5:1, 1965

Chapman LF, Ramos AO, Goodell H, et al: Neurokinin; a polypetide formed during neuronal activity in man. Trans Am Neurol Assoc 85:42, 1960

Cochrane CG: Initiating Events in Immune Complex Injury. Progress in Immunology. New York, Academic Press, Inc, 1971, pp 146–153

Connor RCR: Complicated migraine: A study of permanent neurological and visual defects caused by migraine. Lancet 2:1072, 1962

Curzon G, Theaker P, Phillips BJ: Excretion of 5-hydroxyindole acetic acid in migraine. J Neurol Neurosurg Psychiatry 29:85, 1966

Dalessio DJ: On migraine headache: Serotonin and serotonin antagonism. JAMA 181:318, 1962

Dalessio DJ: Wolff's Headache and Other Head Pain. Third edition. New York, Oxford University Press, Inc, 1972

Dalsgaard-Nielsen T, Genefke IK: Serotonin release and uptake in platelets from healthy persons and migraine patients in attack-free intervals. Headache 14:26, 1974

Diamond S, Baltes BJ: Management of headache by the family physician. Am Fam Physician 5:4, 68, 1972

Dukes HT, Vieth RG: Cerebral arteriography during migraine prodrome and headache. Neurology 14:636, 1964

Edmeads J: Cerebral blood flow in migraine. Headache, in press, 1977

Edmeads J, Hachinski VC, Norris JW: Ergotamine and the cerebral circulation. Hemicrania 7:6, 1976

Ekbom K: Studies on cluster headache. Sundbyberg, Sweden, Solna Tryckeri AB, 1970

Friedman AP, Harter H, Merritt HH: Ophthalmoplegic migraine. Trans Am Neurol Assoc 86:169, 1961

Fog M: Cerebral circulation. 1. Reaction of pial arteries to epinephrine by direct application and by intravenous injection. Arch Neurol Psychiatry 41:109, 1939

Galen: De Compositione Medicamentorum Secundum Locos. In: Opera Omnia. Ed. Kuhn. Lipsiae: C. Cnoblochii. Vol 12, book 2, Cap. III (De hemicrania), p 591, 1826

Fordyce WE: Recent Advances on Pain: Pathophysiology and Clincal Aspects. JJ Bonica, P Procacci, CA Pagni, eds. Springfield, Ill., Charles C Thomas, 1974, pp. 299–312

Gascon G, Barlow C: Juvenile migraine presenting as an acute confusional state. Pediatrics 45:628, 1970

Glista GG, Mellinger JF, Rooke ED: Familial hemiplegic migraine. Mayo Clinic Proc 50:307, 1975

Glover V, Sandler M, Grant E, Rose FC, Orton D, Wilkinson M, Stevens D: Transitory decrease in platelet monoamine oxidase activity during migraine attacks. Lancet, in press

Goodell H, Lewontin R, Wolff HG: The familial occurrence of migraine headache: A study of heredity. Arch Neurol Psychiatry 39:737, 1938

Graham JR: Cluster headache. Headache 11:175, 1972

Graham JR: Seven common headache profiles. Neurology 13:16, 1963

Graham JR, Wolff HG: Mechanism of migraine headache and action of ergotamine tartrate. Arch Neurol Psychiatry 39:737, 1938

Greenblatt SH: Posttraumatic transient cerebral blindness. JAMA 225:1073, 1973

Haas DC, Pineda GS, Lourie H: Juvenile head trauma syndromes and their relationship to migraine. Arch Neurol 32:727, 1975

Haas DC, Sovner RD: Migraine attacks triggered by mild head trauma, and their relation to certain posttraumatic disorders of childhood. J Neurol Neurosurg Psychiatry 32:548, 1969

Hachinski VC, Norris JW, Cooper PW, Edmeads JG: Ergotamine tartrate and cerebral blood flow. Canad J Neurol Sci 2:333, 1975

Hanington E: Preliminary report on tyramine headache. Brit Med J 2:550, 1967

Headache Update, Organon Labs, No's 1, 2, 3, 4, 1976, 77

Hilton BP, Cumings JN: 5-Hydroxytryptamine levels

and platelet aggregation responses in subjects with acute migraine. J Neurol Neurosurg Psychiat 35:505, 1972

Hilton BP, Cumings JM: An assessment of platelet aggregation induced by 5-hydroxytryptamine. J Clin Pathol 24:250, 1971

Horton BT: Histaminic cephalgia: Differential diagnosis and treatment. Mayo Clin Proc 31:325, 1956

Hungerford GD, deBonlay GH, Zilkha KJ: Computerized axial tomography in patients with severe migraine. J Neurol Neurosurg Psychiat 39:990, 1976

Ingvar DH: Pain in the brain—and migraine. Hemicrania 7:2, 1976

Kalendovsky Z, Austin JH: "Complicated migraine." Its association with increased platelet aggregability and abnormal coagulation factors. Headache 15:18, 1975

Kerr FWL: The etiology of trigeminal neuralgia. Arch Neurol 8:15, 1963

Koppman, JW, McDonald RD, Kunzel MG: Voluntary regulation of temporal artery diameter by migraine patients. Headache 14(3):133, 1974

Kugelberg E, Lindblom U: The mechanism of pain in trigeminal neuralgia. J Neurol Neurosurg Psychiatry 22:36, 1959

Lance JW: The mechanism and Management of Headache. London, Butterworth & Co (Publishers) Ltd, 1969

Lance JW, Anthony M, Gonski A: Serotonin, the carotid body, and cranial vessels in migraine. Arch Neurol 16:553, 1967

Lance JW, Curran DA: Treatment of chronic tension headache. Lancet 1:1236, 1964

Lance JW: Migraine. in The Mechanism and Management of Headache, ed 2. London, Butterworth & Co, 1973

Lassen NA, Ingvar DH: The blood flow of the cerebral cortex determined by Krypton 85. Experientia 17:42, 1961

Lepois C: Selectiorum Observationum. Ludg. Batav.: C Boutestein and JA Langerak. De Hemicrania, pp 67–77, 1714

Liveing E: On Megrim. Sick-headache and Some Allied Disorders. London, Churchill, 1873

Lord GDA, Duckworth JW: Immunoglobulin and complement studies in migraine. Headache, 17: 163, 1977

Lovshin LL: Treatment of histaminic cephalalgia with methysergide. Dis Nerv Syst 24:3, 1963

Mathew NT, Hrastnick F, Meyer JS: Regional cerebral blood flow in the diagnosis of vascular headache. Headache 15:252, 1976

Matthews WB: Footballer's migraine. Br Med J 2:326–327, 1972

Medina JL, Diamond S: Migraine and atopy, Headache 16:271, 1976

Meyer JS, Yoshida K, Sakamoto K: Autonomic control of cerebral blood flow measured by electromagnetic flowmeters. Neurology 17:638, 1967

Miller NE: Learning of visceral and glandular responses. Science 163:434, 1969

Nelson E, Rennels M: Neuromuscular contact in intracranial arteries of the cat. Science 167:301, 1970

Nielsen KC, Owman C: Adrenergic innervation of pial arteries related to the circle of Willis in the cat. Brain Res 6:773, 1967

Nielsen KC, Owman C: Contractile response and amine receptor mechanisms in isolated middle cerebral artery of the cat. Brain Res 27:33, 1971

Norris JW, Hachinski VC, Cooper PW: Changes in cerebral blood flow during a migraine attack. Brit Med J 3:676, 1975

Norris JW, Hachinski VC, Cooper PW: Cerebral blood flow changes in cluster headache. Acta Neurol Scand 54:371, 1976

Olesen J: The effect of intracarotid epinephrine, norepinephrine, and angiotensin on the regional cerebral blood flow in man. Neurology 22:978, 1972

Onel Y, Friedman AP, Grossman J: Muscle blood flow studies in muscle-contraction headaches. Neurology 11:935, 1961

Ostfeld AM, Wolff HG: Studies on headache: Arterenol (norepinephrine) and vascular headache of the migraine type. Arch Neurol Psychiatry 74:131, 1955

Pearce J: Migraine, Clinical Features, Mechanisms, and Management. Springfield, Ill, Charles C Thomas, Publisher, 1969

Pickering GW: Experimental observations on headache. Br Med J 1:4087, 1939

Proceedings of the International Headache Symposium, Elsinore, Denmark, May 16–18, 1971; DJ Dalessio, T Dalsgaard-Nielsen, S Diamond. Basel, Switzerland, Sandoz Ltd

Ray BS, Wolff HG: Experimental studies on headache. Pain sensitive structures of the head and their significance in headache. Arch Surg 41:813, 1940

Robb LG: Severe vasospasm following ergot administration. West J Med 123:231, 1975

Rooke, ED: Benign exertional headache. in RE Siekert, ed. The Medical Clinics of North America. Philadelphia, WB Saunders Co, 1968, vol 52

Sacks OW: Migraine, the Evolution of a Common Disorder. Berkeley, University of California Press, 1970

Sandler M, Youdim MBH, Hanington E: A phenylethylamine oxidising defect in migraine. Nature, Lond 250:335, 1974

Sandler M, Youdim, MBH, Southgate J, Hanington, E: The role of tyramine in migraine: some possible biochemical mechanisms in Background to Migraine, Third Migraine Symposium. AL Cochrane, ed. London, Heinemann, 1970, p. 103

Sargent JD, Green EE, Walters ED: The use of autogenic feedback training in a pilot study of migraine and tension headaches. Headache 12:120, 1972

Saxena PR: The effects of antimigraine drugs on the vascular responses evoked by 5-hydroxytryptamine and related biogenic substances on the external carotid bed of dogs: Possible pharmacological implications to their antimigraine action. Headache 12:44, 1972

Schildkraut JJ, Kety SS: Biogenic amines and emotion. Science 156:21, 1967

Schildkraut JJ, Schanberg SM, Breese GR, et al: Norepinephrine metabolism and drugs used in the affective disorders: A possible mechanism of action. Am J Psychiatry 124:56, 1967

Schiller F: The migraine tradition. Bull Hist Med 49:1, 1975

Schuckit M, Robins E, Feighner J: Tricyclic antidepressants and monoamine oxidase inhibitors. Arch Gen Psych 24:509, 1971

Segal J: Biofeedback as a medical treatment. JAMA 232:179, 1975

Sicuteri F: Vasoneuractive substances in migraine. Headaches 6:109, 1966

Sicuteri FA, Testi A, Anselmi B: Biochemical investigations in headache. Int Arch Allergy Appl Immunol 19:55, 1961

Sicuteri F: Mast cells and their active substances; their role in the pathogenesis of migraine. Headache 3:86, 1963

Sicuteri F, Buffoni F, Anselmi B, Bel Bianco PL: An enzyme (MAO) defect on the platelets in migraine. Res Clin Stud Headache 3:245, 1972

Simard D, Paulson OB: Cerebral vasomotor paralysis during migraine attack. Arch Neurol 29:207, 1973

Sjaastad O: Introduction: Chronic Paroxysmal Hemicrania. Proceedings The Bergen Migraine Symposium, Joint Meeting American Association for the Study of Headache and Scandinavian Migraine Society, Bergen Norway June 4-6, 1975

Skinhoj E: Hemodynamic studies within the brain during migraine. Arch Neurol 29:95, 1973

Skinhoj E, Paulson OB: Regional blood flow in internal carotid distribution during migraine attack. Brit Med J 3:569, 1969

Smith GM, Lowenstein, E, Hubbard, JH, Beecher HK: Experimental pain produced by the submaximum effort tourniquet technique: further evidence of validity. J Pharmacol Exp Ther 163:468, 1967

Smith I, Kellow AH, Hanington E: A clinical and biochemical correlation between tyramine and migraine headache. Headache 10:43, 1970

Sovak M, Fronek A, Helland DR, Doyle R: Effects of vasomotor changes in the upper extremities on the hemodynamics of the carotid arterial beds: a possible mechanism of biofeedback therapy of migraine. Proceedings of the San Diego Biomedical Meeting, vol. 15 Academic Press, New York, 1976, p. 363

Sternbach RA, Murphy RW, Timmermans G, Greenhoot JH, Akeson WH: Measuring the severity of clinical pain. In: J J Bonica Ed., Advances in Neurology, Vol. 4, International Symposium on Pain, New York, Raven Press, 1974, pp. 281–288

Sternbach, RA: Pain Patients: Traits and Treatment, New York, Academic Press, 1974

Sternbach R, Deems LM, Timmermans G, Huey L: On the sensitivity of the tourniquet pain test. Pain 3:105, 1977

Symonds CP: Cough headache. Brain 79:557, 1956

Timmermans G, Sternbach RA: Factors of human chronic pain: an analysis of personality and pain reaction variables, Science 184:806, 1974

Tissot SAD: Traité des nerfs et de leurs maladies. Lausanne, Paris, 1873

Walker AE: Chronic post-traumatic headache. Headache 5:67, 1965

Vijayan N: A new post-traumatic headache syndrome: Clinical and therapeutic observations. Headache 17:19, 1977

Welch KMA, Chabi E, Nell JH, et al: Biochemical comparison of migraine and stroke. Headache 16:160, 1976

Woolf AL, Quest IA: Fatal infarction of the brain in migraine. Br Med J 1:225, 1964

Zweifach BW: Microcirculatory aspects of tissue injury. Ann NY Acad Sci 116:831, 1964

Index

Teach Yourself VISUALLY™

Word 2013

29.99

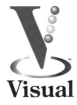

Visual™

Elaine Marmel

WILEY

John Wiley & Sons, Inc.

Teach Yourself VISUALLY™ Word 2013

Published by
John Wiley & Sons, Inc.
10475 Crosspoint Boulevard
Indianapolis, IN 46256

www.wiley.com

Published simultaneously in Canada

Wiley publishes in a variety of print and electronic formats and by print-on-demand. Some material included with standard print versions of this book may not be included in e-books or in print-on-demand. If this book refers to media such as a CD or DVD that is not included in the version you purchased, you may download this material at http://booksupport.wiley.com. For more information about Wiley products, visit www.wiley.com.

Library of Congress Control Number: 2013932108

ISBN: 978-1-118-51769-7

Manufactured in the United States of America

10 9 8 7 6 5 4 3 2

Trademark Acknowledgments

Contact Us

For general information on our other products and services please contact our Customer Care Department within the U.S. at 877-762-2974, outside the U.S. at 317-572-3993 or fax 317-572-4002.

For technical support please visit www.wiley.com/techsupport.

WILEY **Sales** | Contact Wiley at (877) 762-2974 or fax (317) 572-4002.

Credits

Executive Editor
Jody Lefevere

Sr. Project Editor
Sarah Hellert

Technical Editor
Donna Baker

Copy Editor
Gwenette Gaddis

Editorial Director
Robyn Siesky

Business Manager
Amy Knies

Sr. Marketing Manager
Sandy Smith

Vice President and Executive Group Publisher
Richard Swadley

Vice President and Executive Publisher
Barry Pruett

Project Coordinator
Patrick Redmond

Graphics and Production Specialists
Ana Carrillo
Carrie A. Cesavice
Joyce Haughey
Andrea Hornberger
Jennifer Mayberry

Quality Control Technician
Lauren Mandelbaum

Proofreader
Indianapolis Composition Services

Indexer
Potomac Indexing, LLC

About the Author

Elaine Marmel is President of Marmel Enterprises, LLC, an organization that specializes in technical writing and software training. Elaine has an MBA from Cornell University and worked on projects to build financial management systems for New York City and Washington, D.C. This prior experience provided the foundation for Marmel Enterprises, LLC to help small businesses manage the project of implementing a computerized accounting system.

Elaine spends most of her time writing; she has authored and co-authored more than 65 books about Microsoft Excel, Microsoft Word, Microsoft Project, QuickBooks, Peachtree, Quicken for Windows, Quicken for DOS, Microsoft Word for the Mac, Microsoft Windows, 1-2-3 for Windows, and Lotus Notes. From 1994 to 2006, she also was the contributing editor to monthly publications *Inside Peachtree*, *Inside Timeslips*, and *Inside QuickBooks*.

Elaine left her native Chicago for the warmer climes of Arizona (by way of Cincinnati, OH; Jerusalem, Israel; Ithaca, NY; Washington, D.C., and Tampa, FL) where she basks in the sun with her PC, her cross stitch projects, and her dog, Jack.

Author's Acknowledgments

Because a book is not just the work of the author, I'd like to acknowledge and thank all the folks who made this book possible. Thanks to Jody Lefevere for the opportunity to write this book. Thank you, Donna Baker, for doing a great job to make sure that I "told no lies." Thank you, Gwenette Gaddis, for making sure I was understandable and grammatically correct — you made me look very good. And, thank you, Sarah Hellert; your top-notch management of all the players and manuscript elements involved in this book made my life easy and writing the book a pleasure.

Dedication

To Buddy (1995-2012), my constant companion for 17 ½ years. You brought me nothing but joy and I will sorely miss you. And so will Jack.

How to Use This Book

Who This Book Is For

This book is for the reader who has never used this particular technology or software application. It is also for readers who want to expand their knowledge.

The Conventions in This Book

① Steps

This book uses a step-by-step format to guide you easily through each task. **Numbered steps** are actions you must do; **bulleted steps** clarify a point, step, or optional feature; and **indented steps** give you the result.

② Notes

Notes give additional information — special conditions that may occur during an operation, a situation that you want to avoid, or a cross-reference to a related area of the book.

③ Icons and Buttons

Icons and buttons show you exactly what you need to click to perform a step.

④ Tips

Tips offer additional information, including warnings and shortcuts.

⑤ Bold

Bold type shows command names or options that you must click or text or numbers you must type.

⑥ Italics

Italic type introduces and defines a new term.

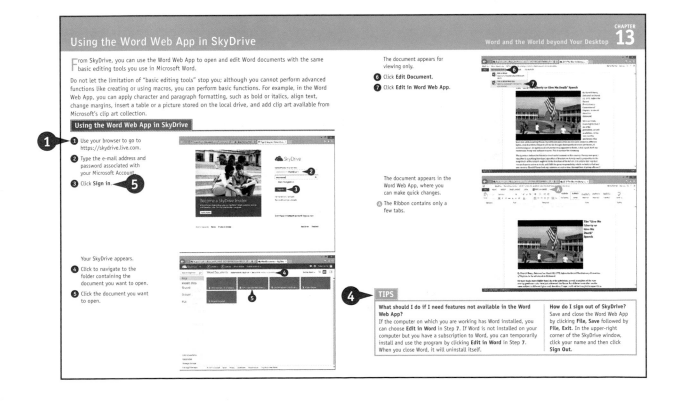

Table of Contents

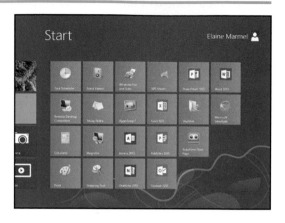

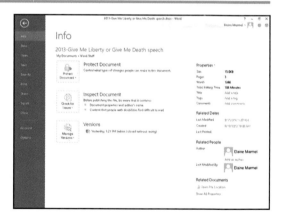

Chapter 3   Editing Text

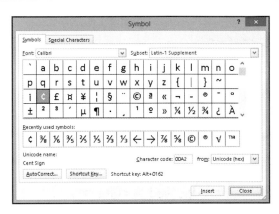

Table of Contents

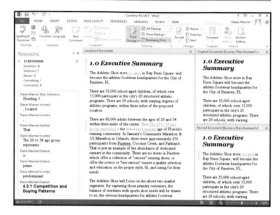

| Chapter 6 | Formatting Paragraphs |

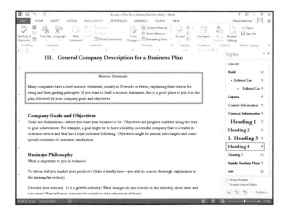

Table of Contents

Chapter 7   Formatting Pages

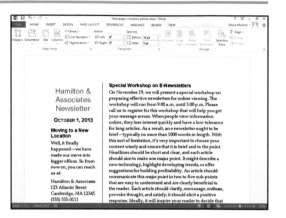

Chapter 8   Printing Documents

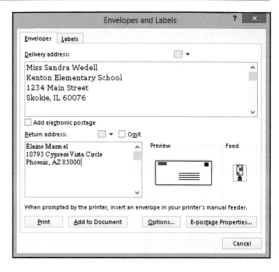

Chapter 9   Working with Tables and Charts

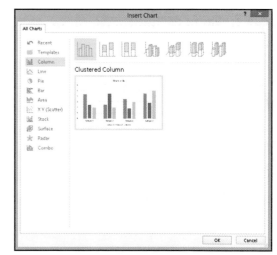

Table of Contents

Chapter 10   Working with Graphics

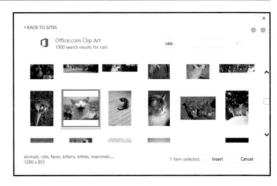

Chapter 11   Customizing Word

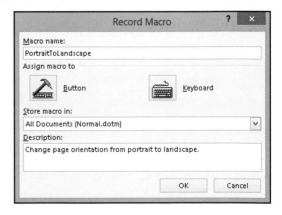

Chapter 12   Working with Mass Mailing Tools

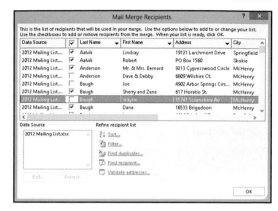

Chapter 13   Word and the World beyond Your Desktop

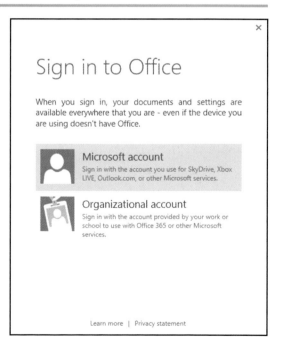

CHAPTER 1

Getting Familiar with Word

Are you ready to get started in Word? In this chapter, you become familiar with the Word working environment, including the Word Start screen and Backstage view, and you learn basic ways to navigate and to enter text using both the keyboard and the mouse. You also learn some basics for using Word on a tablet PC.

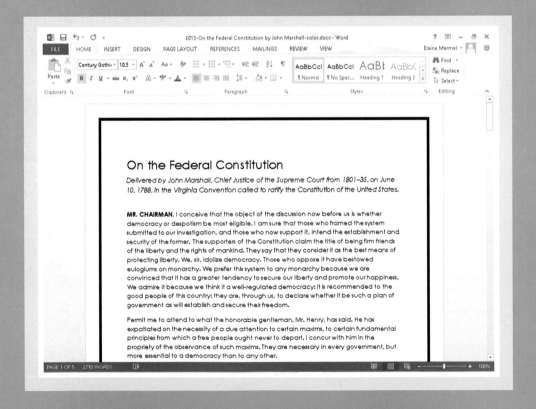

Open Word

Office 2013 runs on a 1 gigahertz (Ghz) or faster x86- or x64-bit processor with 1 or 2 gigabytes of RAM, based on your processor speed, and your system must be running Windows 7, Windows 8, Windows Server 2008 R2, or Windows Server 2012. For additional requirements, visit http://technet.microsoft.com/en-us/library/ee624351%28v=office.15%29.aspx.

This section demonstrates how to open Word from the Windows 8 Start screen. After Word opens, the Word Start screen appears, helping you to find a document on which you recently worked or starting a new document. For other ways to open or start a new document, see Chapter 2.

Open Word

1 On the Windows 8 Start screen, click ▬.

Note: You can start typing the name of the program and then skip to Step **3**.

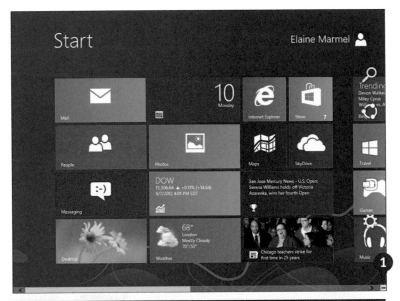

Windows zooms out so that you can see tiles for all installed programs.

2 Click any program tile on the right side of the Start screen.

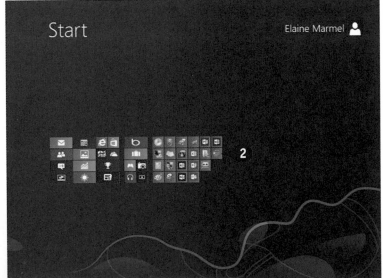

Windows zooms in and enlarges all tiles to their regular size.

③ Click the **Word 2013** tile.

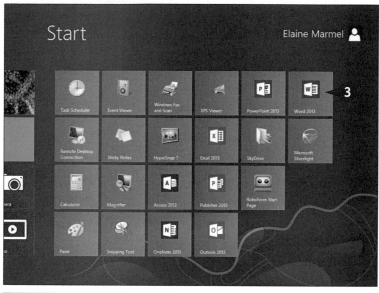

Windows switches to the Desktop and opens Word, displaying the Word Start screen, which helps you open new or existing documents; see Chapter 2 for other ways to open documents.

Ⓐ You can use this panel to open an existing document.

Ⓑ You can use this area to start a new document.

Ⓒ This area indicates whether you have signed in to Office Online.

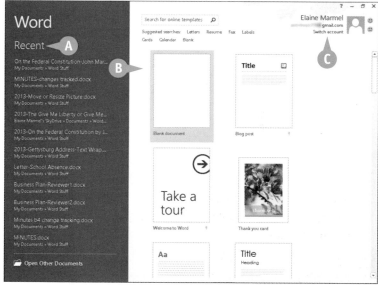

TIPS

How can I open Word if I use Windows 7?
Click the Windows **Start** button, and point at **All Programs**. When Windows 7 displays the All Programs menu, find Word 2013 and click it. In either Windows 7 or Windows 8, you can double-click a Word document to open Word 2013.

What does signing in to Office Online do?
Office Online connects Office 2013 applications to the cloud, providing you with a large set of features that enable you to work on your documents from anywhere. Chapter 13 describes working with Office Online in detail. You do not need to sign in to Office Online unless you need to use online tools such as searching for templates online.

Explore the Word Window

All Office programs share a common appearance and many features, and Word is no different. These features include a Ribbon and a Quick Access Toolbar (QAT). The Ribbon contains commands that Microsoft believes you use most often, and the QAT contains frequently used commands.

A Quick Access Toolbar (QAT)

Contains buttons that perform common actions: saving a document, undoing your last action, or repeating your last action.

B Ribbon

Contains buttons organized in tabs, groups, and commands. **Tabs** appear across the top of the Ribbon and contain groups of related commands. **Groups** organize related commands. **Commands** appear within each group.

C Dialog Box Launcher

Appears in the lower-right corner of many groups on the Ribbon. Clicking this button opens a dialog box or task pane that provides more options.

D Document Area

The area where you type. The flashing vertical bar, called the *insertion point*, represents the location where text will appear when you type.

E Status Bar

Displays document information as well as the insertion point location. This bar contains the number of the page on which the insertion point currently appears, the total number of pages and words in the document, the proofing errors button (⬚), the View buttons, and the Zoom slider.

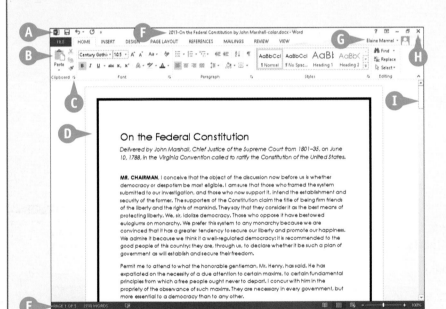

F Title Bar

Shows the program and document titles.

G Office Online Indicator

If you see your name, you are signed in to Office Online. You can click ▼ to display a menu that enables you to change your photo, manage your Microsoft account, or switch to a different Microsoft account. If you are not signed in, this area shows a Sign In link.

H Close Button

Closes the current document. Word closes if no documents are open.

I Scroll Bar

Enables you to reposition the document window vertically. Drag the scroll box within the scroll bar, or click the scroll bar arrows (▲ and ▼).

Work with Backstage View

You can click the **File** tab to display Backstage view, which resembles a menu. Backstage view is the place to go when you need to manage documents or change program behavior. In Backstage view, you find a list of actions — think of them as commands — that you can use to, for example, open, save, print, remove sensitive information, and distribute documents as well as set Word program behavior options. You also can manage the places on your computer hard drive or in your network that you use to store documents and you can manage your Office Online account from Backstage view.

Work with Backstage View

1 Click the **File** tab to display Backstage view.

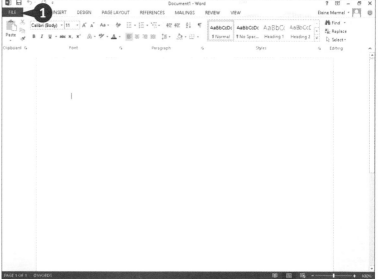

A Commonly used file and program management commands appear here.

B Buttons you can click appear here.

C Information related to the button you click appears here. Each time you click a button, the information shown to the right changes.

Note: The New, Close, and Options commands do not display buttons or information but take other actions. See Chapters 2 and 11 for details on these commands.

2 Click the **Back** button ( ) to return to the open document.

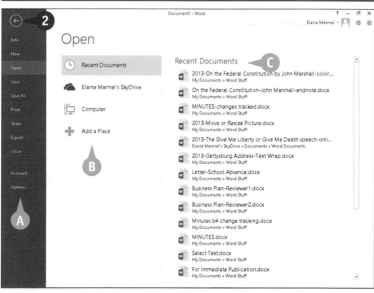

Select Commands

You can keep your hands on your keyboard and select commands from the Ribbon or the Quick Access Toolbar (QAT). Or you can use the mouse to navigate the Ribbon or select a command from the QAT at the top of the window. The method you choose is a matter of personal preference for the task you are performing.

On any particular Ribbon tab, you find groups of related commands. The QAT appears above the File and Home tabs and by default contains the Save, Undo, and Redo commands. To customize the Ribbon or the QAT, see Chapter 11.

Select Commands

Select Commands with the Keyboard

1 If appropriate for the command you intend to use, place the insertion point in the proper word or paragraph.

2 Press **Alt** on the keyboard.

A Shortcut letters and numbers appear on the Ribbon.

Note: The numbers control commands on the Quick Access Toolbar.

3 Press a letter to select a tab on the Ribbon.

This example uses **P**.

Word displays the appropriate tab and letters for each command on that tab.

4 Press a letter or letters to select a command.

If appropriate, Word displays options for the command you selected. Press a letter or use the arrow keys on the keyboard to select an option.

Word performs the command you selected, applying the option you chose.

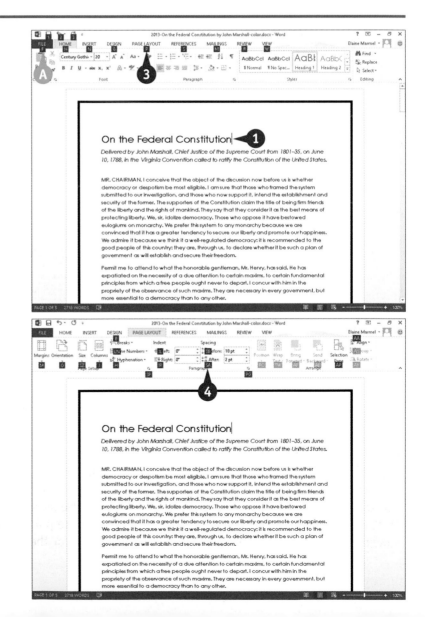

Select Commands with the Mouse

1 Click in the text or paragraph you want to modify.

Note: If appropriate, select the text; see Chapter 3 for details.

2 Click the tab containing the command you want to use.

3 Point to the command you want to use.

B Word displays a ScreenTip describing the function of the button at which the mouse points.

4 Click the command.

C Word performs the command you selected.

Note: If you selected text, click anywhere outside the text to continue working.

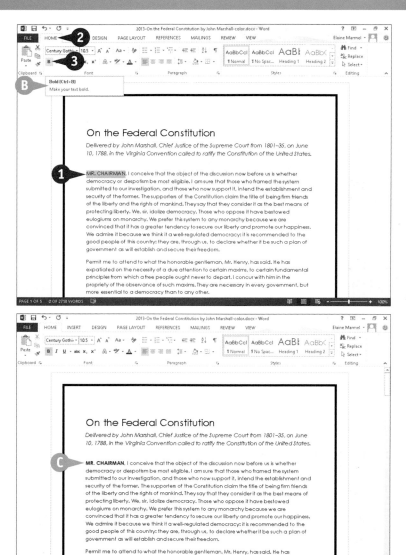

Can I toggle between the document and the Ribbon using the keyboard?
Yes. Each time you press F6, Word changes the focus of the program, switching between the document, the status bar, and the Ribbon, in that order.

What do the small arrows below or beside buttons mean?
When you see a small arrow (▼) on a button, several choices are available for the button. If you click the button directly, Word applies a default choice. However, if you click ▼ , Word displays additional options as either lists or galleries. As you move the mouse pointer over the two parts of the button, Word highlights one or the other to alert you that you have more choices.

Using Word on a Tablet PC

If you are using Word 2013 with Windows 8 on a tablet PC, you need to know some basic touch gestures. Using a tablet PC is a different experience than using a computer with a keyboard and mouse, but Windows 8 was built with the tablet PC in mind, so the touch gestures are intuitive and easy to learn.

On a tablet PC, you use your fingers (or sometimes a stylus, if your tablet comes with one) to run applications, select items, and manipulate screen objects. This may seem awkward at first, but just a little practice of the gestures in this section will make your experience natural and easy.

Using Word on a Tablet PC

Start Word

1 Position your finger or the stylus over a blank spot toward the bottom of the Windows 8 Start screen.

2 Quickly move your finger or the stylus across the tablet screen — called *swiping* — from the right edge to the left edge of the tablet.

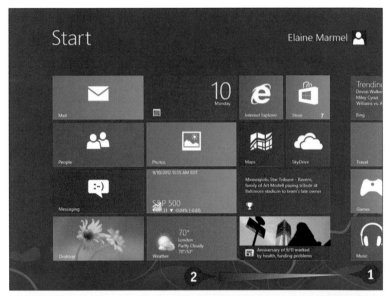

Windows 8 displays the tiles on the right side of the Start screen.

3 Tap the **Word** tile to switch to the Desktop and open Word to the Word Start screen.

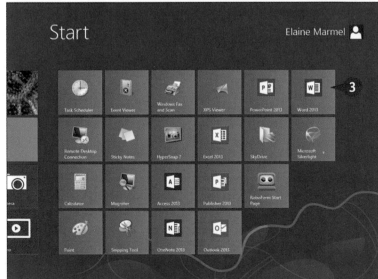

Swipe the Screen

1 Switch to Word's Read Mode view.

Note: See Chapter 3 for details.

2 Swipe left from the right edge of the tablet to read the next page.

3 Swipe right from the left edge of the tablet to read the previous page.

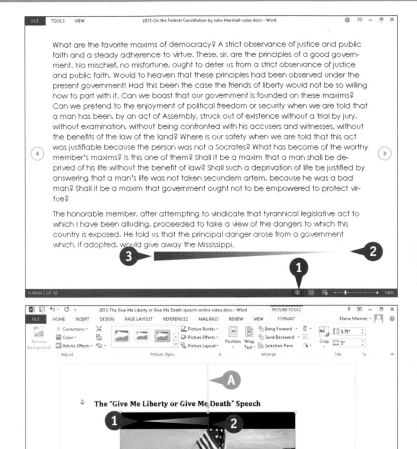

Move an Object

1 Position your finger or the stylus over the item you want to move.

2 Tap and hold the item and begin moving your finger or the stylus.

A The object moves along with your finger or the stylus, and an alignment guide helps you find a position for the object.

3 When the object appears where you want it, lift your finger or the stylus off the screen to complete the move and hide the alignment guide.

TIPS

How do I close Word using gestures?

Position your finger or the stylus at the top edge of the tablet, and then slide it down the screen. At first, you see the Windows 8 application bar for Word, so keep sliding. When you get about halfway, the application becomes a small window. Keep dragging that small window to the very bottom of the screen, and then lift your finger or the stylus. Windows 8 shuts down the application.

How many alignment guides are there?

The Alignment Guide feature uses one vertical and one horizontal alignment guide, and Word displays only one at a time, depending on the position of the object within the document.

Work with the Mini Toolbar and Context Menus

Most of the formatting commands appear on the Home tab in Word, but you have alternatives when you need to format text. You can use the Mini toolbar to format text without switching to the Home tab. The Mini toolbar contains a combination of commands available primarily in the Font group and the Paragraph group on the Home tab.

You also can use the context menu to format text without switching to the Home tab or the Review tab. The context menu contains the Mini toolbar and a combination of commands available primarily in the Font group and the Paragraph group on the Home tab and on the Review tab.

Work with the Mini Toolbar and Context Menus

Work with the Mini Toolbar

1 Select text.

A The Mini toolbar appears transparently in the background.

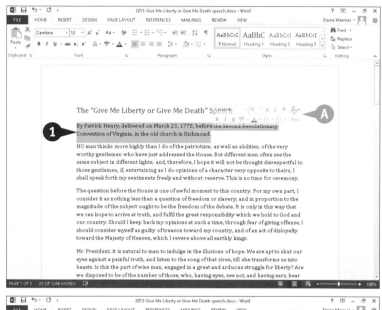

2 Position the mouse pointer close to or over the Mini toolbar.

B The Mini toolbar appears solidly.

3 Click any command or button to perform the actions associated with the command or button.

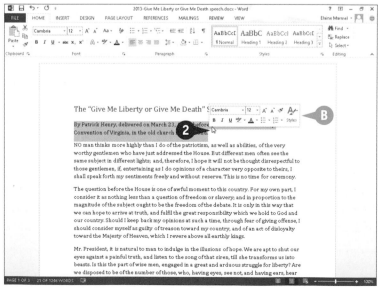

Work with Context Menus

1 Select text.

C The Mini toolbar appears in the background.

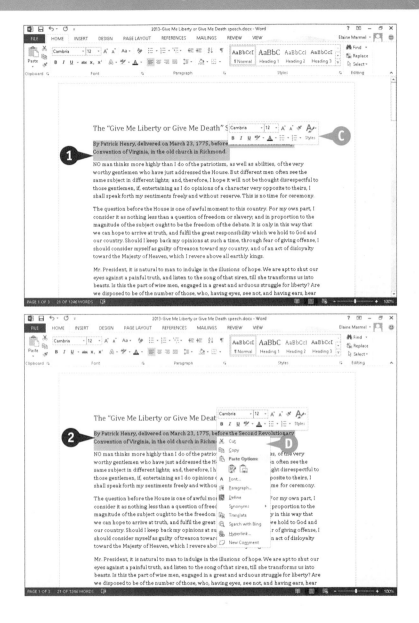

2 Right-click the selected text.

D The context menu appears along with the Mini toolbar.

Note: You can right-click anywhere, not just on selected text, to display the Mini toolbar and the context menu.

3 Click any command or button to perform the actions associated with the command or button.

TIP

Can I turn off the Mini toolbar?
Yes. To do so, click the **File** tab and then click **Options**. The Word Options dialog box appears. On the General tab, deselect **Show Mini Toolbar on selection** (☑ changes to ☐). Click **OK** to close the dialog box.

Enter Text

Word makes typing easy. First, by default, when you start typing, any existing text moves over to accommodate the new text. Further, you do not need to press **Enter** to start a new line. Word calculates for you when a new line should begin and automatically starts it for you, based on the margins you set, the font you use, and the font's size. See Chapter 7 for details on setting margins and Chapter 5 to learn more about choosing a font and setting its size.

To add more than one space between words, use **Tab** instead of **Spacebar**. See Chapter 6 for details on setting tabs.

Enter Text

Type Text

1 Type the text that you want to appear in your document.

A The text appears to the left of the insertion point as you type.

B As the insertion point reaches the end of the line, Word automatically starts a new one.

Press **Enter** only to start a new paragraph.

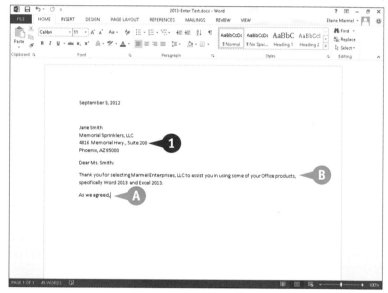

Separate Information

1 Type a word or phrase.

2 Press **Tab**.

To align text properly, you press **Tab** to include more than one space between words.

Several spaces appear between the last letter you typed and the insertion point.

3 Type another word or phrase.

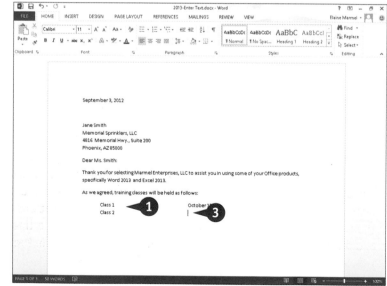

Enter Text Automatically

1 Begin typing a common word, phrase, or date.

The AutoComplete feature suggests common words and phrases based on what you type.

C Word suggests the rest of the word, phrase, or month.

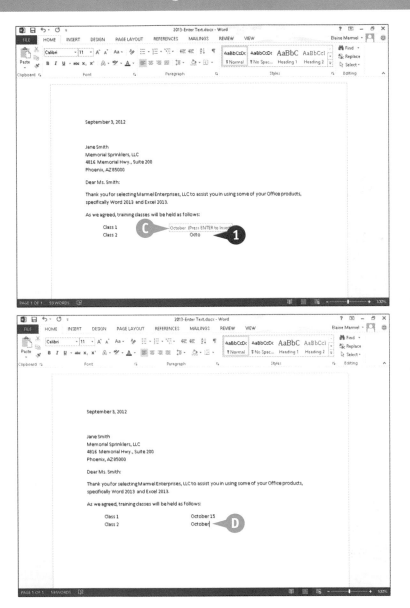

D You can press Enter to let Word finish typing the word, phrase, or month for you.

You can keep typing to ignore Word's suggestion.

TIP

Why should I use Tab instead of Spacebar to include more than one space between words?

Typically, when you include more than one space between words or phrases, you do so to align text in a columnar fashion. Most fonts are proportional, meaning that each character of a font takes up a different amount of space on a line. Therefore, you cannot calculate the number of spaces needed to align words beneath each other. Tabs, however, are set at specific locations on a line, such as 3 inches. When you press Tab, you know exactly where words or phrases appear on a line. Word sets default tabs every .5 inch. To avoid pressing Tab multiple times to separate text, change the tab settings. See Chapter 6 for details.

Move around in a Document

When you edit a large document, you can move the insertion point around the document efficiently using a variety of keyboard shortcuts. Although pressing and holding an arrow key moves the insertion point rapidly in the direction of the arrow, that approach is not efficient when you are viewing page 1 and need to edit text in the middle of the second paragraph on page 5.

You can use many techniques to move the insertion point to a different location in a document; the technique you select depends on the current location of the insertion point and the location to which you want to move.

Move around in a Document

Move by One Character

1 Note the location of the insertion point.

2 Press ➡.

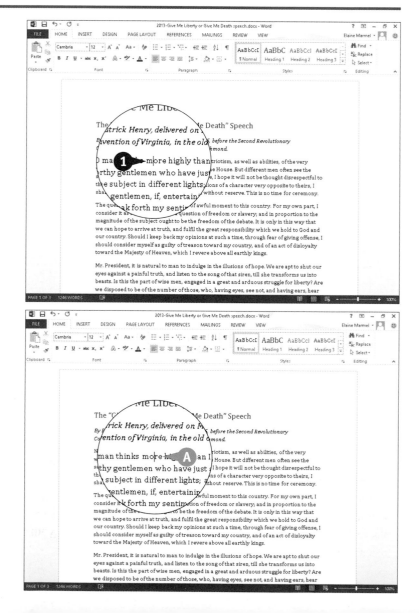

Ⓐ Word moves the insertion point one character to the right.

You can press ⬅, ⬆, or ⬇ to move the insertion point one character left, up, or down.

Holding any arrow key moves the insertion point repeatedly in the direction of the arrow key.

You can press `Ctrl`+➡ or `Ctrl`+⬅ to move the insertion point one word at a time to the right or left.

Move One Screen

1 Note the last visible line on-screen.

2 Press **Page down**.

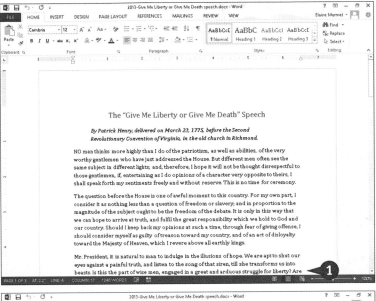

B Word moves the insertion point down one screen.

You can press **Page up** to move the insertion point up one screen.

C You can click ▲ to scroll up or ▼ to scroll down one line at a time in a document.

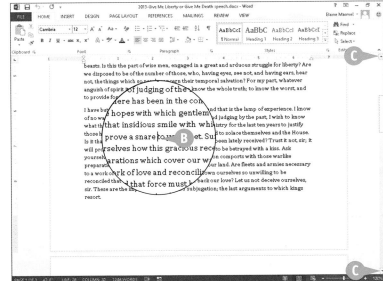

How do I quickly move the insertion point to the beginning or the end of a document or to a specific page?

Press **Ctrl**+**Home** or **Ctrl**+**End** to move the insertion point to the beginning or the end of a document. To land on a specific page, press **F5** to display the Go To dialog box, type the number of the page, and press **Enter**. Press **Shift**+**F5** to move the insertion point to the last place you changed in your document.

Is there a way to move the insertion point to a specific location?

Yes. You can use bookmarks to mark a particular place and then return to it. See Chapter 3 for details on creating a bookmark and returning to the bookmark's location.

CHAPTER 2

Managing Documents

Now that you know the basics, it is time to discover how to navigate among Word documents efficiently. In this chapter, you learn how to manage the Word documents you create, and the tasks in this chapter focus on files stored on your computer; see Chapter 13 to learn about managing documents on SkyDrive.

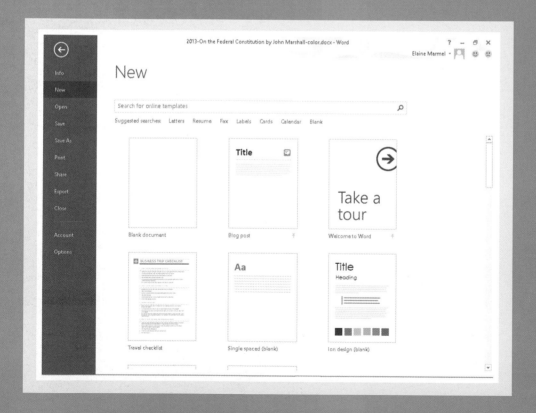

Save a Document to Your Computer

You save documents so that you can use them at another time in Microsoft Word. Word 2013 uses the same XML-based file format that Word 2010 and Word 2007 use, reducing the size of a Word document and improving the likelihood of recovering information from a corrupt file.

After you save a document for the first time, you can click the Save icon on the Quick Access Toolbar (QAT) to save it again. The first time you save a document, Word prompts you for a document name. Subsequent times, when you use the Save button on the QAT, Word saves the document using its original name without prompting you.

Save a Document to Your Computer

Ⓐ Before you save a document, Word displays a generic name in the title bar.

① Click the **File** tab.

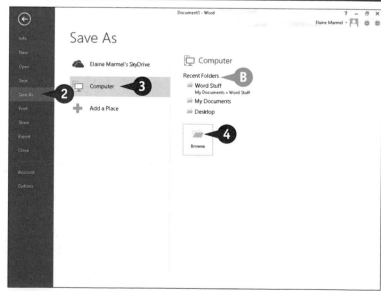

Backstage view appears.

② Click **Save As**.

③ Click **Computer**.

Ⓑ If the folder in which you want to save the document appears here, click it and skip to Step **5**.

④ Click **Browse**.

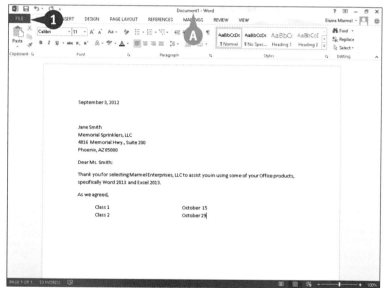

The Save As dialog box appears.

5 Type a name for the document here.

C You can click here to select a location on your computer in which to save the document.

D You can click **New folder** to create a new folder in which to store the document.

6 Click **Save**.

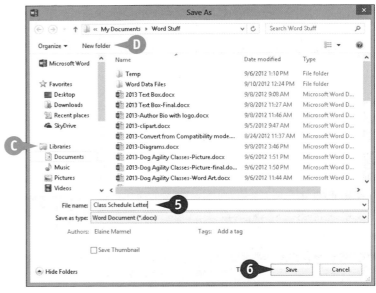

E Word saves the document and displays the name you supplied in the title bar.

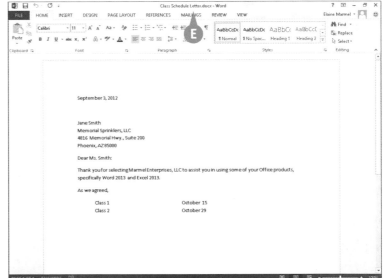

Will my associate, who uses Word 2003, be able to open a document I save in Word 2013?
To make it easier for your associate, you can create the document in Word 2013 but save it in Word 2003 format. See the section "Save a Document to Your Computer in Word 97-2003 Format" for more information.

How can I tell if I am working on a document saved in Word 2013 as opposed to one saved in Word 2003?
Checking the document name in the title bar is the easiest way to identify whether you are working in a document saved in Word 2013 or in any earlier version of Word. The title of a document created in any earlier version of Word appears with "Compatibility Mode" in the title bar.

Reopen an Unsaved Document

You can open documents you created within the last seven days but did not save. It happens: You work on a document and then close it without saving it because you think you will not need it again. And then, a few hours or days later, you find that you do need it.

You can reopen a document you created within the last seven days but did not save because, as you work, Word automatically saves your document even if you take no action to save it.

Reopen an Unsaved Document

1 With any document open, even a blank document, click the **File** tab.

Note: See "Open a Word Document" or "Start a New Document" for details.

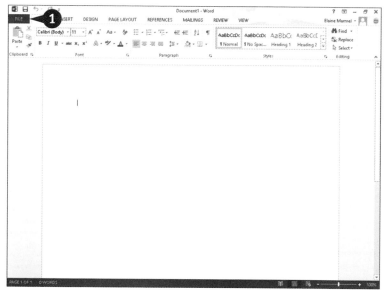

Backstage view appears.

2 Click **Info**.

3 Click **Manage Versions**.

4 Click **Recover Unsaved Documents**.

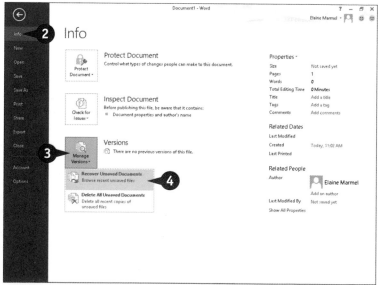

The Open dialog box appears, showing you available files that were auto-saved by Word but not saved as documents by you.

5 Click the unsaved file you want to open.

6 Click **Open**.

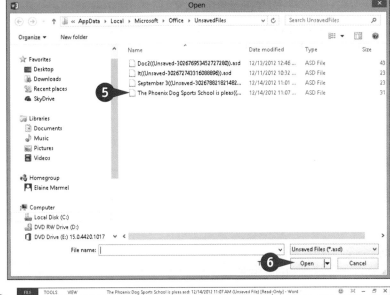

Ⓐ The document appears on-screen in Read Mode view.

Ⓑ The document is a read-only file to which you cannot save changes.

Ⓒ This gold bar identifies the document as a recovered file temporarily being stored on your computer.

7 Click **Save As** to save the file as a Word document.

Note: See the section "Save a Document to Your Computer" for details.

After you save the document, the gold bar disappears.

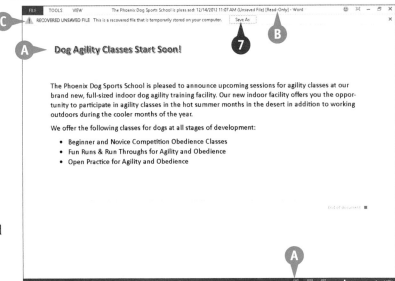

TIPS

How often does Word save a document while I work on it?

By default, Word automatically saves your work — even on documents you have not yet saved — every 10 minutes. You can control the frequency with which Word automatically saves your work; see the section "Set Options for Saving Documents" for details.

Is there another way to open the dialog box that shows unsaved documents?

Yes. Click the **File** tab, and then click **Open**. At the bottom of the Recent Documents list in Backstage view, click **Recover Unsaved Documents** to display the available unsaved documents you can reopen. See the section "Open a Word Document" for more information on the Recent Documents list.

Save a Document to Your Computer in Word 97-2003 Format

You can save documents you create in Microsoft Word in a variety of other formats, such as Word templates, Microsoft Works files, text files, or Word 97-2003 format to share them with people who do not use Microsoft Word 2013.

Although the steps in this section focus on saving a document to Word 97-2003 format, you can use these steps to save a document to any file format Word supports. Be aware that people using Word 2010 or 2007 can open files saved as Word 2013 files; Word 2010 or 2007 users simply cannot use features available in Word 2013.

Save a Document to Your Computer in Word 97-2003 Format

1 Click the **File** tab.

Backstage view appears.

2 Click **Save As**.

3 Click **Computer**.

Ⓐ If the folder in which you want to save the document appears here, click it and skip to Step **5**.

4 Click **Browse**.

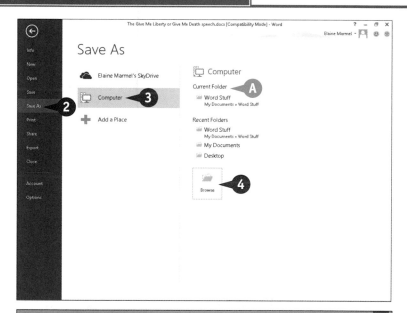

The Save As dialog box appears.

5 Type a name for the document.

6 Click ⌄ to display the formats available for the document, and click **Word 97-2003 Document (*.doc)**.

7 Click **Save**.

Note: If you save a complex document, you might see the Compatibility Checker dialog box, which summarizes changes Word will make when saving your document. Click **OK**.

Word saves the document in the format that you select.

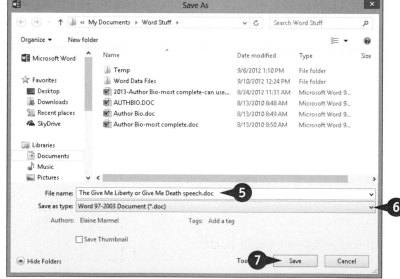

You can save Word documents in PDF or XPS formats. The PDF format is a universal format that any computer user can open using a PDF reader program. There are many free PDF reader programs; perhaps the most well-known one is Adobe Corporation's free Adobe Reader. Windows 8 comes with a built-in PDF reader, making it unnecessary to install your own PDF reader.

XPS is Microsoft's alternative to a PDF file. Windows 8, Windows 7, and Windows Vista come with an XPS viewer; users of other versions of Windows can view XPS documents using Internet Explorer 7 or higher.

Save a Document to Your Computer in PDF or XPS Format

1 Click the **File** tab.

Backstage view appears.

2 Click **Save As**.

3 Click **Computer**.

Ⓐ If the folder in which you want to save the document appears here, click it and skip to Step **5**.

4 Click **Browse**.

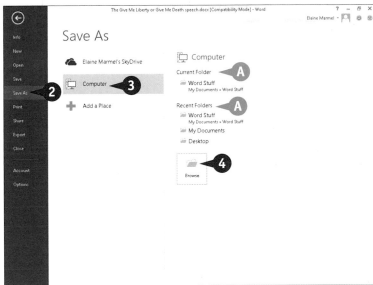

The Save As dialog box appears.

5 Click here to type a name for your document.

6 Click ⌄ to select either **PDF (*.pdf)** or **XPS Document (*.xps)**.

Note: If you choose XPS format, you can opt to save and then open the document.

Ⓑ If you plan to use your document online only, you can select **Minimize size** (○ changes to ◉).

7 Click **Save**.

Word saves the document in the selected format.

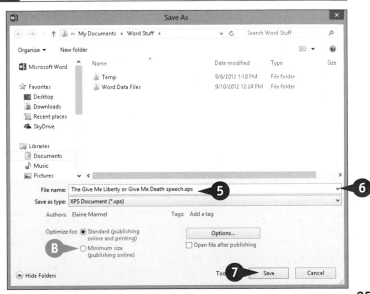

25

Set Options for Saving Documents

You can set a variety of options for saving documents. For example, you can choose to save documents by default in a variety of Word formats other than Word 2013, or you can save documents in any of the following formats: web page, rich text, plain text, XML, OpenDocument, or Microsoft Works. In addition, by default, Word saves documents to SkyDrive and automatically saves your document every 10 minutes while you work on it, even if you have not yet saved it.

You can change any of the Save options to make Word 2013 support the way you work.

Set Options for Saving Documents

Set File-Saving Options

1 Click the **File** tab.

Backstage view appears.

2 Click **Options**.

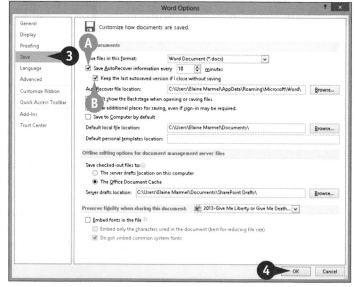

The Word Options dialog box appears.

3 Click **Save**.

Ⓐ You can select **Save AutoRecover information every** (☐ changes to ☑), and specify an interval for saving recovery information.

Ⓑ You can select **Keep the last AutoRecovered file if I close without saving** (☐ changes to ☑) to make sure Word saves unsaved documents.

4 Click **OK** to save your changes.

Set File-Saving Locations

1 Complete Steps **1** to **3** in the subsection "Set File-Saving Options" on the previous page.

2 Click **Browse** next to Default Local File Location.

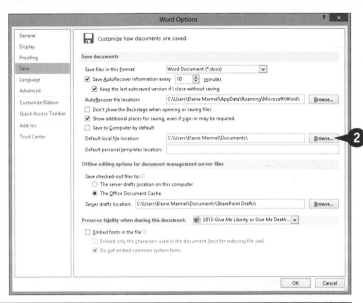

The Modify Location dialog box appears.

3 Click here to navigate to the folder where you want to save Word documents.

4 Click **OK** to close the Modify Location dialog box and redisplay the Word Options dialog box.

You can repeat Steps **2** to **4** to set the AutoRecover File and the Server Drafts locations.

5 Click **OK** in the Word Options dialog box to save your changes.

Word saves your changes.

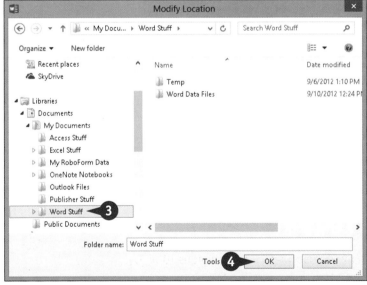

TIPS

How can I make Word automatically save my document to my computer instead of to SkyDrive?
In the Word Options dialog box, select **Save to Computer by default** (☐ changes to ☑).

What happens if I select the Don't Show the Backstage When Opening or Saving Files option?
To take true advantage of this option, you need to add the Open and Save As buttons to the Quick Access Toolbar (QAT). When you opt not to show Backstage view and then click the Open or Save As buttons, Word displays the Open or Save As dialog box without showing Backstage view. If you are comfortable navigating folders, enabling this option saves you time. See Chapter 11 to customize the QAT.

Open a Word Document

You can open documents that you have created and saved previously in order to continue adding data or to edit existing data. Regardless of whether you store a file in a folder on your computer's hard drive or on a CD, you can easily access files using the Open dialog box. If you are not sure where you saved a file, you can use the Open dialog box's Search function to locate it.

When you are finished using a file, you should close it to free up processing power on your computer. See "Close a Document" later in this chapter.

Open a Word Document

1 Click the **File** tab.

Backstage view appears.

2 Click **Open**.

A Recently opened documents appear here. If you see the file you want to open, you can click it to open it and skip the rest of these steps.

Note: You might need to click **Recent Documents** in the list on the left to view recent documents.

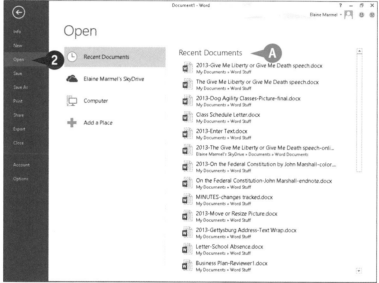

3 Click the place where you believe the document is stored. This section uses **Computer**.

Note: If you choose the wrong place, you can search for the file.

B If the folder containing the document appears here, click it and skip to Step **5**.

4 Click **Browse**.

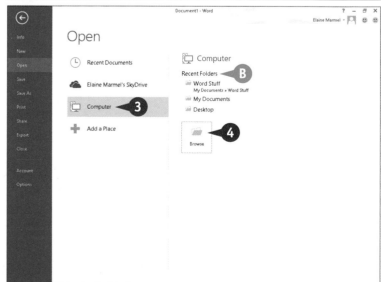

The Open dialog box appears.

5 Click here to navigate to the folder containing the document you want to open.

6 Click the document you want to open.

7 Click **Open**.

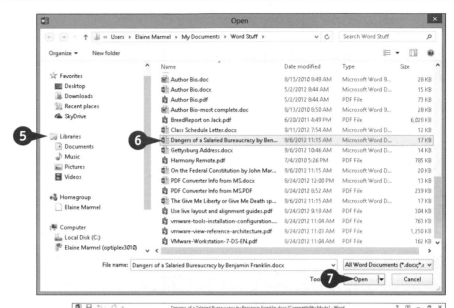

The document appears on-screen.

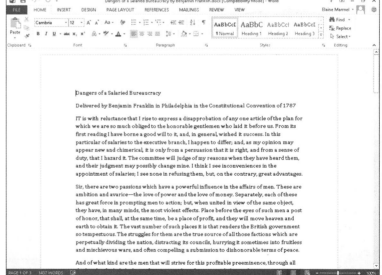

Open a Document of Another Format

You can open and edit documents created by colleagues using several other word-processing programs besides Word. For example, you can open XML, web page, rich text, plain text, OpenDocument, PDF, WordPerfect 5.x or 6.x, or Works 6-9 documents as well as documents created in earlier versions of Word.

Although you can open and edit PDF files, editing PDF files in Word works best if you used Word to originally create the PDF file. If you used a different program to create the PDF file, you will find that Word has difficulty maintaining the file's formatting.

Open a Document of Another Format

1 Click the **File** tab.

Backstage view appears.

2 Click **Open**.

A You can click **Recent Documents** to see a list of recently opened documents. If you see the file you want to open, you can click it to open it and skip the rest of these steps.

3 Click the place where you believe the document is stored. This section uses **Computer**.

Note: If you choose the wrong place, you can search for the file.

B If the folder containing the document appears here, click it and skip to Step **5**.

4 Click **Browse**.

The Open dialog box appears.

5 Click here to navigate to the folder containing the document you want to open.

6 Click ☑ to select the type of document you want to open.

7 Click the file you want to open.

8 Click **Open**.

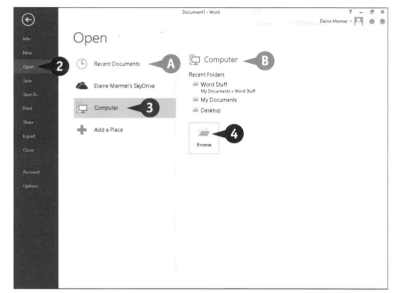

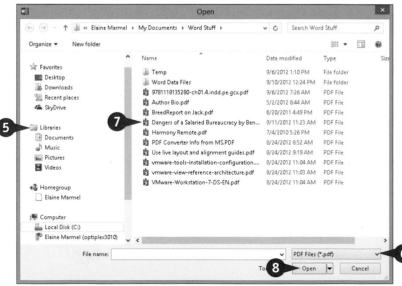

If you open a PDF file, Word displays a message indicating that it is converting your PDF file to an editable Word document; click **OK** to continue.

Note: You may be prompted to install a converter to open the file; click **Yes** or **OK** to install the converter and open the file.

Ⓒ Word opens the file.

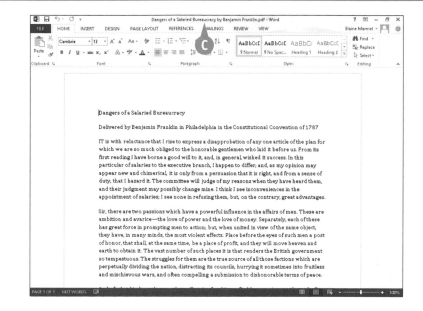

How do I open an XPS file?

Although you can create an XPS file in Word, you cannot open the file in Word. Instead, you must use an XPS viewer. Word 2013 under Windows 8 comes with a built-in XPS viewer; to open an XPS file, find it using File Explorer and double-click it.

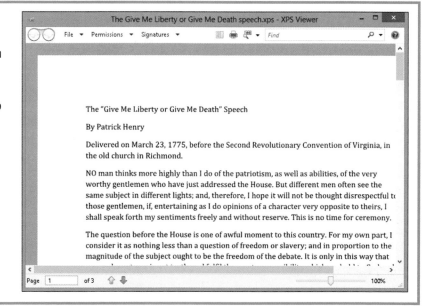

Start a New Document

Each time you open Word, the Word start screen offers you a variety of choices to begin a new document. But you do not need to close and reopen Word to start a new document. This section demonstrates how to start a new document while you are already working in Word.

You can use a variety of *templates* — documents containing predefined settings that save you the effort of creating the settings yourself — as the foundation for your documents. Word 2013 displays a variety of templates on the Word Start screen and also when you choose to start a new document while working in Word.

Start a New Document

1 With a document already open in Word, click the **File** tab.

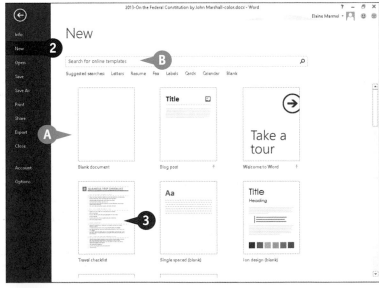

Backstage view appears.

2 Click **New**.

Ⓐ Templates appear here.

Ⓑ You can search for templates online at Office.com.

3 Click a template.

Note: This example uses Travel checklist.

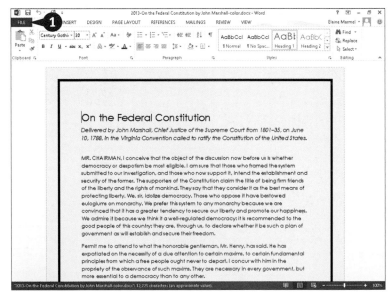

A preview of the template appears.

4 Click **Create**.

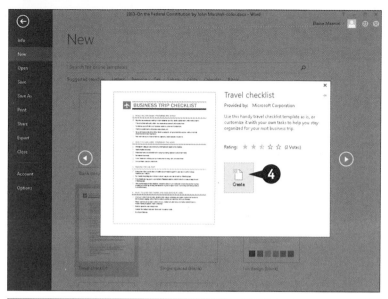

C The new document based on the template you chose appears.

You can edit this document any way you choose.

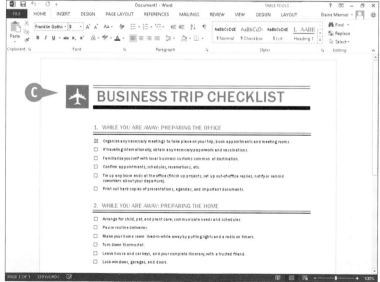

BUSINESS TRIP CHECKLIST

1. WHILE YOU ARE AWAY: PREPARING THE OFFICE

☒ Organize any necessary meetings to take place on your trip; book appointments and meeting rooms.
☐ If traveling internationally, obtain any necessary paperwork and vaccinations.
☐ Familiarize yourself with local business customs common at destination.
☐ Confirm appointments, schedules, reservations, etc.
☐ Tie up any loose ends at the office (finish up projects; set up out-of-office replies; notify or remind coworkers about your departure).
☐ Print out hard copies of presentations, agendas, and important documents.

2. WHILE YOU ARE AWAY: PREPARING THE HOME

☐ Arrange for child, pet, and plant care; communicate needs and schedules.
☐ Pause routine deliveries.
☐ Make your home seem lived-in while away by putting lights and a radio on timers.
☐ Turn down thermostat.
☐ Leave house and car keys, and your complete itinerary, with a trusted friend.
☐ Lock windows, garages, and doors.

TIPS

When I save the document, am I overwriting the settings in the template?
No. The document contains the settings found in the template, but saving the document has no effect on the template. The next time you choose to use that template, it will contain its original information. Think of it this way: A blank document is based on the Normal template, which contains no text, but it contains other settings such as fonts, font sizes, line spacing settings, and margins.

What should I do if I change my mind about the template I chose in Step 3?
Instead of performing Step **4**, you can click ✕ in the upper-right corner of the preview. Word redisplays Backstage view showing the choices when you click New.

Switch between Open Documents

When you have multiple documents open, you can switch between them to, for example, copy information from one document to another. You can open as many documents as you need, and you can switch between them from within Word or by using the Windows taskbar. You use the View tab in Word, or you can use the Windows taskbar to switch documents. By default, Word 2013 displays each document in its own window, and the Desktop identifies each open window by displaying a button on the Windows taskbar.

Switch between Open Documents

Switch Documents Using Word

1 Click the **View** tab.

2 Click **Switch Windows**.

Ⓐ A list of all open documents appears at the bottom of the menu. A check mark (✓) appears beside the currently active document.

3 Click the document you want to view.

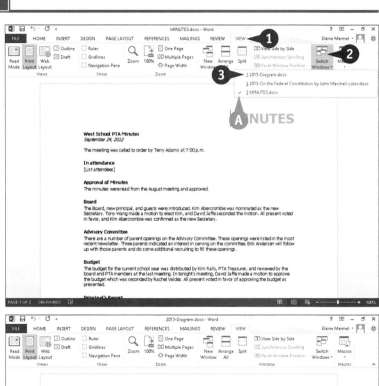

The selected document appears.

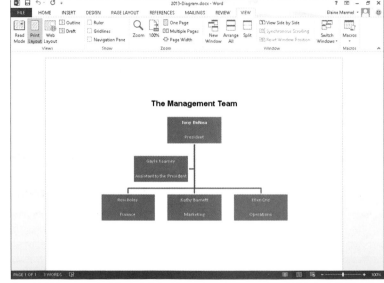

Switch Documents Using the Windows Taskbar

1 Open all the documents you need.

Note: See "Open a Word Document" or "Open a Document of Another Format" for details.

2 Point the mouse at the Word buttons in the Windows taskbar.

B Preview thumbnails appear for each open document. The document at which you point the mouse also previews in Word.

C You can click a preview thumbnail's ⊠ to close the document.

3 To view a document, click its preview.

The document appears.

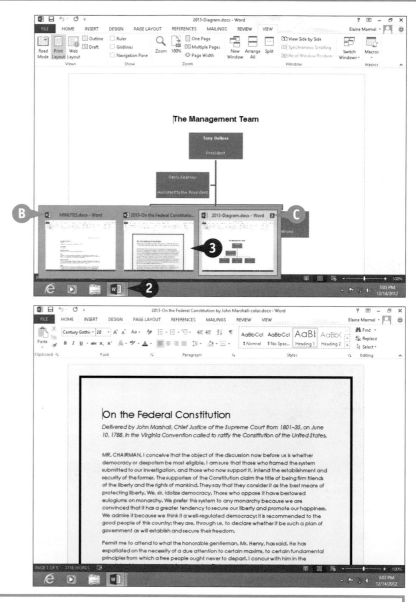

TIP

Is there a way to keep the taskbar buttons separate from each other instead of stacked on top of each other?

Yes. Right-click a blank spot on the taskbar, and click **Properties** in the menu that appears. The Taskbar Properties dialog box appears. Click the **Taskbar buttons** ⊡ and choose **Combine when taskbar is full** or **Never combine** (**A**). Click **OK** to save your changes.

Compare Documents Side by Side

You can view two open documents side by side to compare their similarities and differences. Although you could open both documents in their own windows and switch between them, that process can be cumbersome if you want to compare them. Switching between documents is the more effective tool when you want to copy or move text from one document to another. Viewing documents side by side is the more effective tool for comparing document content.

Using the technique described in this section, you can scroll through both documents simultaneously.

Compare Documents Side by Side

Compare Documents

1 Open the two documents you want to compare.

Note: See "Open a Word Document" or "Open a Document of Another Format" for details.

2 Click the **View** tab.

3 Click **View Side by Side**.

Word displays the documents in two panes beside each other.

4 Drag either document's scroll bar.

Word scrolls both documents simultaneously.

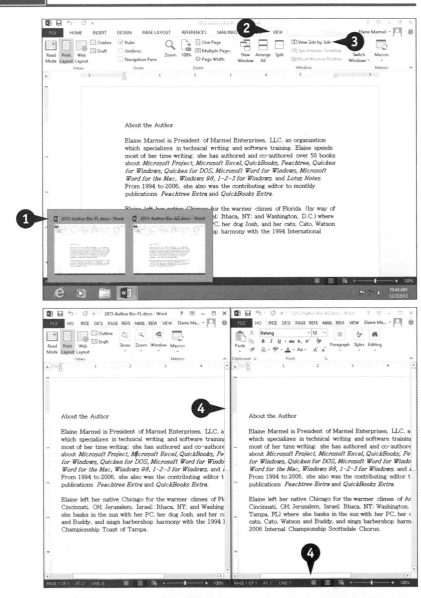

Stop Comparing Documents

1 Click **Window** in the document on the left.

A Options drop down from the Window button.

2 Click **View Side by Side**.

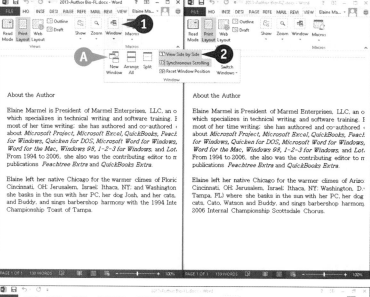

Word redisplays the document in a full screen.

B The second document is still open. You can see preview thumbnails for both documents in the Windows taskbar, and you can click a preview thumbnail to switch to the other document.

Note: For details on this technique, see the section "Switch between Open Documents" earlier in this chapter.

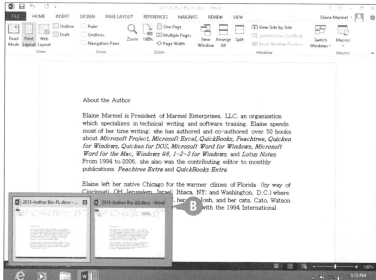

See Chapter 4 for details.

TIPS

Is there a way to compare two documents with their differences highlighted?

Yes. When you have sent the same document to several people for review, each will return the document with his or her comments. You can compare the different document versions to see their differences. See Chapter 4 for details.

What does the Reset Window Position button do?

With respect to comparing documents side by side, the **Reset Window Position** button has no effect. But you can use **Arrange All** to place one window above the other, each in its own separate pane. To return to side-by-side viewing, click **Reset Window Position**.

Work with Document Properties

You can use the Document Properties panel to supply information about a document such as the document's title, keywords that appear in the document, the category in which a document falls, or even comments about the document.

After you save document property information, you can use it when you search for documents in Windows Explorer (Windows Vista and Windows 7) or File Explorer (Windows 8). Windows Explorer and File Explorer display a Search box in the upper-right corner; after selecting the most likely folder that contains the document, type a search word or phrase in the box.

Work with Document Properties

1 Click the **File** tab.

Backstage view appears.

2 Click **Info**.

Ⓐ The Information panel appears.

3 Click **Properties**.

4 Click **Show Document Panel** to display the properties that you can fill in above the document.

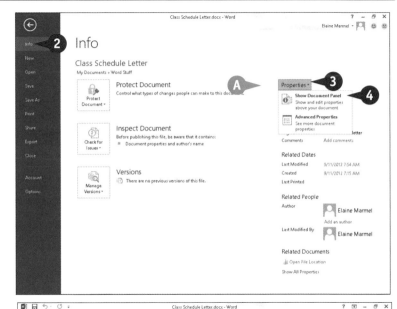

Ⓑ The Document Properties panel appears above the document.

5 Click in a box, and type information.

6 Repeat Step **5** as needed.

7 Click × in the Document Properties panel to save your changes and return to editing the document.

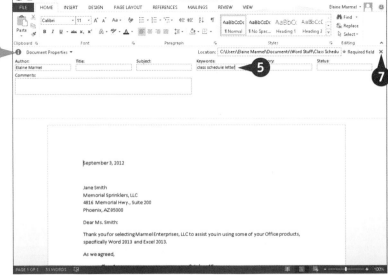

Close a Document

When you finish working with a document, you close it to remove it from the Word window and prepare to work with another document or perform some other task. Closing a document when you finish using it makes your Word working area easier to navigate. If you made any changes to the document, Word prompts you to save them before closing the document. If you did not make any changes before closing the document, Word removes the document from the Word window. If you need to work in the document again, open it; see the section "Open a Word Document."

Close a Document

1 Click the **File** tab.

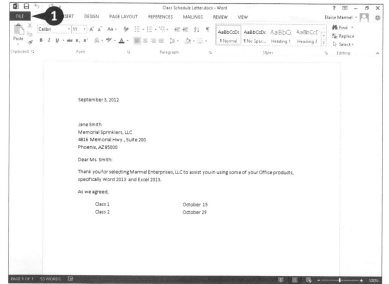

Backstage view appears.

2 Click **Close**.

Word removes the document from your screen.

If you had other documents open, Word displays the last document you used; otherwise, you see a blank Word window.

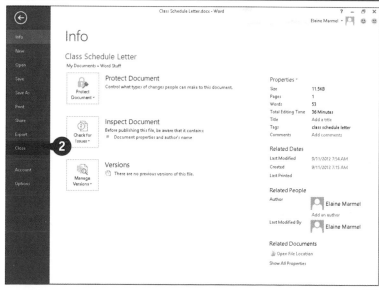

Inspect a Document before Sharing

Y ou can remove any personal information that Word stores in a document. For issues of privacy, you may want to remove this information before you share a document with anyone.

The Document Inspector searches your document for comments, revision marks, versions, and ink annotations. It searches document properties for hidden metadata and personal information. It inspects for task pane apps saved in the document as well as text that has been collapsed under a heading. If your document contains custom XML data, headers, footers, watermarks, or invisible content, the Document Inspector alerts you.

Inspect a Document before Sharing

1 Click the **File** tab.

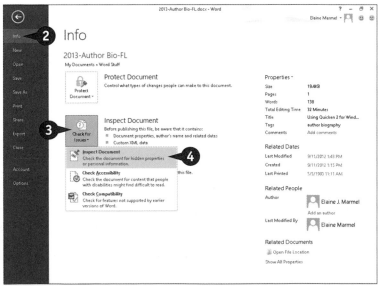

Backstage view appears.

2 Click **Info**.

3 Click **Check for Issues**.

4 Click **Inspect Document**.

Note: If you have unsaved changes, Word prompts you to save the document, which you do by clicking **Yes**.

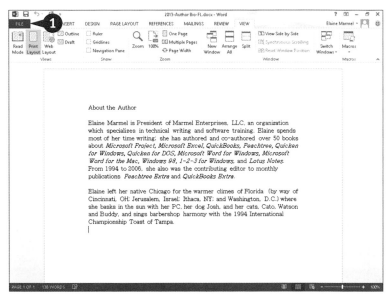

40

The Document Inspector window appears.

Ⓐ You can deselect these options (☑ changes to ☐) to avoid inspecting for these elements.

5 Click **Inspect**.

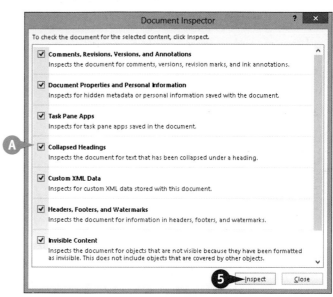

The Document Inspector looks for the information you specified and displays the results.

Ⓑ You can remove any identified information by clicking **Remove All** beside that element.

Ⓒ You can click **Reinspect** after removing identifying information.

6 Click **Close**.

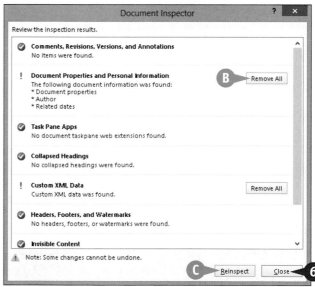

Can I review the information that the Document Inspector displays before I remove it?

No. The only way to review the information before you remove it is to close the Document Inspector *without* removing information, use the appropriate Word features to review the information, and then rerun the Document Inspector as described in this section.

What happens if I remove information and then decide that I really want that information?

You cannot undo the effects of removing the information using the Document Inspector. However, to restore removed information, you can close the document *without* saving changes and then reopen it.

Work with Protected Documents

You can limit the changes others can make to a document by protecting it with a password. Word offers two kinds of protection: Password and User Authentication. User authentication, not shown in this section, relies on Windows authentication.

You can limit the styles available to format the document, the kinds of changes users can make, and the users who can make changes.

Work with Protected Documents

1 Click the **Review** tab.

2 Click **Restrict Editing**.

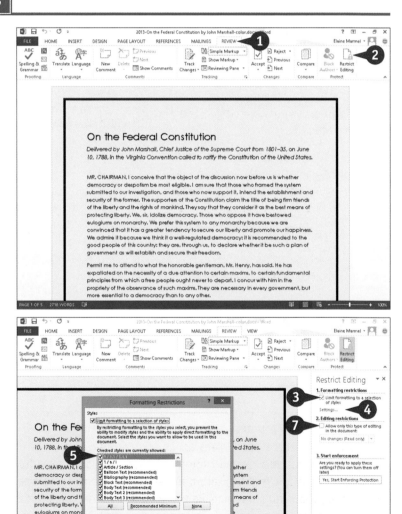

The Restrict Formatting and Editing pane appears.

3 Select this option to limit document formatting to the styles you select (☐ changes to ☑).

4 Click the **Settings** link.

The Formatting Restrictions dialog box appears.

5 Deselect the styles you want unavailable (☑ changes to ☐).

6 Click **OK**.

7 Select this option to specify editing restrictions (☐ changes to ☑).

8 Click ▼ , and select the type of editing to permit.

You can select parts of the document to make them available for editing.

9 Select this option to identify users who are allowed to edit the selected parts of the document (☐ changes to ☑).

10 Click **Yes, Start Enforcing Protection**.

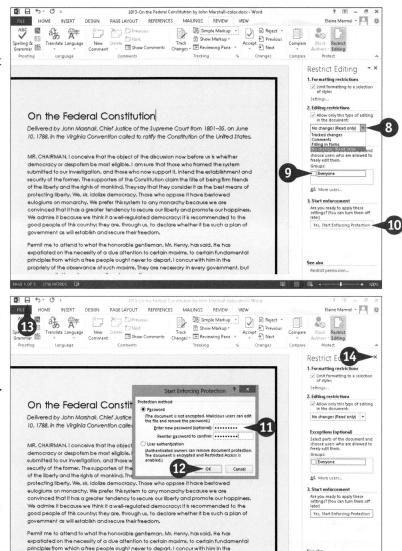

11 In the Start Enforcing Protection dialog box, type a password, and then retype it.

Note: If your computer uses Information Rights Management (IRM), you can opt to use User Authentication, which also encrypts your document; only users you specify can remove document protection.

12 Click **OK**.

13 Click the **Save** button (🖫).

Word protects the document and saves the protection.

14 Click × to close the Restrict Editing pane.

TIPS

How do I open a protected document and work in it?
You open a protected document as you would open any other document. Areas you can edit are highlighted. If you try to change an area that is not highlighted, a message appears in the status bar, explaining that you cannot make the modification because that area of the document is protected. Follow Steps **1** and **2** in this section to display the Protect Document pane, and click **Show All Regions I Can Edit** to find areas you can change. To turn off protection, you need the protection password.

How do I stop protecting a document?
Click the **Stop Protection** button at the bottom of the Restrict Editing pane. Supply the password, and then deselect (☑ changes to ☐) any editing restrictions in place. Click 🖫 to save the document.

Mark a Document as Final

When you mark a document as final, Word makes the document read-only; you cannot make changes to it or inspect it.

Marking a document as final is not a security feature; instead, it is a feature that helps you focus on reading rather than editing because it makes editing unavailable. If you want to focus on security, consider assigning a password to the document that others must supply to open the document. Alternatively, you can assign a digital signature to indicate that a document has not changed since you signed it, or you can restrict editing as described in "Work with Protected Documents."

Mark a Document as Final

Mark the Document

1 Click the **File** tab.

Backstage view appears.

2 Click **Info**.

3 Click **Protect Document.**

4 Click **Mark As Final**.

A message explains that Word will mark the document as final and then save it.

5 Click **OK**.

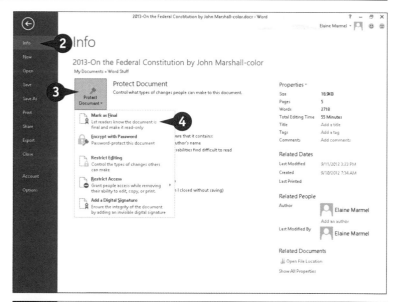

A Word saves the document and displays another message confirming that the document has been marked as final and editing commands are unavailable. If you do not want to see this message again, select this option (☐ changes to ☑).

6 Click **OK**.

Backstage view highlights the Protect Document button to draw your attention.

7 Click the **Back** button (⬅).

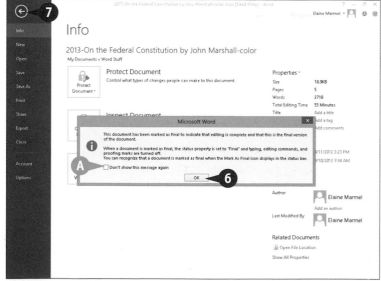

Edit a Final Document

B The document is now read-only, and commands on the QAT become unavailable.

C Word hides the Ribbon buttons because most editing commands are not available.

D This gold bar appears, indicating that the document has been marked as final.

8 Click **Edit Anyway** in the gold bar at the top of the document.

E Word no longer marks the document as read-only.

F Word redisplays and makes available all Ribbon buttons.

G QAT buttons are available.

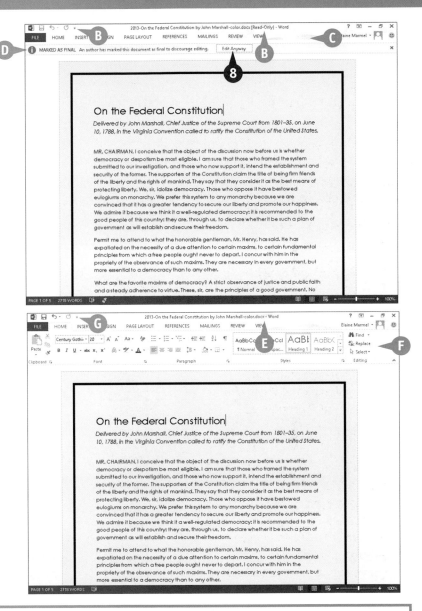

TIPS

Can any user remove the "Marked As Final" status from a document?

Yes. If you absolutely do not want others to edit or change your document, consider other security options. For example, you can restrict editing and protect the document with a password. You also can consider saving your document as a PDF or XPS document, as described in "Save a Document to Your Computer in PDF or XPS format."

Why is the Protect Document button in Backstage view highlighted in yellow?

This draws your attention to the fact that some protection has been applied to the document. When you mark a document as final, you can still restrict editing with a password or add a digital signature, but you cannot require a password to open the document.

Convert Word Documents from Prior Versions to Word 2013

Y ou can convert existing Word 97-Word 2003 documents to the new format introduced by Word 2007. You also can convert Word 2007 and Word 2010 documents to Word 2013 documents.

It is helpful to convert documents created in older versions of Word to Word 2013 format when you want to take advantage of tools that are available in Word 2013 but not in earlier versions of Word. For example, you can open a Word 2010 document that contains an image and you can move the image, but you will not see alignment guides during the move unless you convert the Word 2010 document to Word 2013.

Convert Word Documents from Prior Versions to Word 2013

1 Open any prior version Word document; this example uses a Word 2003 document.

Note: See "Open a Word Document" or "Open a Document of Another Format" for details.

A In the title bar, Word indicates that the document is open in Compatibility Mode.

2 Click the **File** tab.

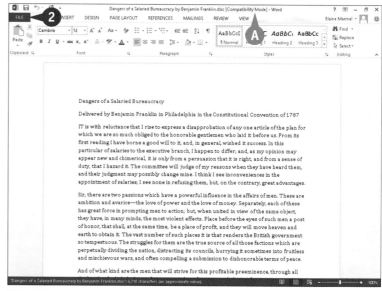

Backstage view appears.

3 Click **Info**.

4 Click **Convert**.

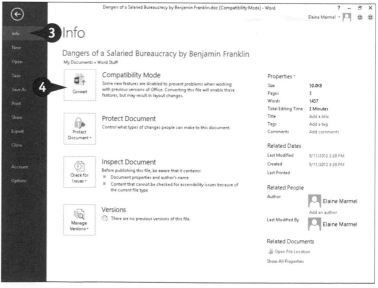

Word closes Backstage view and displays a message indicating it will convert the document to the newest file format.

Ⓑ If you do not want to view this message in the future when you convert documents, select this option (☐ changes to ☑).

5 Click **OK**.

Ⓒ Word converts the document and removes the Compatibility Mode indicator from the title bar.

6 Click the **Save** button (🖫).

The Save As dialog box appears.

Ⓓ Word suggests the same file name but the new file format extension .docx.

7 Click **Save**.

Word saves the document in Word 2013 format.

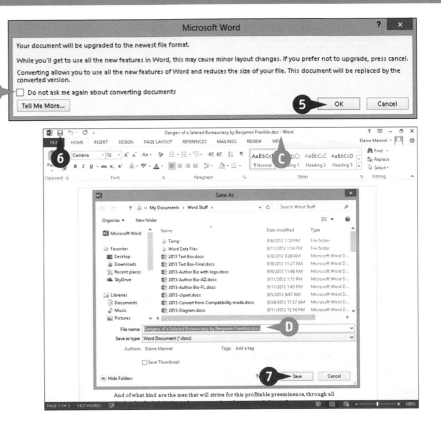

TIPS

Do I need to convert my documents from earlier versions of Word before I work on them in Word 2013?

No. You can work on a document created in an older version of Word and even incorporate Word 2013 features not available in earlier versions of Word. You only need to convert documents in which you expect to include features available only in Word 2013.

Is there any difference between using the method described in this section and opening a Word 97-Word 2003 document and then using the Save As command?

Not really. If you use the Save As method and choose Word Document (*.docx), Word prompts you to convert the older version document to the Word 2013 format using the Convert command as described in this section.

CHAPTER 3

Editing Text

After you know how to navigate around Word, it is time to work with the text that you type on a page. In this chapter, you learn editing techniques that you can use to change text in documents you create.

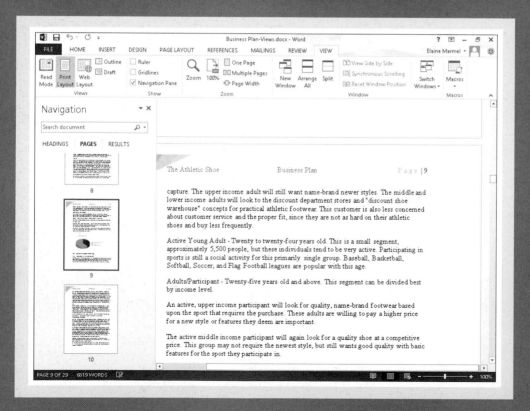

Insert Text

Word makes typing easy; you can quickly type a letter, memo, or report in Word. You can insert text into a document by adding to existing text or replacing existing text. By default, Word is set to Insert mode; when you start typing, Word moves any existing text to the right to accommodate the new text. In Overtype mode, Word replaces existing text to the right of the insertion point, character for character. If you have set up Word to toggle between Insert mode and Overtype mode, you can press **Insert** to switch between Insert and Overtype modes.

Insert Text

Insert and Add Text

1 Click the location where you want to insert text.

The insertion point flashes where you clicked.

You can press ←, →, ↑, or ↓ to move the insertion point one character or line.

You can press **Ctrl**+→ or **Ctrl**+← to move the insertion point one word at a time to the right or left.

2 Type the text you want to insert.

Word inserts the text to the left of the insertion point, moving existing text to the right.

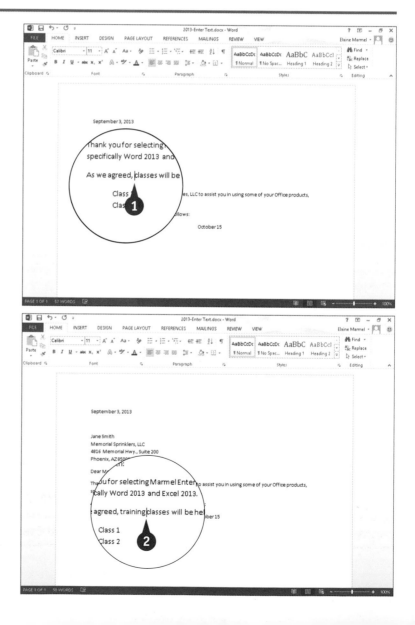

Insert and Replace Text

1 Position the insertion point where you want to replace existing text

2 Right-click the status bar.

3 Click **Overtype** to display a check beside it.

A An indicator appears in the status bar.

4 Click the indicator to switch to Overtype mode.

B The indicator switches to Overtype.

Note: Each time you click the indicator, you switch between Overtype and Insert mode.

5 Type the new text.

As you type, Word replaces the existing text with the new text you type.

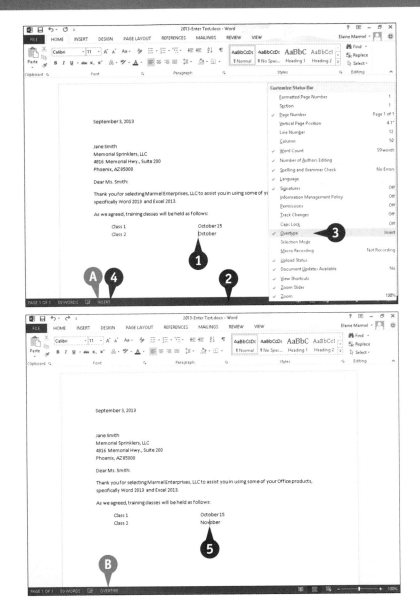

TIP

How can I use the keyboard to control switching between Insert mode and Overtype mode?
Perform the steps that follow. Click the **File** tab and click **Options** to display the Word Options dialog box. Click **Advanced** and select **Use the Insert key to control overtype mode** (☐ changes to ☑). Click **OK**, and then press **Insert**. Word switches between Insert mode and Overtype mode.

Delete Text

When you make a mistake or simply change your mind about text you have already typed, you can easily remove the text from your document. Whether you have a large or a small amount of text to remove, you use either `Delete` or `Backspace` on your keyboard. This section demonstrates how to remove one character at a time. Note that when you need to delete a larger amount of text, you do not need to remove it one character at a time, but you use the same basic technique demonstrated here.

Delete Text

Using the Delete Key

1 Click to the left of the location where you want to delete text.

The insertion point flashes where you clicked.

You can press ←, →, ↑, or ↓ to move the insertion point one character or line.

You can press `Ctrl`+→ or `Ctrl`+← to move the insertion point one word at a time to the right or left.

2 Press `Delete` on your keyboard.

A Word deletes the character immediately to the right of the insertion point.

You can press and hold `Delete` to repeatedly delete characters to the right of the insertion point.

You can press `Ctrl`+`Delete` to delete the word to the right of the insertion point.

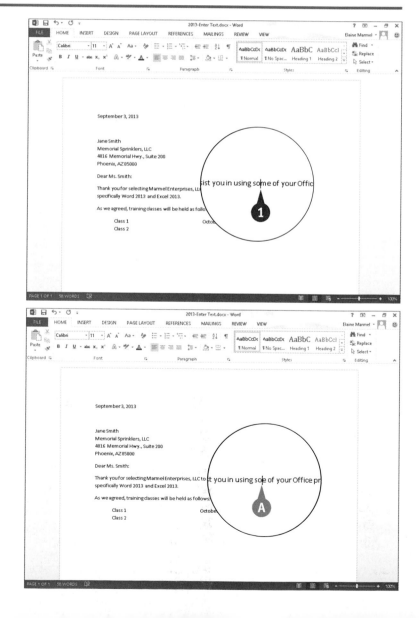

Using the Backspace Key

1 Click to the right of the location where you want to delete text.

The insertion point flashes where you clicked.

2 Press **Backspace** on your keyboard.

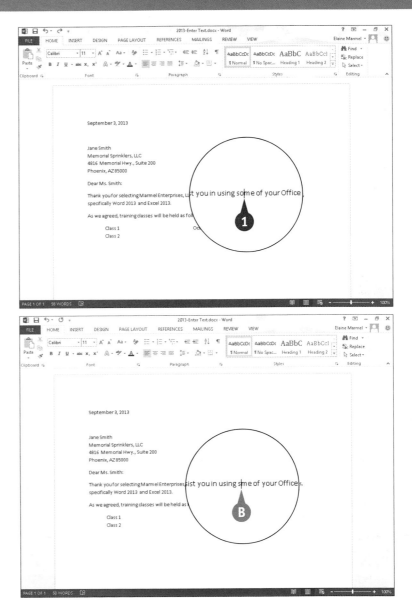

B Word deletes the character immediately to the left of the insertion point.

You can press and hold **Backspace** to repeatedly delete characters to the left of the insertion point.

You can press **Ctrl** + **Backspace** to delete the word to the left of the insertion point.

TIPS

Do I have to delete a large block of text one character or one word at a time?

No, and, in fact, to work efficiently, you should not delete a large block one character or word at a time. You can select the block of text and then press either **Delete** or **Backspace**; either key deletes selected text. For details on selecting text, see the section "Select Text" later in this chapter.

What should I do if I mistakenly delete text?

You should use the Undo feature in Word to restore the text you deleted. For details on how this feature works, see the section "Undo Changes" later in this chapter.

Insert Blank Lines

You can insert blank lines in your text to signify new paragraphs by inserting paragraph marks or line breaks. Word stores paragraph formatting in the paragraph mark shown in this section. When you start a new paragraph, you can change the new paragraph's formatting without affecting the preceding paragraph's formatting.

You use line breaks to start a new line without starting a new paragraph; typically, when you type the inside address of a letter, you use line breaks. For more information on styles and displaying paragraph marks, see Chapter 6.

Insert Blank Lines

Start a New Paragraph

1 Click where you want to start a new paragraph.

2 Press **Enter**.

A Word inserts a paragraph mark and moves any text to the right of the insertion point into the new paragraph.

3 Repeat Steps **1** and **2** for each blank line you want to insert.

Insert a Line Break

1 Click where you want to start a new paragraph.

2 Press **Shift** + **Enter**.

B Word inserts a line break.

Note: Any text on the line to the right of the insertion point moves onto the new line.

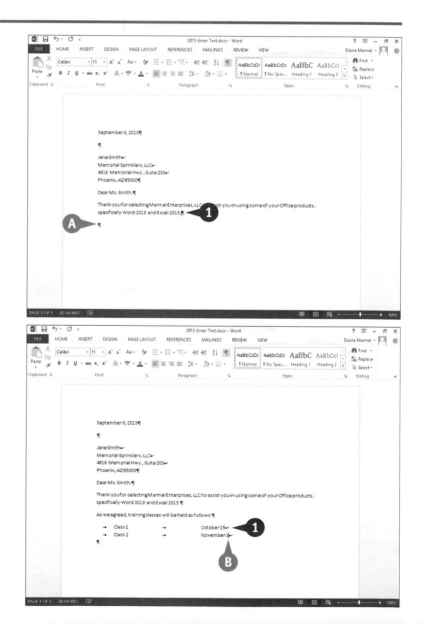

Undo Changes

You can use the Undo feature to reverse actions you take while working in a document. For example, suppose that you accidentally delete text that you meant to keep instead of deleting other text. In this case, you can use the Undo feature to recover the text you accidentally deleted.

You also can use the Undo feature to remove formatting you might have applied, particularly if you decide that you do not like the look of the formatting. Rather than take steps to remove the formatting, simply undo your actions.

Undo Changes

Note: The position of the insertion point does not affect using the Undo feature.

1 Click the **Undo** button (↺ ▾).

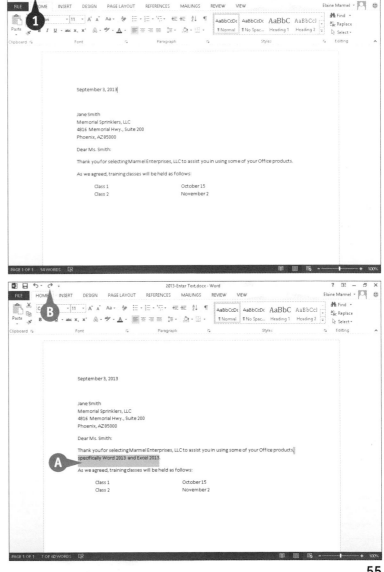

Ⓐ Word reverses the effects of the last change you made.

You also can press Ctrl + Z to reverse an action.

Note: You can repeatedly click the **Undo** button (↺ ▾) to reverse each action you have taken, from last to first.

Ⓑ If you decide not to reverse an action after clicking the **Undo** button (↺ ▾), click the **Redo** button (↻), which reverses the action of the Undo button (↺ ▾).

Select Text

Before performing many tasks in Word, you identify the existing text on which you want to work by selecting it. For example, you select existing text to underline it, align it, change its font size, or apply color to it.

You can take advantage of shortcuts using the keyboard and the mouse together to select a word, a sentence, or your entire document, and the text you select does not need to appear together in one location. If you like to keep your hands on the keyboard as much as possible, you can select text using only the keyboard.

Select Text

Select a Block of Text

1 Position the mouse pointer to the left of the first character you want to select.

2 Click and drag to the right and down over the text you want to select and release the mouse button.

A The selection appears highlighted, and the Mini toolbar appears.

Note: This example hides the Mini toolbar so that you can see the beginning and end of the selection.

To cancel a selection, you can click anywhere on-screen or press ⬅, ➡, ⬆, or ⬇.

Select a Word

1 Double-click the word you want to select.

B Word selects the word, and the Mini toolbar appears.

You can slide the mouse pointer away from the Mini toolbar to make it disappear.

Note: See Chapter 1 for details on using the Mini toolbar.

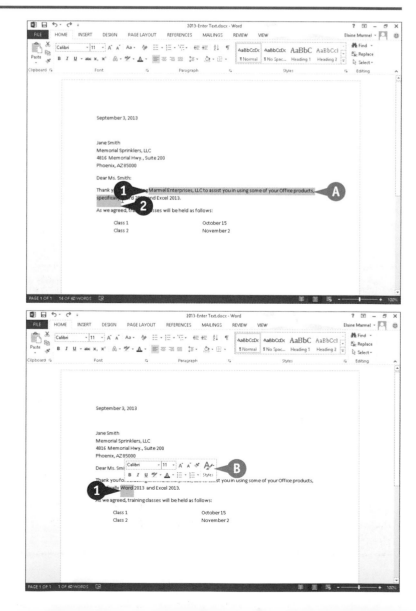

Select a Sentence

1 Press and hold **Ctrl**.

2 Click anywhere in the sentence you want to select.

C Word selects the entire sentence, and the Mini toolbar appears.

You can slide the mouse pointer away from the Mini toolbar to make it disappear.

Note: See Chapter 1 for details on using the Mini toolbar.

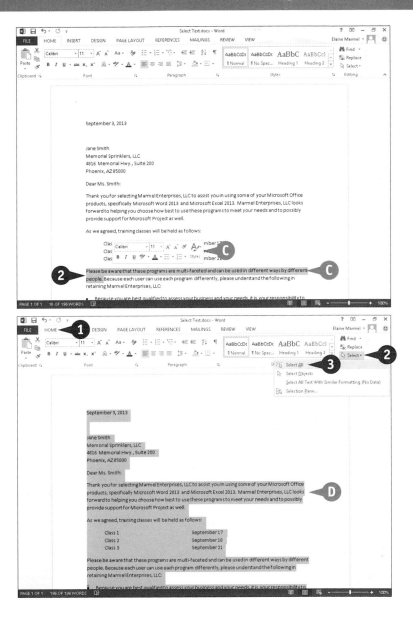

Select the Entire Document

1 Click the **Home** tab.

2 Click **Select**.

3 Click **Select All**.

D Word selects the entire document.

You also can press and hold **Ctrl** and press **A** to select the entire document.

To cancel the selection, click anywhere.

TIPS

Can I select text using the keyboard?
Yes. Press and hold **Shift** while pressing ←, →, ↑, or ↓. You also can press **Shift**+**Ctrl** to select, for example, several words in a row. If you press and hold **Shift**+**Ctrl** while pressing → five times, you select five consecutive words to the right of the insertion point.

How can I select noncontiguous text?
You select the first area using any of the techniques described in this section. Then press and hold **Ctrl** as you select the additional areas. Word selects all areas, even if text appears between them.

Mark and Find Your Place

When you want to mark your place in a document as you edit it so that you can easily return to it later, you can use the Bookmark feature. You can also use bookmarks to identify text that, for example, you plan to change but do not have the time to do so at the present. You can place the text in a bookmark so that you can easily locate it when you do have time to change it.

Bookmark indicators do not appear by default, but you can choose to display them as shown in this section. Bookmark indicators do not print.

Mark and Find Your Place

Mark Your Place

① Click the location you want to mark.

Note: If you select text instead of clicking at the location you want to mark, Word creates a bookmark containing text.

② Click the **Insert** tab.

③ Click **Links**.

④ Click **Bookmark**.

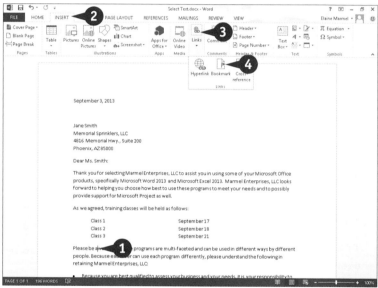

The Bookmark dialog box appears.

⑤ Type a name for the bookmark.

Note: Do not include spaces in a bookmark name.

⑥ Click **Add**.

Word saves the bookmark and closes the Bookmark dialog box.

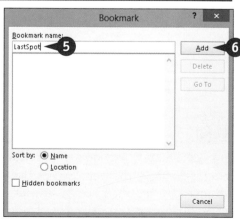

Find Your Place

1 Click the **Home** tab.

2 Click ▼ beside Find.

3 Click **Go To**.

The Go To tab of the Find and Replace dialog box appears.

4 Click **Bookmark**.

5 Click ▼, and select a bookmark.

6 Click **Go To**.

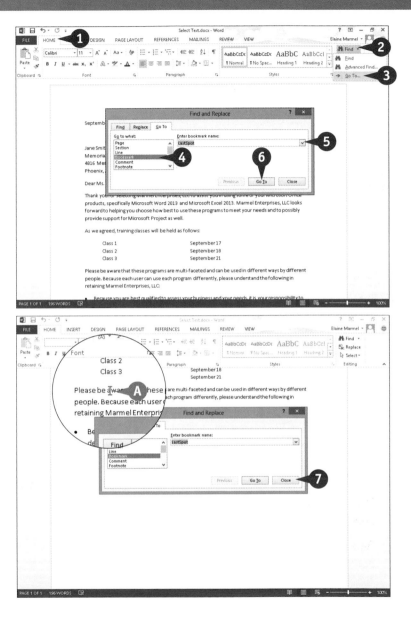

Ⓐ Word moves the insertion point to the bookmark.

Note: If the bookmark contains text, Word selects the text in the bookmark.

7 Click **Close**, or press `Esc`.

Word closes the Find and Replace dialog box.

TIP

How can I display bookmarks in my document?

Perform the steps that follow. Click the **File** tab and then click **Options**. In the Options dialog box, click **Advanced**. In the Show document content section, select **Show bookmarks** (☐ changes to ☑). Click **OK**, and Word displays open and close brackets representing the bookmark. A bookmark that marks a location looks like an I-beam (I).

Move or Copy Text

You can move information in your document by cutting and then pasting it. You also can repeat text by copying and then pasting it. For example, you might cut or copy information in a document and paste it elsewhere in the same document.

When you move text, the text disappears from the original location and appears in a new one. When you copy and paste text, it remains in the original location and also appears in a new one. You can move or copy information in two ways: using buttons on the Ribbon or using the drag-and-drop method.

Move or Copy Text

Using Ribbon Buttons

1. Select the text you want to move or copy.

Note: To select text, see the section "Select Text."

2. Click the **Home** tab.

3. To move text, click the **Cut** button (✂); to copy text, click the **Copy** button (📋).

Note: If you cut text, it disappears from the screen.

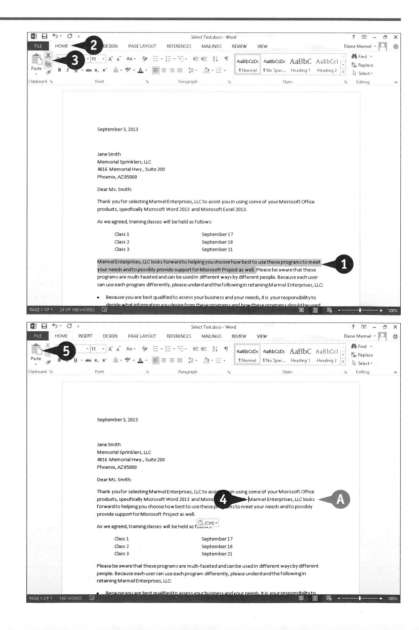

4. Click to place the insertion point at the location where you want the text to appear.

5. Click the **Paste** button.

A. The text appears at the new location.

Drag and Drop

1 Select the text you want to move or copy.

2 Position the mouse pointer over the selected text ($\text{I}^\equiv$ changes to $\mathbb{k}$).

3 Either move or copy the text.

To move text, drag the mouse ($\mathbb{k}$ changes to $\mathbb{k}$).

To copy text, press and hold Ctrl and drag the mouse ($\mathbb{k}$ changes to $\mathbb{k}$).

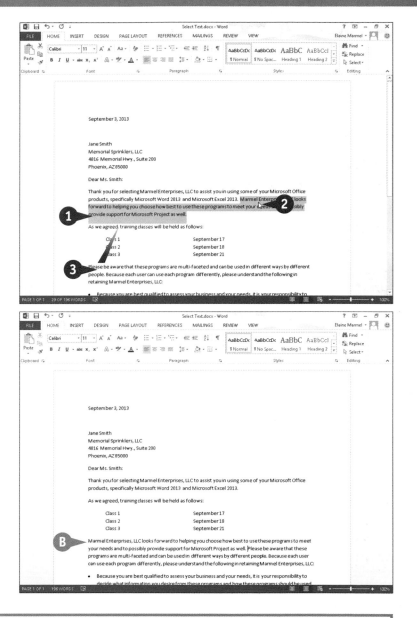

Ⓑ The text appears at the new location.

TIPS

Can I can move or copy text using menus?
Yes. Select the text that you want to move or copy, and then right-click it. The context menu and the Mini toolbar appear; click **Cut** or **Copy**. Then place the insertion point at the location where you want the text to appear, and right-click again. From the context menu, click **Paste**.

Can I copy or move information other than text?
Yes. You can copy or move any element that you can select, such as text, pictures, tables, graphics, and so on. You also can copy or move text from one Word document to another; see the next section, "Share Text between Documents."

Share Text between Documents

You can move or copy information both within the current document and between two or more documents. For example, suppose that you are working on a marketing report and some colleagues provide you with background information for your report. You can copy and paste the information from the colleagues' documents into your document.

Any text that you cut disappears from its original location. Text that you copy continues to appear in its original location and also appears in the new location you choose.

Share Text between Documents

1 Open the documents you want to use to share text.

2 Select the text you want to move or copy.

Note: For details on selecting text, see the section "Select Text."

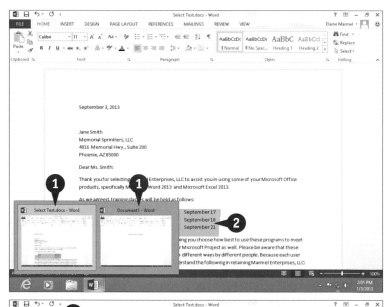

3 Click the **Home** tab.

4 Click ✂ to move text, or click 🗐 to copy text.

5 Switch to the other document by clicking its button in the Windows taskbar.

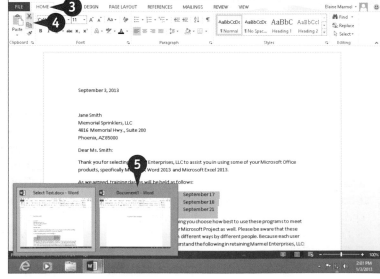

The other document appears.

6 Place the insertion point at the location where the text you are moving or copying should appear.

7 Click the **Paste** button.

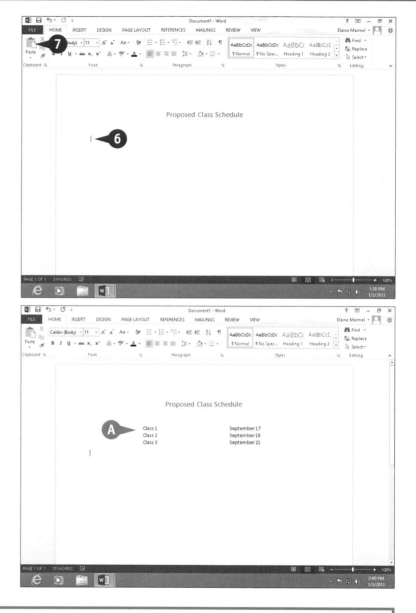

A The text appears in the new location.

TIPS

Why do I see a button when I paste?
Word displays the Paste Options button (🅱(Ctrl)▾) to give you the opportunity to determine how to handle the formatting of the selection you are pasting. See the section "Take Advantage of Paste Options" for details on how to use Paste options.

What format will Word use by default for text I paste?
The default appearance of pasted text depends on options set in the Word Options dialog box. To view or set the default appearance, click the **Paste Options** button (🅱(Ctrl)▾), click **Set Default Paste** to display the Word Options dialog box, and set options in the Cut, Copy, and Paste section.

Move or Copy Several Selections

Using the Office Clipboard, you can move or copy several selections at the same time. The Office Clipboard is the location where Word stores information you cut or copy until you paste it. By default, Word only stores the last information you cut or copied, making only that information available when you paste. However, if you open the Office Clipboard, Word can save up to the last 24 selections that you cut or copied. You can paste the items from the Office Clipboard into a single document or multiple documents in any order you want.

Move or Copy Several Selections

1 Click the **Home** tab.

2 Click the Clipboard group dialog box launcher (🗔).

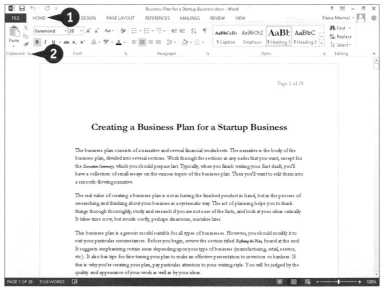

Ⓐ The Office Clipboard pane appears.

Note: If you cut or copied anything prior to this time, an entry appears in the Clipboard pane.

3 Select the text or information you want to move or copy.

4 Click the **Cut** button (✂) or the **Copy** button (🗐).

Ⓑ An entry appears in the Clipboard pane.

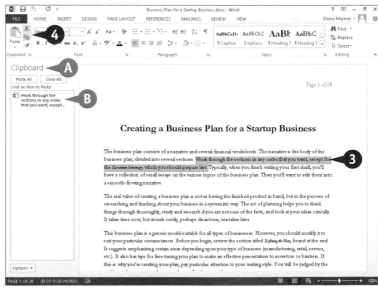

5 Repeat Steps **3** and **4** for each selection you want to move or copy.

C Word adds each entry to the Clipboard pane; the newest entry appears at the top of the pane.

6 Click in the document or in a different document where you want to place text you cut or copied.

7 Click a selection in the Clipboard pane to place it in the document.

D The entry appears in the document.

8 Repeat Steps **6** and **7** to paste other items from the Clipboard.

E If you want to place all the items in one location and the items appear in the Clipboard pane in the order you want them in your document, you can click **Paste All**.

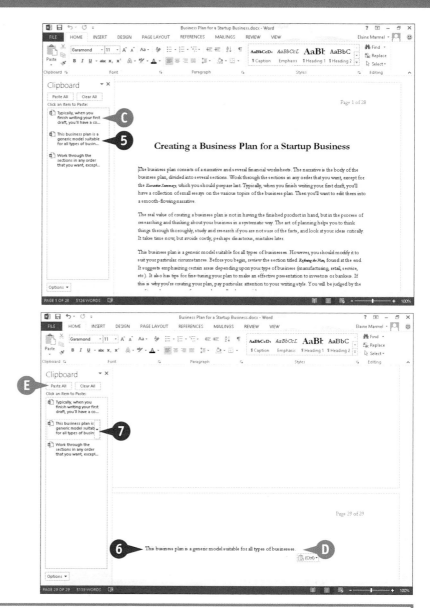

Why does a down arrow appear when I point at an item in the Clipboard pane?

If you click ▼ , a menu appears. From this menu, you can click **Paste** to add the item to your document, or you can click **Delete** to remove the item from the Clipboard pane.

Must I display the Office Clipboard to collect copied elements?

No. Click the **Options** button at the bottom of the Clipboard pane, and then click **Collect Without Showing Office Clipboard**. As you cut or copy, a message appears in the lower-right corner of your screen, telling you how many elements are stored on the Office Clipboard. You must display the Office Clipboard to paste any item except the one you last cut or copied.

Take Advantage of Paste Options

Sometimes, when you move or copy information, the formatting at the original location is not the formatting that you want to use at the destination location. Using Paste Options, you can choose the formatting Word applies to the selection at its new location. You can preview the formatting for a particular paste option without actually applying that formatting. The formatting options available depend upon the information you copy. This section shows how to paste information from an Excel workbook into a Word document; in this scenario, you see several options that might not appear if you paste information from one Word document to another.

Take Advantage of Paste Options

1 Make a selection; this example uses an Excel spreadsheet selection, but you can select text in a Word document.

2 Click the **Copy** button (📋) or the **Cut** button (✂).

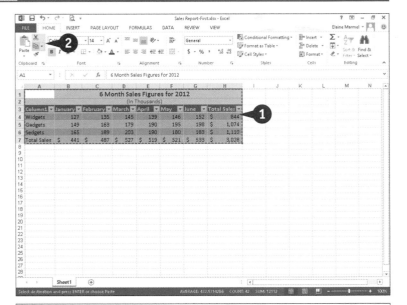

3 Position the insertion point in your Word document where you want to paste the information.

4 Click the bottom half of the **Paste** button.

A Buttons representing paste options appear.

5 To preview formatting for the selection, point at the **Keep Source Formatting** button (📋).

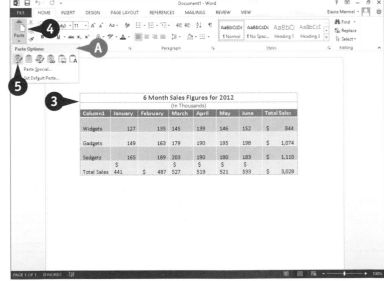

6 To preview formatting for the selection, point at the **Use Destination Styles** button ().

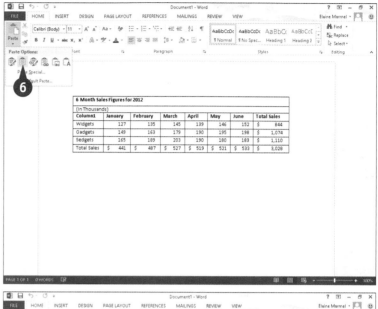

7 To preview formatting for the selection, point at the **Keep Text Only** button ().

8 Click a **Paste Options** button to paste the selection and specify its format in your Word document.

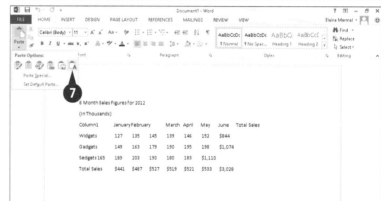

What do the various Paste Options buttons mean?

Button	Function	Button	Function
	Uses the formatting of the selection you copied or cut.		Formats the selection using the style of the location where you paste the selection and links the selection at the new location to the selection at the original location.
	Formats the selection using the style of the location where you paste the selection.		Formats the selection as a graphic that you cannot edit in Word.
	Uses the formatting of the selection you cut or copied and links the selection at the new location to the selection at the original location.		Applies no formatting to the selection; only text appears.

Switch Document Views

You can view a document five ways. The view you use depends entirely on what you are doing at the time; select the view that best meets your needs. For example, if you are working with a long document that has headings and sub-headings, and you want to work on the document's organization, Outline view might work best for you. On the other hand, if you are reviewing a document, consider Read Mode view, which has been updated to support tablet PC motions.

For more on the various views, see the section "Understanding Document Views."

Switch Document Views

1 Click the **View** tab.

2 Click one of the buttons in the Views group on the Ribbon: **Read Mode**, **Print Layout**, **Web Layout**, **Outline**, or **Draft**.

Word switches your document to the view you selected.

Note: In this example, the document switches from Print Layout view to Outline view, showing four outline levels, each representing a heading style.

Ⓐ Outline view displays its own tab of outline-related tools.

Ⓑ Buttons for three of the views also appear at the right edge of the status bar; position the mouse pointer over each button to see its function, and click a button to switch views:

📖 — Read Mode

📄 — Print Layout

📑 — Web Layout

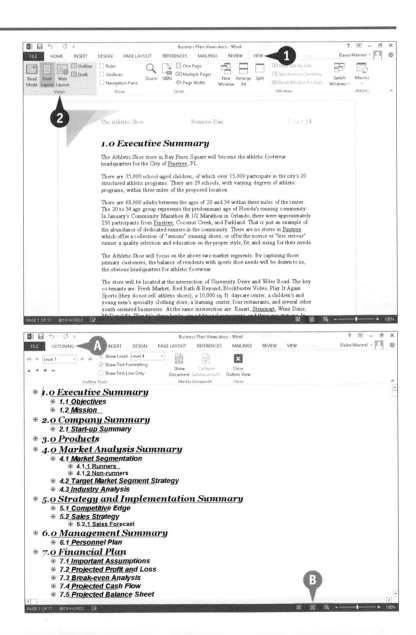

Understanding Document Views

Y ou can control the way that you view your document by choosing from five different views: Read
Mode, Print Layout, Web Layout, Outline, and Draft. The view you choose depends on what you
are doing. If you are reviewing a document and only doing minor editing, Read Mode works well.

Read Mode View

Read Mode, which supports tablet motions, view optimizes your document for
easier reading and helps minimize eye strain when you read a document
on-screen. This view removes most toolbars. To return to another view, click
View and then click **Edit Document** or press Esc .

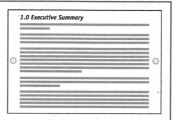

Print Layout View

Print Layout view presents a "what you see is what you get" view of your
document. In Print Layout view, you see elements of your document that
affect the printed page, such as margins, headers, and footers.

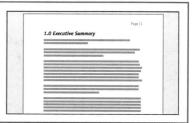

Web Layout View

Web Layout view is useful when you are designing a web page because it
displays a web page preview of your document.

Draft View

Draft view is designed for editing and formatting; it does not display your
document the way it will print. Instead, you can view elements such as the
Style Area — which shows the formatting style for each paragraph — on the
left side of the screen, but you cannot view certain document elements such as
graphics or the document's margins, headers, and footers.

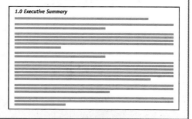

Outline View

Outline view helps you work with the organization of a
document. Word indents text styled as headings based
on the heading number; you can move or copy entire
sections of a document by moving or copying the
heading. You also can display the Style Area, as
shown here.

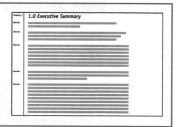

Heading 1 ⊕ **1.0 Executive Summary**
Heading 2   ⊕ *1.1 Objectives*
Heading 2   ⊕ *1.2 Mission*
Heading 1 ⊕ **2.0 Company Summary**
Heading 2   ⊕ *2.1 Start-up Summary*
Heading 1 ⊕ **3.0 Products**
Heading 1 ⊕ **4.0 Market Analysis Summary**
Heading 2   ⊕ *4.1 Market Segmentation*

Work with the Navigation Pane

If you are working with a very long document, using the scroll bar on the right side of the screen or the Page Up and Page Down keys on your keyboard to locate a particular page in that document can be time-consuming. To rectify this, you can use the Navigation Pane to navigate through a document. This pane can display all the headings in your document or a thumbnail image of each page in your document. You can then click a heading or a thumbnail image in the Navigation pane to view the corresponding page.

Work with the Navigation Pane

Navigate Using Headings

Note: To navigate using headings, your document must contain text styled with Heading styles. See Chapter 6 for details on styles.

1 Click the **View** tab.

2 Select **Navigation Pane**
(☐ changes to ✔).

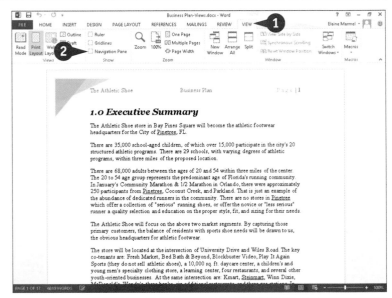

A The Navigation Pane appears.

B Heading 1 styles appear at the left edge of the Navigation Pane.

C Word indents Heading 2 styles slightly and each subsequent heading style a bit more.

D This icon (◢) represents a heading displaying subheadings; you can click it to hide subheadings.

E This icon (▷) represents a heading hiding subheadings; you can click it to display subheadings.

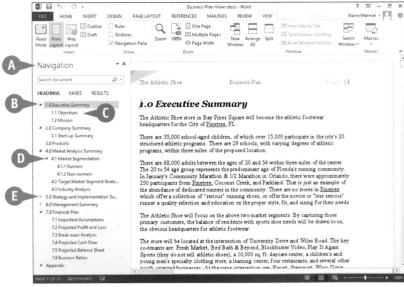

3 Click any heading in the Navigation Pane to select it.

F Word moves the insertion point to it in your document.

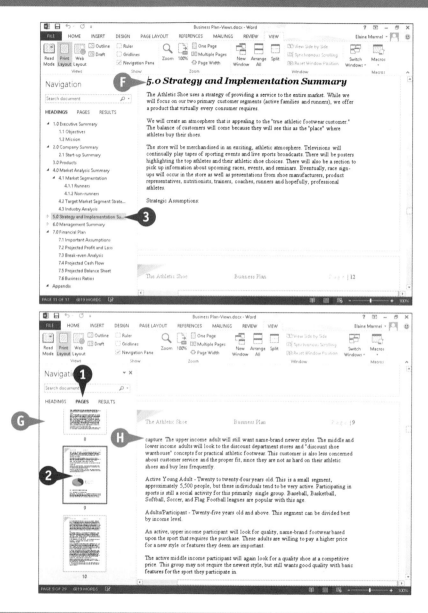

Navigate by Page

1 Click **Pages**.

G Word displays each page in your document as a thumbnail.

2 Click a thumbnail.

H Word selects that page in the Navigation Pane and moves the insertion point to the top of that page. Word surrounds the current page's thumbnail with a heavy blue border.

What do I do with the Search Document box?

You can use the Search Document box to find text in your document; see Chapter 4 for details on using this box and on other ways you can search for information in your document.

Can I control the headings that appear?

Yes. While viewing headings, right-click any heading in the Navigation pane. From the menu that appears, point at **Show Heading Levels** and, from the submenu that appears, click the heading level you want to display, such as **Show Heading 1**, **Show Heading 2**, and so on through **Show Heading 9**.

Insert Symbols

From time to time, you might need to insert a symbol such as a mathematical symbol or special character into your Word document. From the Symbol Gallery, you can insert many common symbols, including mathematical and Greek symbols, architectural symbols, and more. If you do not find the symbol you need in the Symbol Gallery, you can use the Symbol dialog box. The Symbol dialog box displays a list of recently used symbols as well as hundreds of symbols in a variety of fonts. You also can use the Symbol dialog box to insert special characters.

Insert Symbols

1 Click the location in the document where you want the symbol to appear.

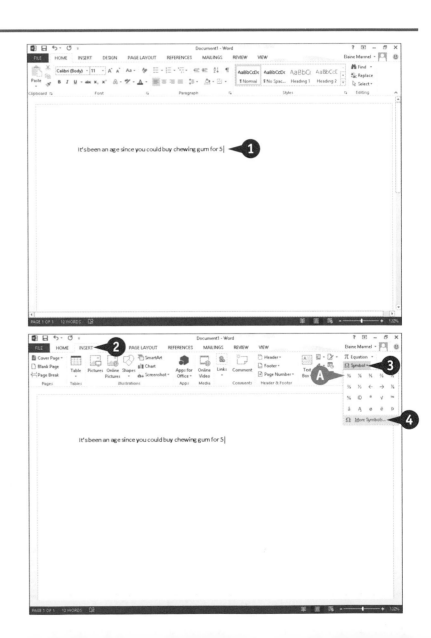

2 Click the **Insert** tab.

3 Click **Symbol**.

Ⓐ A gallery of commonly used symbols appears. If the symbol you need appears in the gallery, you can click it and skip the rest of these steps.

4 Click **More Symbols**.

The Symbol dialog box appears.

5 Click ⌄ to select the symbol's font.

The available symbols change to match the font you selected.

B You can click ⌃ and ⌄ to scroll through available symbols.

6 Click a symbol.

7 Click **Insert**.

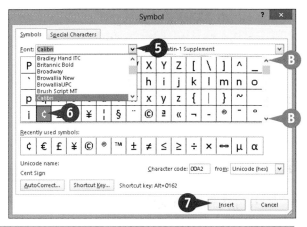

C The symbol appears at the current insertion point location in the document.

Note: You can control the size of the symbol the same way you control the size of text; see Chapter 6 for details.

The dialog box remains open so that you can add more symbols to your document.

8 When finished, click **Close**.

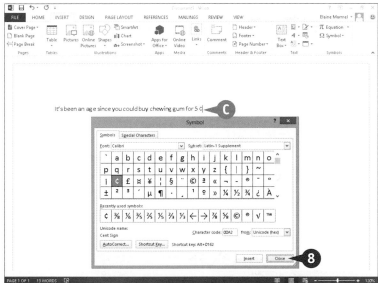

How do I add a special character?

To add a special character, open the Symbol dialog box and click the **Special Characters** tab. Locate and click the character you want to add, and then click **Insert**. Click **Close** to close the dialog box.

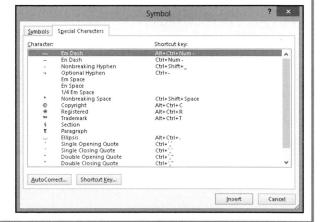

Work with Equations

You can easily create complex equations in Word 2013. The Equations Gallery contains many commonly used equations, such as the area of a circle or, for you physicists out there, the Fourier Series. If you do not see the equation you want, you might find it on Office.com.

If you add a structure to an equation, Word supplies dotted box placeholders for you to click and substitute constants or variables. Using the Equation Tools Design tab on the Ribbon, you can select formatting choices for your equation. Note that the Equation feature does not function when you work in Compatibility Mode.

Work with Equations

Insert an Equation

1 Position the insertion point where you want to insert an equation.

2 Click the **Insert** tab.

3 Click ▼ beside Equation.

Ⓐ The Equation Gallery, a list of commonly used equations, appears.

You can click an equation to insert it and then skip Steps **4** and **5**.

4 Click **Insert New Equation**.

Ⓑ Word inserts a blank equation box.

Ⓒ The Equations Tools Design tab appears on the Ribbon.

5 Type your equation.

You can click the tools on the Ribbon to help you type the equation.

6 Press ➡, or click outside the equation box.

Word hides the equation box, and you can continue typing.

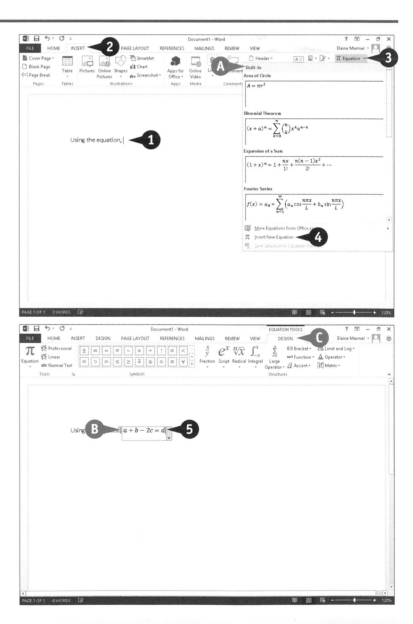

Delete an Equation

① Click anywhere in the equation to display it in the equation box.

② Click the three dots on the left side of the box.

Word highlights the contents of the equation box.

③ Press **Delete**.

Word deletes the equation from your document.

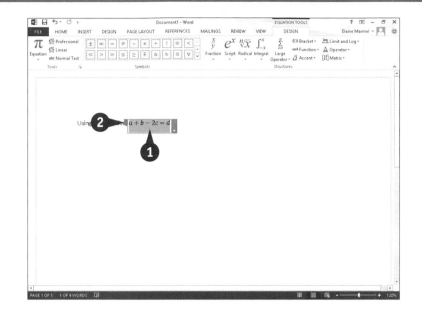

Can I save an equation that I use regularly so I do not have to create it each time I need it?

Yes. Follow these steps:

① Click anywhere in the equation.

② Click the three dots on the left side of the box.

③ Click the **Equation Tools Design** tab.

④ Click **Equation**.

⑤ Click **Save Selection to Equation Gallery**.

⑥ In the Create New Building Block dialog box that appears, click **OK**.

The next time you display the Equation Gallery, your equation appears on the list.

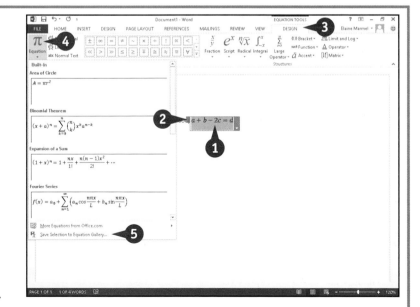

Zoom an Object

In Read Mode view, you can enlarge an image to get a better view of it. You can enlarge any type of image, including pictures, shapes, clip art, and inserted online videos, and you can zoom images in Word documents or in PDF files that you open in Word.

When you zoom an object, you can enlarge it twice from its original size; the first zoom level magnifies the image some, and the second zoom level makes the image fill the majority of your screen. Note that, although you can zoom inserted online videos, you can zoom them only to the first zoom level.

Zoom an Object

1. Open a document containing an image of any type.

2. Click 📖 to switch to Read Mode view.

3. Double-click the image.

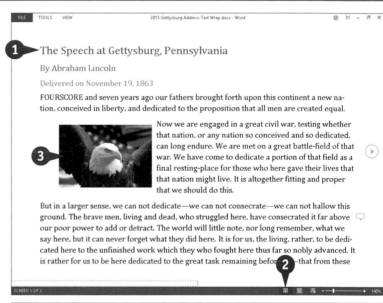

A. Word enlarges the image.

4. Click the Zoom arrow (🔍) in the upper-right corner of zoomed image.

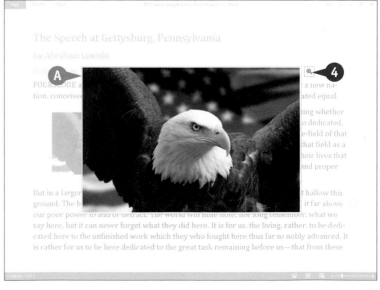

B Word enlarges the image even further.

C You can click the Zoom arrow (🔍) again, and Word switches between the first and second levels of zoom.

5 Press Esc, or click anywhere outside the image

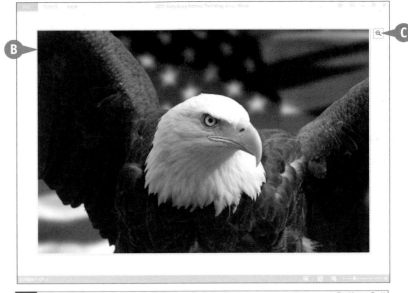

D Word redisplays the image in its original size, with the image selected; handles (⬜ and 🔄) surround the image.

Note: See Chapter 10 for details on working with images.

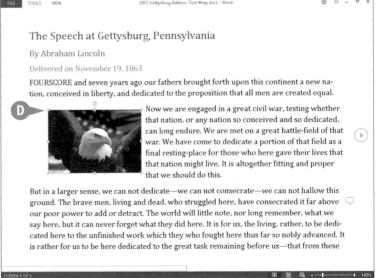

TIP

I tried to zoom an image in a PDF file, but more than just the image zoomed; why?
In all probability, the PDF file you opened was not created in Word. Although you can open a PDF file in Word, if the file was not created in Word, the original PDF layout will probably not translate properly. Word tends to read the PDF file content as objects rather than text and images, so in all likelihood, Word zoomed the image as well as text surrounding it that were part of the original PDF file layout.

Zoom In or Out

The Zoom feature controls the magnification of your document on-screen; you can use it to enlarge or reduce the size of the text. Zooming in enlarges text. Zooming out reduces text, providing more of an overview of your document. Zooming does not affect the printed size of your text; it simply makes text larger or smaller on-screen.

You can zoom using the Zoom dialog box, as shown in this section, or for less precise zooming, you can use the Zoom slider bar located in the lower-right corner of the Word window.

Zoom In or Out

1 Click the **View** tab.

2 Click **Zoom**.

The Zoom dialog box appears.

3 Click a zoom setting.

Ⓐ You can click the **Many pages** button and select to display multiple pages.

Note: The number of pages you can view depends on the resolution you set for your monitor.

Ⓑ A preview of the settings you choose appears here.

4 Click **OK**.

The document appears on-screen using the new zoom setting.

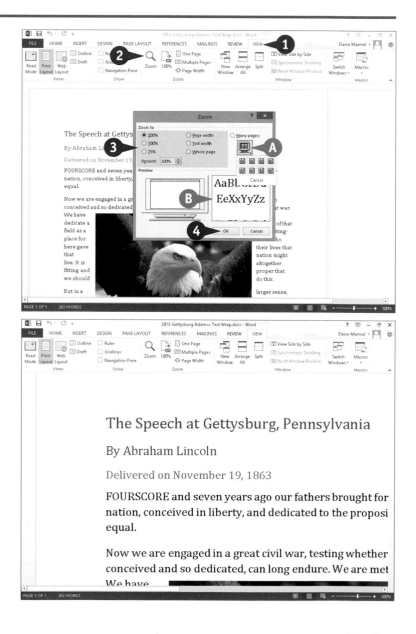

Translate Text

You can translate a word from one language to another using language dictionaries installed on your computer. If you are connected to the Internet, the Translation feature searches the dictionaries on your computer as well as online dictionaries.

You can choose Translate Document from the Translate drop-down menu to send the document over the Internet for translation, but be aware that Word sends documents as unencrypted HTML files. If security is an issue, do not choose this route; instead, consider hiring a professional translator.

Translate Text

1 Select a phrase to translate.

2 Click the **Review** tab.

3 Click **Translate**.

4 Click **Translate Selected Text**.

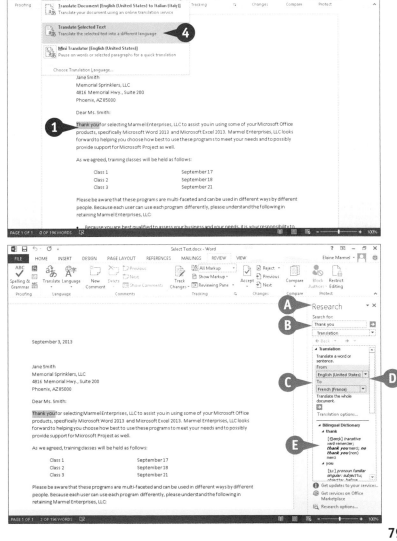

Ⓐ The Research pane appears.

Ⓑ The phrase you selected appears here.

Ⓒ The current translation languages appear here.

Ⓓ You can click ▼ to display available translation languages.

Ⓔ The translation appears here.

Set Options for Additional Actions

The Additional Actions feature provides you with a way to save time. When you enable this feature, Word recognizes certain types of context-sensitive information, such as an address or a date, and gives you the opportunity to use the information to take extra steps. For example, for an address, you can display a map or driving directions or add the information to Outlook contacts. For a date, you can display your Outlook Calendar.

You can control the kinds of information Word recognizes and identifies for additional actions that can save you time. You also can turn off additional action recognition entirely.

Set Options for Additional Actions

1 Click the **File** tab.

Backstage view appears.

2 Click **Options**.

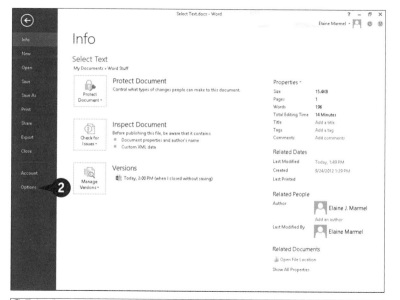

The Word Options dialog box appears.

3 Click **Proofing**.

4 Click **AutoCorrect Options**.

The AutoCorrect dialog box appears.

5 Click the **Actions** tab.

6 You can select this option (☐ changes to ☑) to turn on recognition of additional actions.

7 Turn additional action recognition on (☑) or off (☐).

8 Click **OK** to close the AutoCorrect dialog box.

9 Click **OK** to close the Word Options window.

Word saves your preferences.

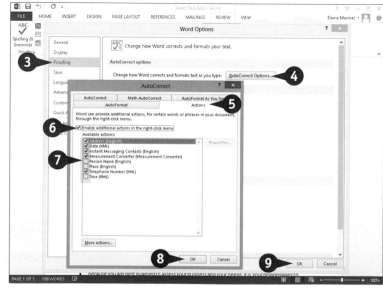

Using Additional Actions

You can use the Additional Actions feature to save time. Using this feature, Word recognizes certain context-sensitive information and provides extra information. With this feature, Word can convert measurements, add a person or telephone number to Outlook Contacts, schedule a meeting, display a map of a location, or get you driving directions to that location.

This feature may not be on by default; see the previous section, "Set Options for Additional Actions." This section shows you how to use the Additional Actions feature.

Using Additional Actions

1 Right-click text for which you have enabled additional actions. In this example, an address is used.

A A context menu appears.

2 Click **Additional Actions**.

B Word displays a list of actions you can take using the text.

3 Click an action.

Word performs the action, or the program that performs the action you selected appears on-screen.

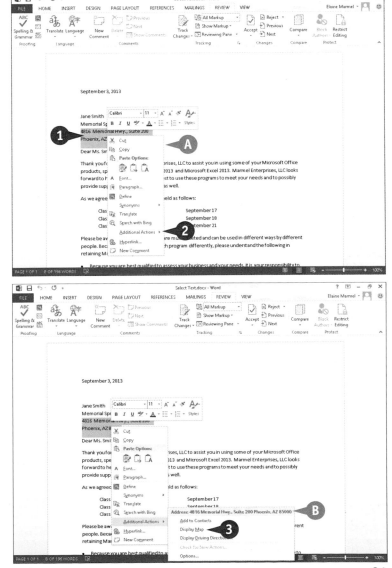

CHAPTER 4

Proofreading

This chapter shows you how to handle proofreading tasks in Word. You can search through text to find something in particular or to replace text. Word contains some features to help you define words and address spelling and grammar issues. This chapter also shows you how to track revisions and work with revisions and comments provided by reviewers.

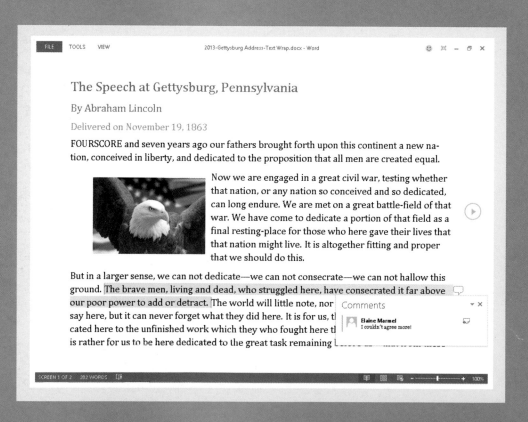

Work in Read Mode View

Read Mode view optimizes your document for easier reading and helps minimize eye strain when you read a document on-screen. This view removes most toolbars. Read Mode view supports mouse, keyboard, and tablet motions. To move from page to page in a document using your mouse, you can click the arrows on the left and right sides of the pages or use the scroll wheel. To navigate using the keyboard, you can press the Page Up, Page Down, space bar, and Backspace keys on the keyboard, or press any arrow key. If you use a tablet or other touch pad device, swipe left or right with your finger.

Work in Read Mode View

Look Up Information Using Define

1. Click 📖 to display the document in Read Mode.

2. Select the word you want to look up, and right-click.

3. From the menu that appears, click **Define**.

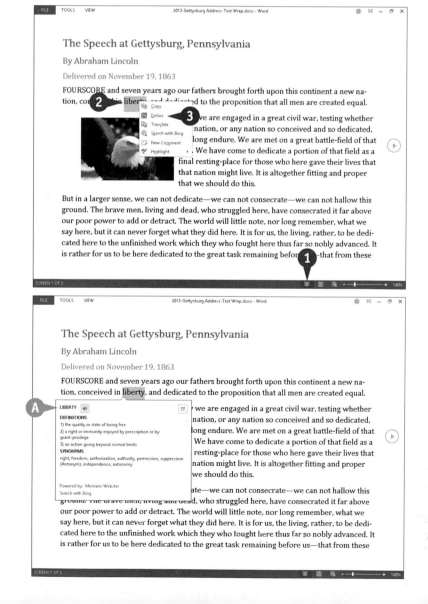

Note: If you have not yet installed a dictionary, a pane appears, giving you dictionary choices. See Chapter 13 for details on downloading and installing a dictionary.

Ⓐ Word displays a balloon containing definition information.

You can click anywhere outside of the balloon to close it.

Search for Information Using Bing

1 Click 📖 to display the document in Read Mode.

2 Select the word or phrase you want to look up, and right-click.

3 From the menu that appears, click **Search with Bing**.

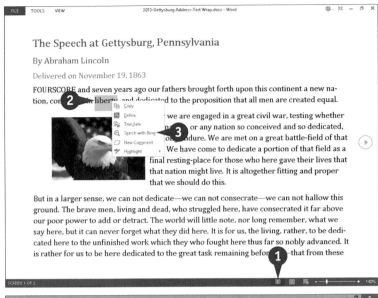

Your browser opens, displaying search results for the word you selected in Step **2**.

4 Close the browser window by clicking ⊠ in the upper-right corner to redisplay your document in Word.

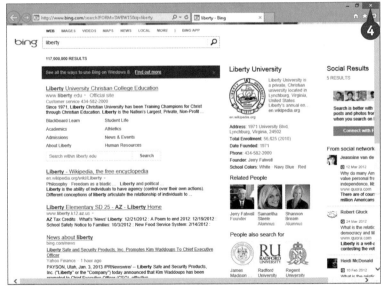

TIP

Can I change the color of the page?
Yes. Follow these steps:

1 Click **View**.

2 Click **Page Color**.

3 Choose a page color.

This example uses Sepia.

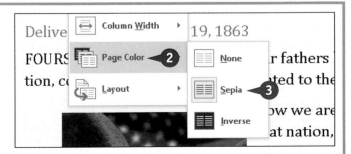

continued ▶

Read Mode view offers more than just minimized eye strain; while you work in Read Mode view, you can look up words in the dictionary, search the Internet for a word or phrase, highlight important text, and insert comments in documents you are reviewing. If you are viewing a long document in Read Mode view, you also can use the Navigation pane to move around the document. You can open the Navigation pane from the Tools menu in Read Mode view; for details on using the Navigation pane, see Chapter 3.

Work in Read Mode View (continued)

Highlight Important Text

1 Click 📖 to display the document in Read Mode.

2 Select the words you want to highlight, and right-click.

3 From the menu that appears, click **Highlight**.

4 Click a highlight color.

A Word highlights the selected text in the color you chose.

You can click anywhere outside the highlight to see its full effect and continue working.

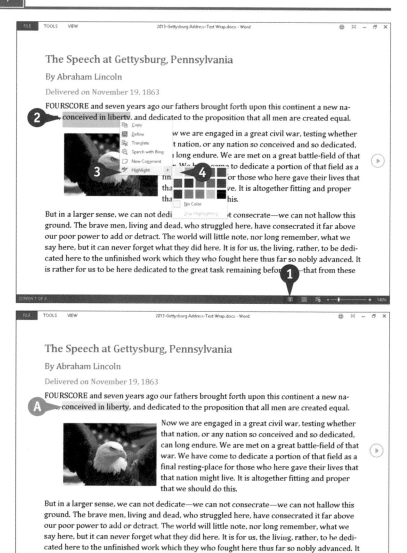

Insert a Comment

1 Click 📖 to display the document in Read Mode.

2 Select the words about which you want to comment, and right-click.

3 From the menu that appears, click **New Comment**.

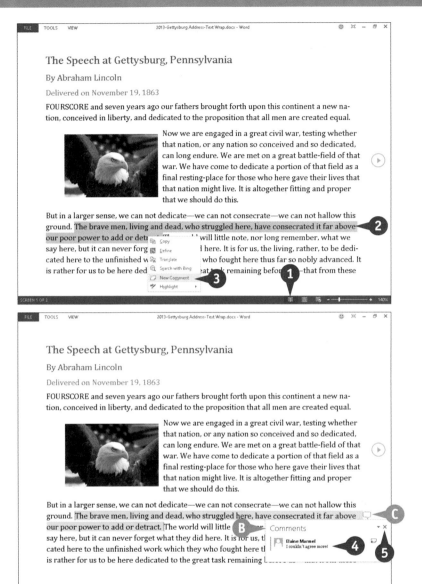

B Word changes the color used to select the text and displays a comment block containing the insertion point.

4 Type your comment.

5 Click × to close the comment block.

C This symbol represents your comment; click it at any time to view the comment.

TIPS

What are some of the different views available in Read Mode?

To display all comments in the document click **View** and then click **Show Comments**. To view your document as if it were printed on paper, click **View** and then click **Layout**. From the menu that appears, click **Paper Layout**.

Can I change the column width?

Yes. Click **View**, and then click **Column Width**. From the menu that appears, choose **Narrow** or **Wide**; click **Default** to return to the original column view. Note that on a standard monitor, Default and Wide look the same; Wide takes effect on wide-screen monitors.

Search for Text

Occasionally, you need to search for a word or phrase in a document. For example, suppose you want to edit a paragraph in your document that contains a specific word or phrase. You can use Word's Find tool to search for the word or phrase instead of scrolling through your document to locate that paragraph. You can search for all occurrences simultaneously or for each single occurrence in the order in which they occur from the current position of the insertion point.

This section focuses on finding text; see the next section, "Substitute Text," for information on finding and replacing text.

Search for Text

Search for All Occurrences

1. Click the **Home** tab.

2. Click **Find**.

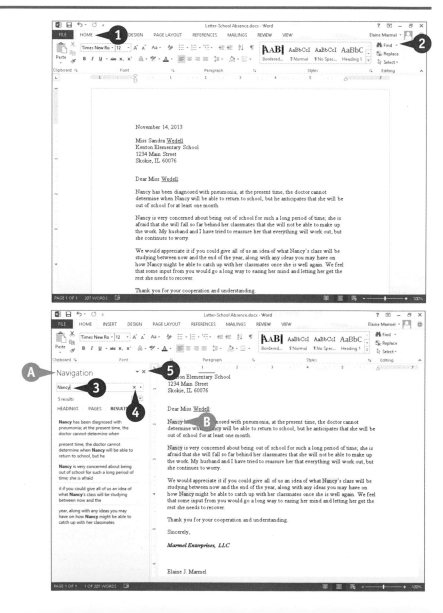

A. The Navigation pane appears.

3. Type the word or phrase for which you want to search.

B. Word highlights all occurrences of the word or phrase in yellow.

4. Click × to clear the search and results.

5. Click × to close the Navigation pane.

Search for One Occurrence at a Time

1 Press **Ctrl** + **Home** to position the insertion point at the beginning of your document.

2 Click the **Home** tab.

3 Click ▼ beside the Find button.

4 Click **Advanced Find** to display the Find and Replace dialog box.

5 Type the word or phrase for which you want to search.

C You can click **More** (More changes to Less) to display additional search options.

D You can click **Reading Highlight** and then click **Highlight All** to highlight each occurrence.

E You can click **Find in** to limit the search to the main document or the headers and footers.

6 Click **Find Next** to view each occurrence.

7 When Word finds no more occurrences, a dialog box appears telling you that the search is finished; click **OK**.

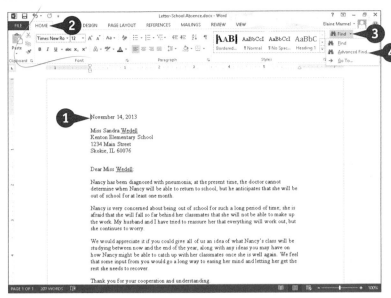

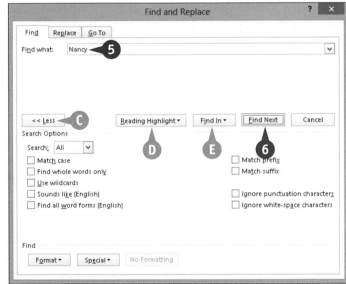

TIPS

How can I set options to limit my search in the Navigation pane?

Complete Steps **1** and **2** in the subsection "Search for All Occurrences" to open the Navigation pane. Click ▼ in the search box. Click **Options** to display the Find Options dialog box, where you can set the same options you set when following the steps in the subsection "Search for One Occurrence at a Time."

Can I search for elements other than words?

Yes. Complete Steps **1** and **2** in the subsection "Search for All Occurrences" to open the Navigation pane. Click ▼ in the search box. From the menu that appears, you can search for graphics, tables, equations, footnotes or endnotes, and comments.

Substitute Text

Often, you want to find a word or phrase because you need to substitute some other word or phrase for it. For example, suppose you complete a long report, only to discover that you have misspelled the name of a product you are reviewing. You do not need to hunt through the document to change each occurrence; you can use the Replace tool to substitute a word or phrase for all occurrences of the original word or phrase.

On the other hand, you can selectively substitute one word or phrase for another — a particularly useful tool when you have overused a word.

Substitute Text

1 Press **Ctrl**+**Home** to position the insertion point at the beginning of your document.

2 Click the **Home** tab.

3 Click **Replace**.

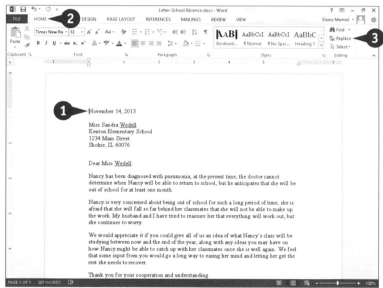

The Find and Replace dialog box appears.

4 Type the word or phrase you want to replace here.

5 Type the word or phrase you want Word to substitute here.

A You can click **More** to display additional search and replace options (More changes to Less).

6 Click **Find Next**.

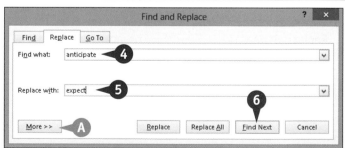

B Word highlights the first occurrence of the word or phrase that it finds.

C If you do not want to change the highlighted occurrence, you can click **Find Next** to ignore it.

7 Click **Replace**.

D To change all occurrences in the document, you can click **Replace All**.

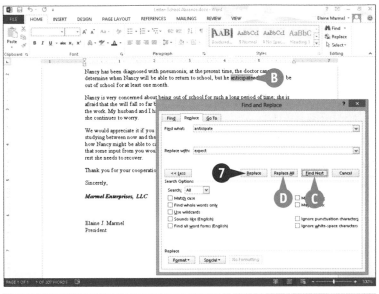

E Word replaces the original word or phrase with the word or phrase you specify as the substitute.

8 Repeat Steps **6** and **7** as needed.

9 When Word finds no more occurrences, a dialog box appears telling you that the search is finished; click **OK**.

F The Cancel button in the Find and Replace dialog box changes to Close.

10 Click **Close** to close the Find and Replace dialog box.

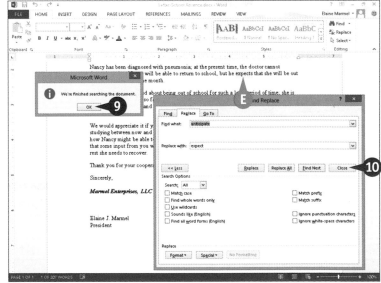

TIPS

Can I find italic text and change it to boldface text?

Yes. Follow Steps **1** to **3**, and click **More** to expand the window. Follow Steps **4** and **5**, but, instead of typing text, click **Format** and then click **Font**. In the Font style list of the Font dialog box that appears, click **Italic** for Step **4** and **Bold** for Step **5**. Then complete Steps **6** to **10**.

Can I search for and replace special characters such as tabs or paragraph marks?

Yes. Follow Steps **1** to **3**, and click **More** to expand the window. Then follow Steps **4** and **5**, but instead of typing text, click **Special** to display a menu of special characters. For Step **4**, select the special character you want to find. For Step **5**, select the special character you want to substitute. Then complete Steps **6** to **10**.

Count Words in a Document

You can count the number of words in a selection, sentence, paragraph, or document or in any portion of a document. Suppose, for example, that your history teacher just assigned you to write a paper describing the First Continental Congress, and the paper must be at least 500 words long. You can use the Word Count feature.

This feature also comes in particularly handy when you must limit the number of words in a section of a document. For example, college application essays often require that you write no more than 500 words.

Count Words in a Document

Display the Word Count

1 Right-click the status bar.

Ⓐ The Status Bar Configuration menu appears.

Ⓑ The number of words in the document appears here.

2 If no check mark appears beside Word Count, click **Word Count**; otherwise, skip this step.

3 Click anywhere outside the menu.

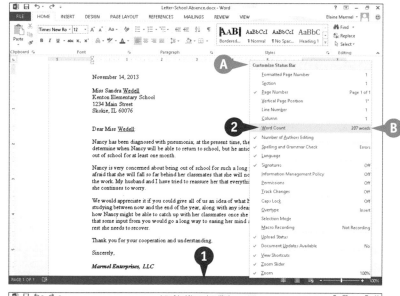

Ⓒ Word closes the menu, and the number of words in the document appears on the status bar.

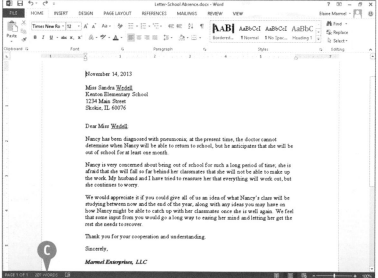

Display Count Statistics

1 Click the word count on the status bar.

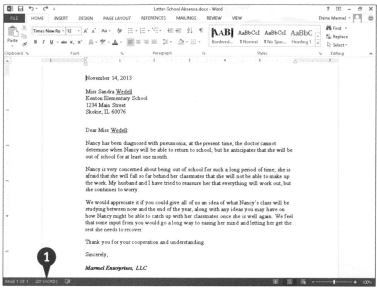

The Word Count dialog box appears.

The Word Count dialog box reports the number of pages, words, characters with and without spaces, paragraphs, and lines in your document.

2 When you finish reviewing count statistics, click **Close**.

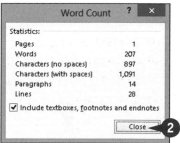

TIP

Can I count the number of words in just one paragraph?

Yes. Do the following:

1 Select the text containing the words you want to count.

A Both the number of words in the selection and the total words in the document appear in the Word Count box on the status bar.

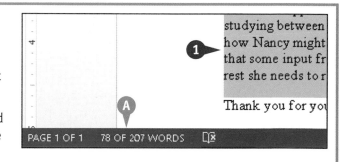

Automatically Correct Mistakes

Using the AutoCorrect feature, Word automatically corrects hundreds of common typing and spelling mistakes as you work, using a preset list of misspellings.

To speed up your text-entry tasks, you can add your own problem words — ones you commonly misspell — to the list. The next time you mistype the word, AutoCorrect fixes your mistake for you. If you find that AutoCorrect consistently changes a word that is correct as is, you can remove that word from the AutoCorrect list. If you would prefer that AutoCorrect not make any changes to your text as you type, you can disable the feature.

Automatically Correct Mistakes

1 Click the **File** tab.

Backstage view appears.

2 Click **Options**.

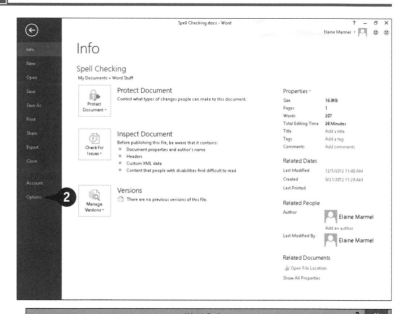

The Word Options dialog box appears.

3 Click **Proofing** to display proofing options.

4 Click **AutoCorrect Options**.

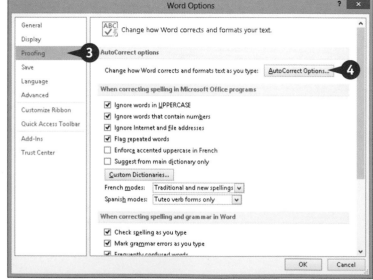

The AutoCorrect dialog box appears.

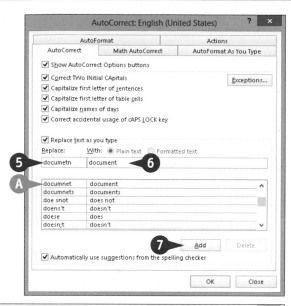

A The corrections Word already makes automatically appear in this area.

5 Click here, and type the word you typically mistype or misspell.

6 Click here, and type the correct version of the word.

7 Click **Add**.

B Word adds the entry to the list to automatically correct.

You can repeat Steps **5** to **7** for each automatic correction you want to add.

8 Click **OK** to close the AutoCorrect dialog box.

9 Click **OK** to close the Word Options dialog box.

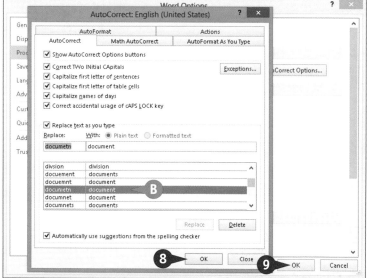

How does automatic correction work?

As you type, if you mistype or misspell a word stored as an AutoCorrect entry, Word corrects the entry when you press Spacebar, Tab, or Enter.

What should I do if Word automatically replaces an entry that I do not want replaced?

Position the insertion point at the beginning of the AutoCorrected word, and click the **AutoCorrect Options** button (🏷). From the list that appears, click **Change back to**. To make Word permanently stop correcting an entry, follow Steps **1** to **4**, click the stored AutoCorrect entry in the list, and then click **Delete**.

Automatically Insert Frequently Used Text

Suppose you repeatedly type the same text in your documents — for example, your company name. You can add this text to Word's Quick Parts Gallery; then, the next time you need to add the text to a document, you can select it from the gallery instead of retyping it.

In addition to creating your own Quick Parts for use in your documents, you can use any of the wide variety of preset phrases included with Word. You access these preset Quick Parts from Word's Building Blocks Organizer window. (See the tip at the end of this section for more information.)

Automatically Insert Frequently Used Text

Create a Quick Parts Entry

1 Type the text that you want to store, including all formatting that should appear each time you insert the entry.

2 Select the text you typed.

3 Click the **Insert** tab.

4 Click the **Quick Parts** button (⊞ ▾).

5 Click **Save Selection to Quick Part Gallery**.

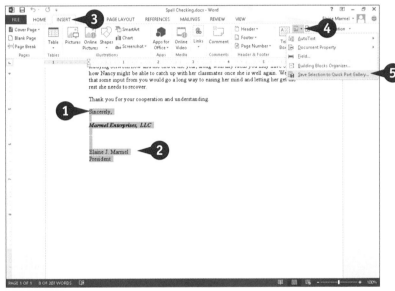

The Create New Building Block dialog box appears.

6 Type a name that you want to use as a shortcut for the entry.

A You can also assign a gallery, a category, and a description for the entry.

7 Click **OK**.

Word stores the entry on the Quick Part Gallery.

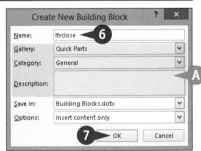

Insert a Quick Part Entry

1 Click in the text where you want to insert a Quick Part.

2 Click the **Insert** tab.

3 Click the **Quick Parts** button (▣ ▾).

All building blocks you define as Quick Parts appear on the Quick Part Gallery.

4 Click the entry that you want to insert.

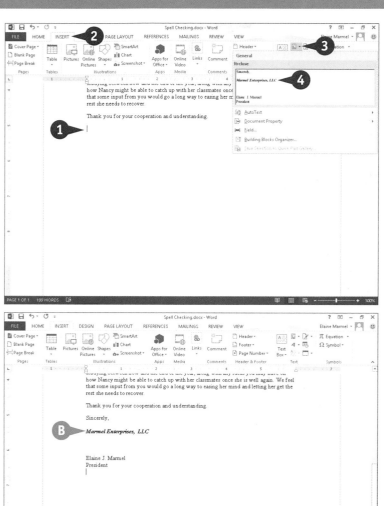

B Word inserts the entry into the document.

Note: You can use the Quick Part without using the mouse by typing the name you assigned to the entry and then pressing **F3**.

TIPS

How can I find and use an AutoText entry?
Click **Insert**, and then click **Quick Parts**. Below the Quick Parts Gallery, point at **AutoText**. A gallery of all the AutoText entries appears.

How do I remove a Quick Parts entry?
To remove a Quick Parts entry from the Building Blocks Organizer, open the Organizer (see the preceding tip for help), locate and select the entry you want to remove, click **Delete**, and click **Yes** in the dialog box that appears.

Check Spelling and Grammar

Word automatically checks for spelling and grammar errors as you type. Misspellings appear underlined with a red wavy line, and grammar errors are underlined with a blue wavy line. If you prefer, you can turn off Word's automatic Spelling and Grammar Check features, as described in the next section.

If you prefer, you can review your entire document for spelling and grammatical errors all at one time. To use Word's Spelling and Grammar checking feature, you must install a dictionary; see Chapter 13 for details on installing apps for Word.

Check Spelling and Grammar

Correct a Mistake

1 When you encounter a spelling or grammar problem, right-click the underlined text.

2 Click a correction from the menu that appears.

A To ignore the error, you can click **Ignore All**.

B To make Word stop flagging a word as misspelled, click **Add to Dictionary**.

Run the Spell Checker

1 Click at the beginning of your document.

2 Click the **Review** tab.

3 Click **Spelling & Grammar**.

C Word selects the first spelling or grammar mistake and displays the Spelling or Grammar pane.

D The spelling or grammar mistake appears here.

E Suggestions to correct the error appear here.

F Definitions of the error and the highlighted suggestion appear here.

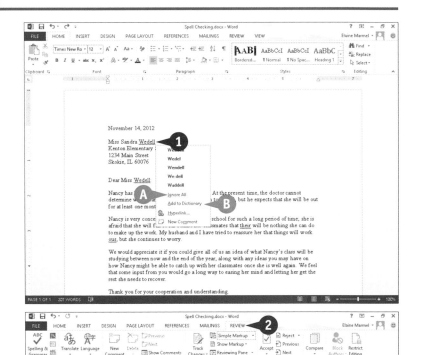

4 Click the suggestion you want to use.

5 Click **Change**.

G To correct all misspellings of the same word, you can click **Change All**.

H You can click **Ignore** or **Ignore All** to leave the selected word or phrase unchanged.

6 Repeat Steps **4** and **5** for each spelling or grammar mistake.

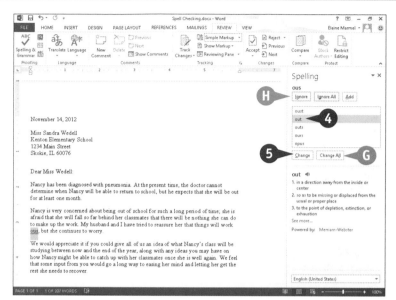

Word displays a dialog box when it finishes checking for spelling and grammar mistakes.

7 Click **OK**.

Note: To check only a section of your document, select that section.

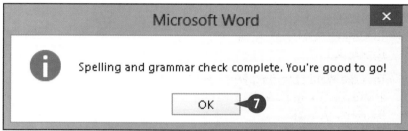

TIP

When should I use the Add to Dictionary button?

Word identifies misspellings by comparing words in your document to whichever dictionary you chose to install. (See Chapter 13 for details on downloading and installing apps like the dictionary for Word.) When a word you type does not appear in the dictionary being used by Word, Word flags the word as misspelled. The word might be a term that you use regularly; if so, click **Add to Dictionary** so that Word stops flagging the word as a misspelling.

Disable Grammar and Spell Checking

By default, Word automatically checks spelling and grammar by displaying red and blue squiggly lines whenever it identifies a spelling or grammar mistake. If the red and blue squiggly underlines annoy you, you can turn off automatic spelling and grammar checking. When you turn off automatic spelling and grammar checking, Word no longer displays red and blue squiggly lines under words or phrases it does not recognize. You can always check spelling and grammar after you complete your work on your document but before you send it to the recipient or to co-workers for review.

Disable Grammar and Spell Checking

1 Click the **File** tab.

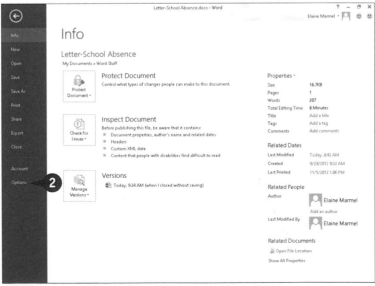

Backstage view appears.

2 Click **Options**.

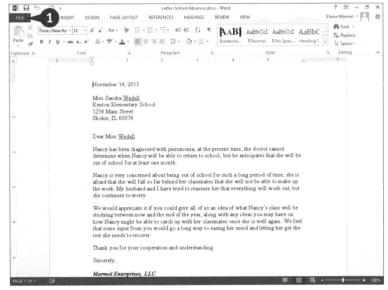

The Word Options dialog box appears.

3 Click **Proofing**.

4 Deselect **Check spelling as you type** (☑ changes to ☐) to disable automatic spell checking.

5 Deselect **Mark grammar errors as you type** (☑ changes to ☐) to disable automatic grammar checking.

6 Click **OK**.

Ⓐ Word no longer identifies the spelling and grammar errors in the current document.

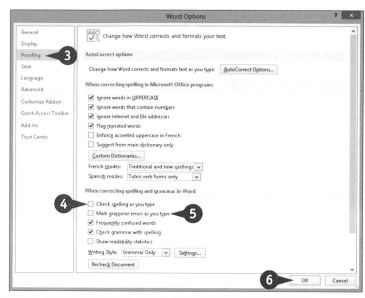

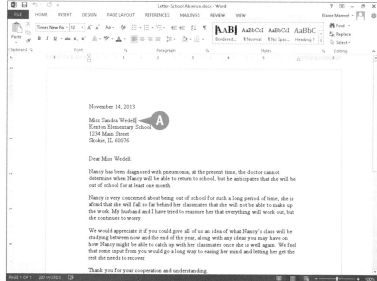

TIPS

If I disable automatic spelling and grammar checking, how do I check spelling and grammar?
Use the procedure described in the section "Check Spelling and Grammar." When you follow the procedure in that section, you disable only the portion of the feature where Word automatically identifies misspellings or grammar mistakes with squiggly red or blue underlines.

What should I do if I change my mind and decide that I want to see the red and blue squiggly lines?
Repeat the steps in this section, selecting the options you deselected previously (☐ changes to ☑).

Find a Synonym or Antonym with the Thesaurus

If you are having trouble finding just the right word or phrase, you use Word's thesaurus to find a more suitable word than the word you originally chose. The thesaurus can help you find a synonym — a word with a similar meaning — for the word you originally chose, as well as an antonym, which is a word with an opposite meaning.

Word displays synonyms and antonyms as major headings in the Thesaurus pane; you can identify a major heading because a carat appears beside it. Each word under a major heading is a synonym or antonym that you can substitute in your document.

Find a Synonym or Antonym with the Thesaurus

① Click the word for which you want to find an opposite or substitute.

② Click the **Review** tab.

③ Click the **Thesaurus** button (▥).

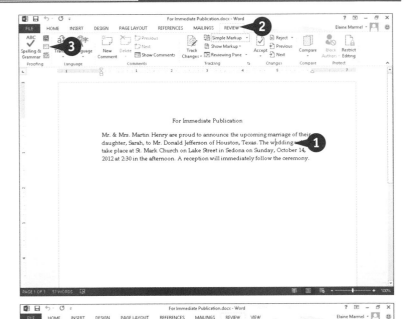

Ⓐ The Thesaurus pane appears.

Ⓑ The word you selected appears here.

Ⓒ Each word with a carat on its left and a part of speech on its right represents a major heading.

Note: You cannot substitute major headings for the word in your document.

Ⓓ Each word listed below a major heading is a synonym or antonym for the major heading.

Ⓔ Antonyms are marked.

4 Point the mouse at the word you want to use in your document, and click the ▼ that appears.

5 Click **Insert**.

F Word replaces the word in your document with the one in the Thesaurus pane.

6 Click × to close the Thesaurus pane.

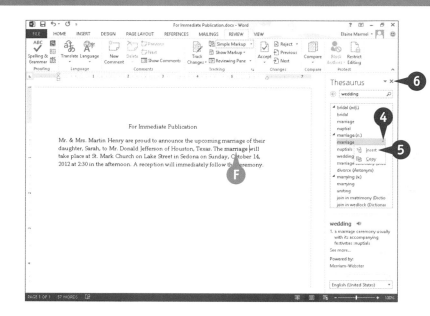

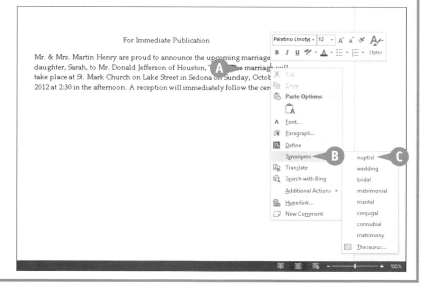

Is there a faster way I can display synonyms and antonyms?

Yes. You can use the keyboard shortcut **Shift** + **F7** to open the Thesaurus pane, or you can perform the steps that follow. Click the word for which you want a synonym or antonym (**A**). Right-click the word and click **Synonyms** (**B**) from the menu that appears. Click a choice to replace the word in your document (**C**).

Find a Definition

You can look up the definition of a word at any time from any Word view. You can see a definition of a word at the bottom of the Thesaurus pane; refer to the section "Find a Synonym or Antonym with the Thesaurus" for details.

If you prefer, you can bypass the thesaurus and use a dictionary; Word 2013 does not come with a dictionary installed. Instead, you must download a dictionary from the Office App store and install it; see Chapter 13 for details on how to download and install an Office app.

Find a Definition

1 Click anywhere in the word for which you want a definition.

2 Click the **Review** tab.

3 Click the **Define** button ( ).

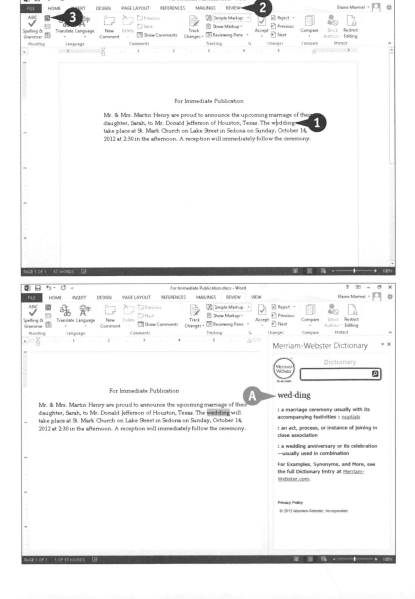

Ⓐ A pane appears on the right side of the screen, displaying various definitions for the word you selected.

Track Document Changes During Review

Word can track the editing and formatting changes made to your document. This feature is particularly useful when more than one person works on the same document. When Word tracks document revisions, it uses different colors to track the changes made and who made them, so that you can easily identify who did what to a document. By default, Word displays changes in Simple Markup view, which indicates, in the left margin, areas that have changes. If you prefer to see changes as you make them, you can view all changes as you work by switching to All Markup view.

Track Document Changes During Review

① Click the **Review** tab.

② Click **Track Changes** to enable change tracking.

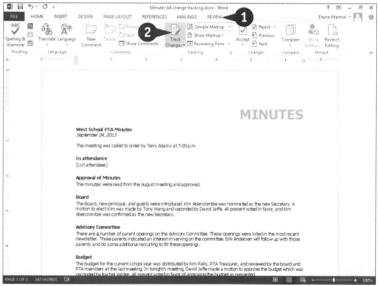

③ Make changes to the document as needed.

Ⓐ A red vertical bar appears in the left margin beside lines containing changes.

Ⓑ If you prefer to view changes as you work, click ▼ beside Simple Markup and choose **All Markup**.

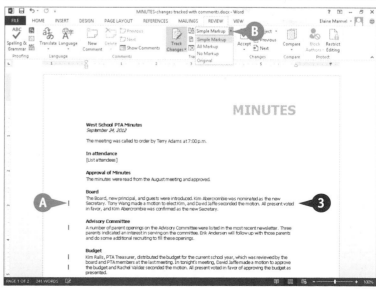

Lock and Unlock Tracking

You can control who can turn change tracking on and off using the Lock Tracking feature, which requires a password to turn off change tracking. You no longer need to deal with the situation where you turn on change tracking and send out a document for review. Then, when you get the document back, it contains no change markings because the reviewer turned the Track Changes feature off.

In the past, you needed to use the Compare Documents feature to determine how the reviewed document differed from the original. But now, you can lock change tracking.

Lock and Unlock Tracking

Lock Tracked Changes

1 In the document you want to lock tracked changes, click the **Review** tab.

2 Click **Track Changes** to turn on change tracking.

3 Click the bottom half of the **Track Changes** button.

4 Click **Lock Tracking**.

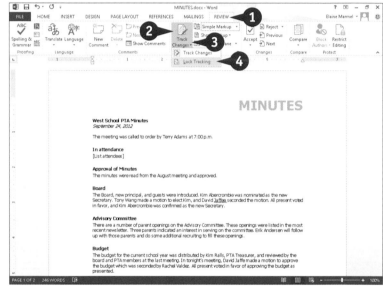

The Lock Tracking dialog box appears.

5 Type a password.

6 Retype the password.

7 Click **OK**.

Note: Make sure you remember the password or you will not be able to turn off the Track Changes feature.

Word saves the password, and the Track Changes button appears gray and unavailable.

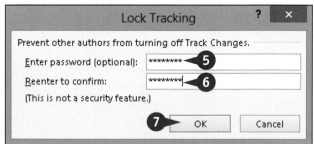

Unlock Tracked Changes

1 Open a document with tracked changes locked.

2 Click the **Review** tab.

3 Click the bottom half of the **Track Changes** button.

4 Click **Lock Tracking**.

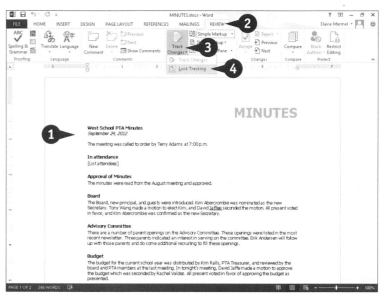

The Unlock Tracking dialog box appears.

5 Type the password.

6 Click **OK**.

The Track Changes button becomes available again, so that you can click it and turn off the Track Changes feature.

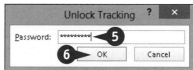

TIP

What happens if I supply the wrong password?

This message box appears. You can retry as many times as you want. If you cannot remember the password, you can create a new version that contains all revisions already accepted, which you can then compare to the original to identify changes. Press **Ctrl**+**A** to select the entire document. Then press **Shift**+**←** to deselect just the last paragraph mark in the document. Then press **Ctrl**+**C** to copy the selection. Start a new blank document, and press **Ctrl**+**V** to paste the selection.

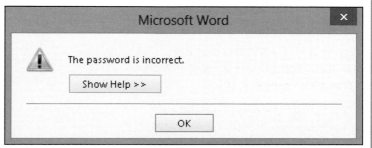

Work with Comments

You can add comments to your documents. For example, when you share your documents with other users, you can use comments to leave feedback about the text without typing directly in the document and others can do the same.

To indicate that a comment was added, Word displays a balloon in the right margin near the commented text. When you review comments, they appear in a block. Your name appears in comments you add, and you can easily review, reply to, or delete a comment, or you can indicate that you have addressed a comment.

Work with Comments

Add a Comment

1. Click or select the text about which you want to comment.

2. Click the **Review** tab.

3. Click **New Comment**.

A. A comment balloon appears, marking the location of the comment.

B. A Comments block appears.

4. Type your comment.

5. Click anywhere outside the comment to continue working.

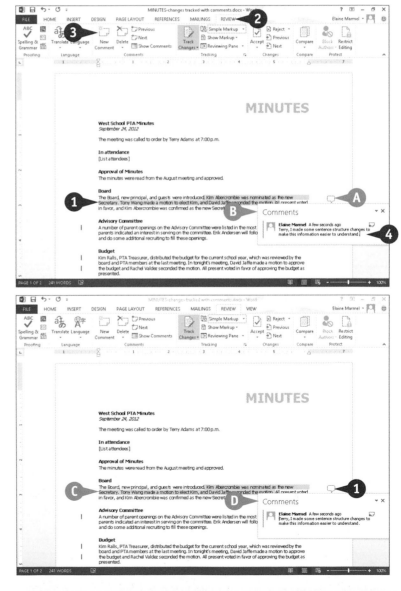

Review a Comment

1. While working in Simple Markup view, click a comment balloon.

C. Word highlights the text associated with the comment.

D. Word displays the Comments block and the text it contains.

Note: To view all comments along the right side of the document, click **Show Comments** in the Comments group on the Review tab.

2. Click anywhere outside the comment to hide the Comments block and its text.

Reply to a Comment

1 While working in Simple Markup view, click a comment balloon to display its text.

2 Click the **Reply to Comment** button ( ).

E Work starts a new comment, indented under the first comment.

3 Type your reply.

4 Click anywhere outside the comment to continue working.

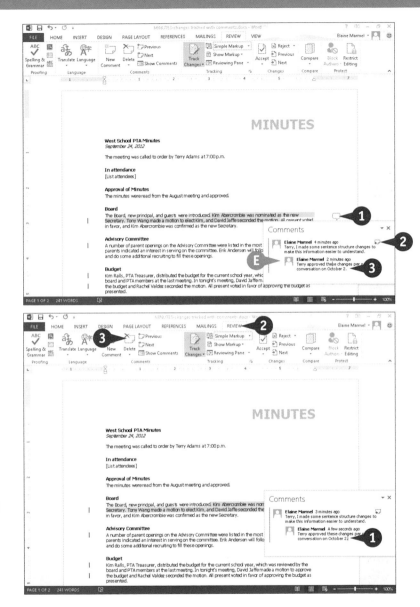

Delete a Comment

1 Click the comment that you want to remove.

2 Click the **Review** tab.

3 Click the **Delete** button.

Note: You can also right-click a comment and click **Delete Comment**. And you can delete all comments in the document by clicking the bottom of the **Delete** button and then clicking **Delete All Comments in Document**.

Word deletes the comment.

TIP

How can I indicate that I have addressed a comment without deleting it?
You mark the comment as done. Right-click the text of the comment, and choose **Mark Comment Done**. Word fades the comment text to light gray.

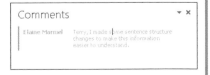

Review Tracked Changes

When you review a document containing tracked changes, you decide whether to accept or reject the changes. As you accept or reject changes, Word removes the revision marks.

When Word tracks revisions, it uses different colors to track the changes made and who made them so that you can easily identify who did what to a document. By default, Word displays changes in Simple Markup view, which indicates, in the left margin, areas that have changes. You can use the Reviewing pane to identify who made each change, or you can hide the pane and work directly with the revisions.

Review Tracked Changes

Display the Reviewing Pane

1 Open a document in which changes were tracked.

2 Click the **Review** tab.

3 Click **Reviewing Pane**.

Ⓐ In the Revisions pane, Word displays the reviewer's name, the date, time, and the details of each change.

Ⓑ You can click ⏶ to hide the summary of revisions and view only the details of each revision.

Ⓒ You can click ✕ to close the pane.

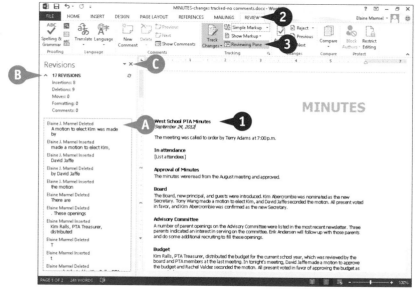

Review Changes

Note: Documents containing tracked changes open in Simple Markup view. Red vertical bars appear in the left margin to indicate locations where changes were made.

1 Click any vertical bar in the left margin.

All vertical bars turn gray, and Word changes the view to All Markup and displays all changes in the document.

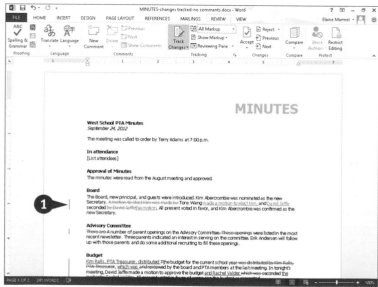

D Deleted text appears in color with strikethrough formatting.

E Added text appears underlined and in color.

Note: Each reviewer's changes appear in a different color.

2 Press Ctrl+Home to place the insertion point at the beginning of the document.

3 Click **Next** to review the first change.

F Word highlights the change.

You can click **Next** again to skip over the change without accepting or rejecting it.

4 Click **Accept** to incorporate the change into the document or **Reject** to revert the text to its original state.

G Word accepts or rejects the change, removes the revision marks, and highlights the next change.

5 Repeat Step **4** to review all revisions.

H If you need to move backward to a change you previously skipped, you can click **Previous**.

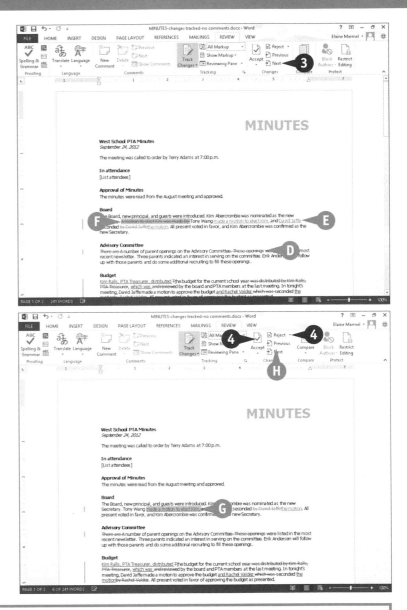

TIP

Can I print revisions?

Yes, you can print revisions in the document by simply printing the document. Or you can print a separate list of revisions by performing the steps that follow. Click the **File** tab to display Backstage view, and then click **Print**. Click the button below **Settings** (**A**). From the menu that appears, click **List of Markup** (**B**). Click **Print**.

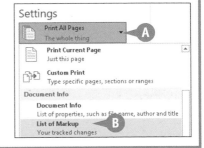

Combine Reviewers' Comments

Suppose that two different reviewers review a document, but they review simultaneously using the original document. When they each return the reviewed document, you have two versions of the original document, each containing potentially different changes. You can combine the documents so that you can work from the combined changes of both reviewers.

When you combine two versions of the same document, Word creates a third file that flags any discrepancies between the versions using revision marks like you see when you enable the Track Changes feature. You can then work from the combined document and evaluate each change.

Combine Reviewers' Comments

Note: To make your screen as easy to understand as possible, close all open documents.

1 Click the **Review** tab.

2 Click **Compare**.

3 Click **Combine**.

The Combine Documents dialog box appears.

4 Click the **Open** button ( ) for the first document you want to combine.

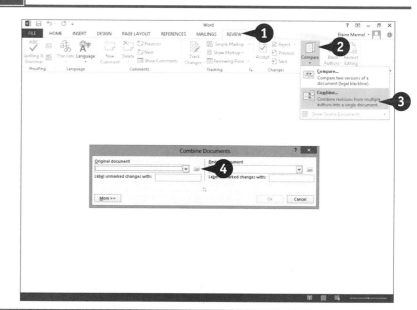

The Open dialog box appears.

5 Navigate to the folder containing the first file you want to combine.

6 Click the file.

7 Click **Open**.

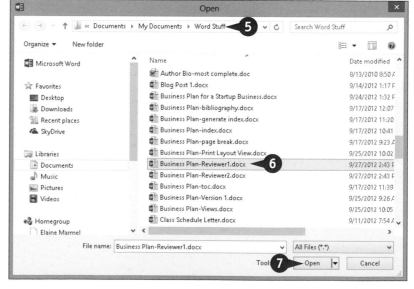

112

The Combine Documents dialog box reappears.

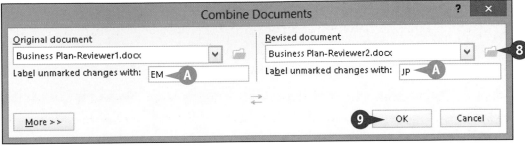

8 Repeat Steps **4** to **7**, clicking the **Open** button (📁) for the second document you want to compare.

Ⓐ You can type a label for changes to each document in these boxes.

9 Click **OK**.

Word displays four panes.

Ⓑ The left pane contains a summary of revisions.

Ⓒ The center pane contains the result of combining both documents.

Ⓓ The top-right pane displays the document you selected in Step **6**.

Ⓔ The bottom-right pane displays the document you selected in Step **8**.

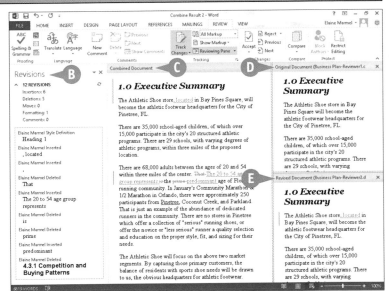

Two reviewers reviewed the same document, but they forgot to track changes; can I somehow see their changes?

Follow the steps in this section, but in Step **3**, click **Compare**. Word again displays four panes; the summary appears in the left pane, results of comparing the two documents appears in the center pane, while the document you select in Step **6** appears in the top-right pane, and the document you select in Step **8** appears in the bottom-right pane.

How do I save the combined document?

The same way you save any Word document; see Chapter 2 for details.

CHAPTER 5

Formatting Text

You can format text for emphasis and for greater readability. And although the individual types of formatting are discussed separately, you can perform each of the tasks in this chapter on a single selection of text.

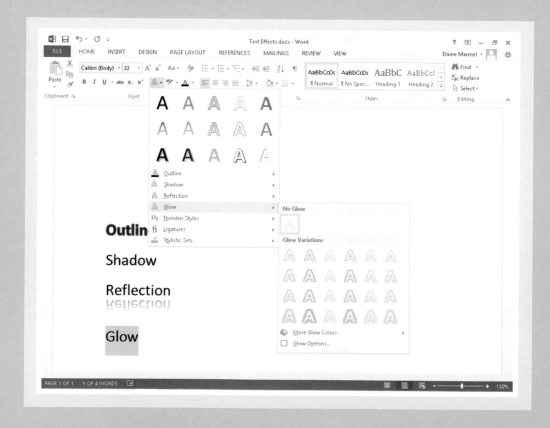

Change the Font

You can change the typeface that appears in your document by changing the font. Changing the font can help readers better understand your document.

Use *serif* fonts — fonts with short lines stemming from the bottoms of the letters — to provide a line that helps guide the reader's eyes along the line, making reading easier with less eye strain. Most readers are not even aware that the short line along the bottom of the letters helps guide their eyes. Use *sans serif* fonts — fonts without short lines stemming from the bottoms of the letters — for headlines.

Change the Font

1 Select the text that you want to format.

A If you drag to select, the Mini toolbar appears in the background, and you can use it by moving ⌖ toward the Mini toolbar.

2 To use the Ribbon, click the **Home** tab.

3 Click the **Font** ▼ to display a list of the available fonts on your computer.

Note: Word displays a sample of the selected text in any font at which you point the mouse.

4 Click the font you want to use.

B Word assigns the font to the selected text.

You can click anywhere outside the selection to continue working.

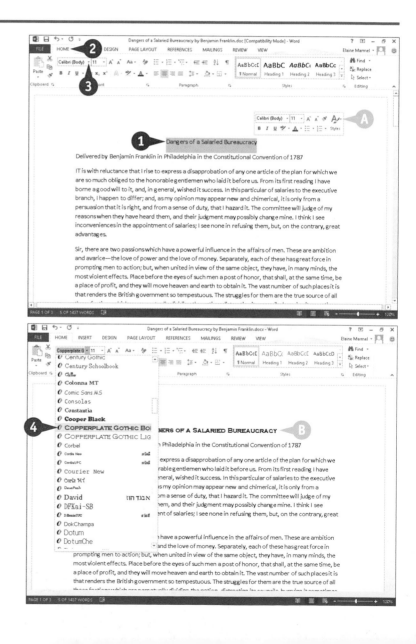

Change Text Size

You can increase or decrease the size of the text in your document. Increase the size to make reading the text easier; decrease the size to fit more text on a page.

Fonts are measured in *points*; the term originates in typography as a fraction of a pica, but desktop publishing redefined the point in the 1980s and 1990s as 1/72 inches. In both typography and desktop publishing, 12 points equal a pica, the standard font size used for reading.

Change Text Size

1 Select the text that you want to format.

A If you drag to select, the Mini toolbar appears in the background, and you can use it by moving toward the Mini toolbar.

2 To use the Ribbon, click the **Home** tab.

3 Click the **Font Size** ▼ to display a list of the possible sizes for the current font.

Note: Word displays a sample of the selected text in any font size at which you point the mouse.

4 Click a size.

B Word changes the size of the selected text.

This example applies a 24-point font size to the text.

Note: You also can change the font size using the **Grow Font** and **Shrink Font** buttons (A˄ and A˅) on the Home tab. Word increases or decreases the font size with each click of the button.

You can click anywhere outside the selection to continue working.

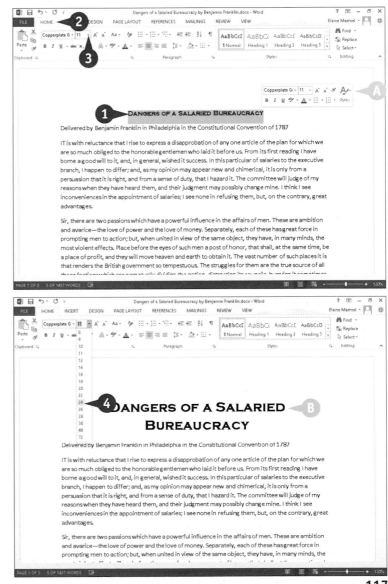

Emphasize Information with Bold, Italic, or Underline

You can apply italics, boldface, or underlining to add emphasis to text in your document. Each technique distinguishes text in a different way.

Boldface changes the brightness of the text, making the text darker than surrounding text. Italic applies a script-line appearance to text, slanting it the way handwriting slants. Underlining is not often used in printed material because it is considered to be too distracting to the reader; instead, you might find underlining appearing in handwritten materials to emphasize a point.

Emphasize Information with Bold, Italic, or Underline

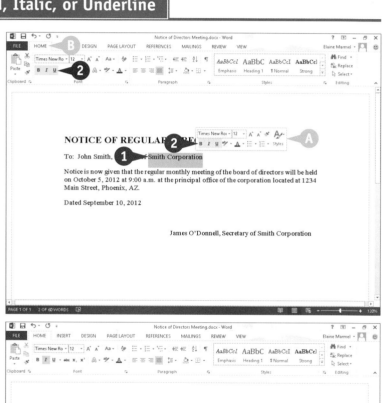

1 Select the text that you want to emphasize.

Ⓐ If you drag to select, the Mini toolbar appears in the background, and you can use it by moving ▷ toward the Mini toolbar.

Ⓑ If you want to use the Ribbon, click the **Home** tab.

2 Click the **Bold** button (**B**), the **Italic** button (*I*), or the **Underline** button (U ˅) on the Ribbon or the Mini toolbar.

Ⓒ Word applies the emphasis you selected.

This example shows the text after italic is selected.

You can click anywhere outside the selection to continue working.

Superscript or Subscript Text

You can assign superscript or subscript notation to text. A superscript or subscript is a number, figure, or symbol that appears smaller than the normal line of type and is set slightly above or below it; superscripts appear above the baseline of regular text, while subscripts appear below the baseline. Subscripts and superscripts are perhaps best known for their use in formulas and mathematical expressions, but they are also used when inserting trademark symbols.

Superscript or Subscript Text

1 Type and select the text that you want to appear in superscript or subscript.

A If you drag to select, the Mini toolbar appears in the background.

2 Click the **Home** tab.

3 Click the **Superscript** button (x^2) or the **Subscript** button (x_2).

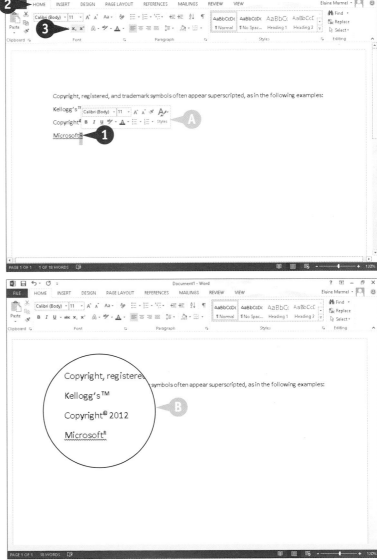

B Word adds superscripts or subscripts to the selected text.

You can click anywhere outside the selection to continue working.

Change Text Case

You ou can change the case of selected text instead of retyping it with a new case applied. You can apply five types of case to your text. You can apply lowercase to selected text, which uses no capital letters. You can apply uppercase to selected text, which uses all capital letters. Using sentence case, you capitalize the first letter of the selected phrase while all other words in the phrase appear lowercase. You can capitalize each word in a selected phrase, or you can toggle case, which changes uppercase letters to lowercase and lowercase letters to uppercase in selected text.

Change Text Case

1 Select the text to which you want to assign a new case.

   If you drag to select, the Mini toolbar appears in the background.

2 Click the **Home** tab.

3 Click the **Change Case** button (Aa ▾).

4 Click the case you want to use.

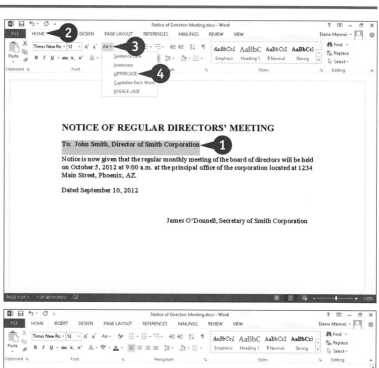

Ⓐ The selected text appears in the new case.

   You can click anywhere outside the selection to continue working.

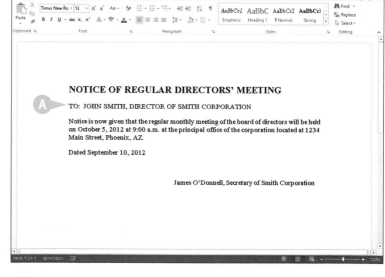

Change Text Color

You can change the color of selected text for emphasis. For example, if you are creating a report for work, you might make the title of the report a different color from the information contained in the report or even color-code certain data in the report.

Color is effective when you view your document on-screen, save it as a PDF or an XPS file, or print it using a color printer.

Change Text Color

1 Select the text that you want to change to a different color.

A If you drag to select, the Mini toolbar appears faded in the background, and you can use it by moving ⯈ toward the Mini toolbar.

2 To use the Ribbon, click the **Home** tab.

3 Click ▼ next to the Font Color button (**A** ▾), and point the mouse at a color.

Word displays a preview of the selected text.

4 Click a color.

B Word assigns the color to the text.

This example applies a blue color to the text.

You can click anywhere outside the selection to continue working.

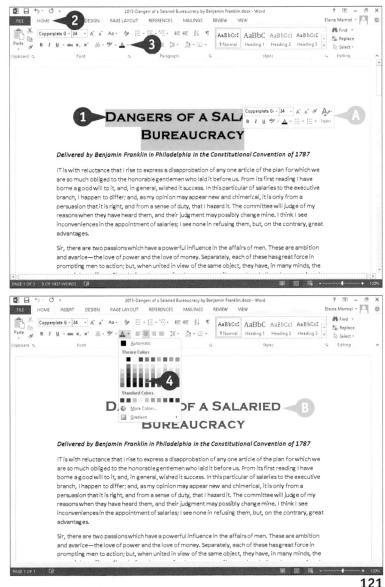

Apply Text Effects

Y ou can use a text effect to draw a reader's eye to the text. Text effects go beyond typical techniques you use for emphasis, such as boldface, italics, or underlining. (You can read about these emphasis techniques in the section "Emphasize Information with Bold, Italic, or Underline" earlier in this chapter.) Using text effects, you can apply outlines, shadows, reflections, and glows to text or WordArt. Text effects accomplish your goal of drawing the reader's eye most successfully if you apply them sparingly and limit your use of them to headlines or titles.

Apply Text Effects

1 Type and select the text to which you want to apply an effect.

2 Click the **Home** tab.

3 Click the **Text Effects** button (A ∙).

A The Text Effects Gallery appears.

4 Point the mouse at the type of text effect you want to apply.

B Word displays a gallery of options available for the selected text effect; you can preview any text effect by pointing the mouse at it.

5 Click an option from the gallery to apply it.

C Word applies your choice to the selected text.

You can click anywhere outside the selection to continue working.

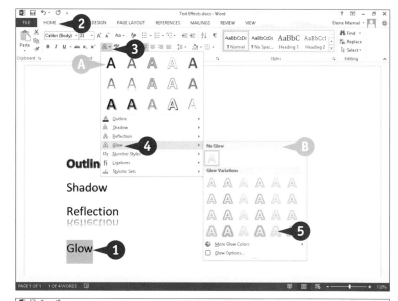

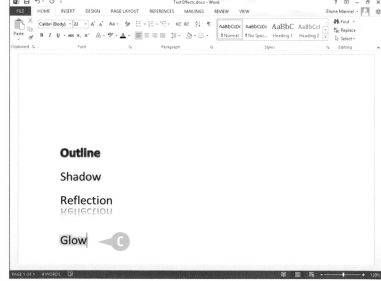

Apply a Font Style Set

You can use font style sets to enhance the appearance of OpenType fonts. Font style sets can add just the right mood to a holiday card by adding flourishes to the letters in the font set.

The OpenType font structure adds several options to its predecessor TrueType that enhance the OpenType font's typographic and language support capabilities. OpenType fonts use an extension of .otf or .ttf; the .ttf form includes PostScript font data. OpenType fonts store all information in a single font file and have the same appearance on Macs and PCs.

Apply a Font Style Set

1 Select an OpenType font.

This example uses Gabriola.

2 Type some text, and select it.

If you drag to select, the Mini toolbar appears faded in the background.

3 Click the **Text Effects** button (Ⓐ ▾).

Ⓐ The Text Effects Gallery appears.

4 Point the mouse at **Stylistic Sets**.

Ⓑ Word displays a gallery of options available for Stylistic Sets; you can preview any set by pointing the mouse at it.

5 Click an option from the gallery to apply it.

Ⓒ Word applies the font style set to the text you selected.

You can click anywhere outside the selection to continue working.

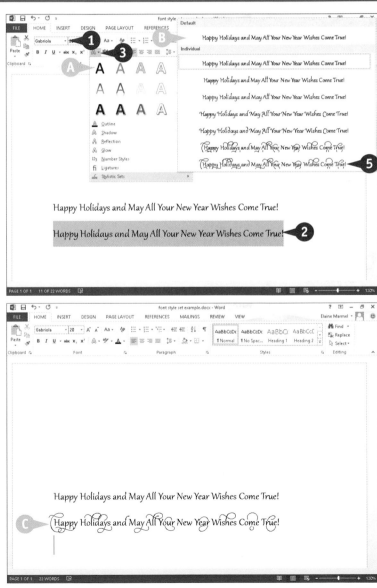

123

Apply Highlighting to Text

You can use color to create highlights in a document to draw attention to the text. You can help your reader be an active reader and understand and remember what you have written if you highlight a keyword or a small phrase. Highlighting is effective when viewing the document on-screen or when you print the document using a color printer.

Do not be tempted to overuse highlighting. If you highlight every other sentence or even all the headings in a document, your reader will learn to ignore the highlighting.

Apply Highlighting to Text

1. Select the text that you want to highlight.

   If you drag to select, the Mini toolbar appears in the background, and you can use it by moving ⊳ toward the Mini toolbar.

2. To use the Ribbon, click the **Home** tab.

3. Click ▼ beside the Text Highlight Color button (✏) on the Ribbon or the Mini toolbar, and point at a color.

Ⓐ A palette of color choices appears.

   You can point the mouse at any color, and Word displays a sample of the selected text highlighted in that color.

4. Click a color.

Ⓑ Word highlights the selected text using the color you choose.

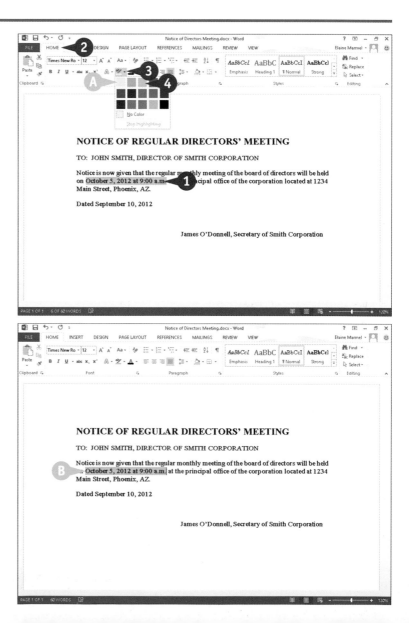

Apply Strikethrough to Text

You can use the Strikethrough feature to draw a line through text you propose to delete. Strikethrough formatting is often used in the legal community to identify text a reviewer proposes to delete; this formatting has developed a universal meaning and has been adopted by reviewers around the world. However, if you need to track both additions and deletions and want to update the document in an automated way, use Word's review tracking features as described in Chapter 4.

Apply Strikethrough to Text

1 Select the text to which you want to apply strikethrough formatting.

If you drag to select, the Mini toolbar appears in the background.

2 Click the **Home** tab.

3 Click the **Strikethrough** button (abc).

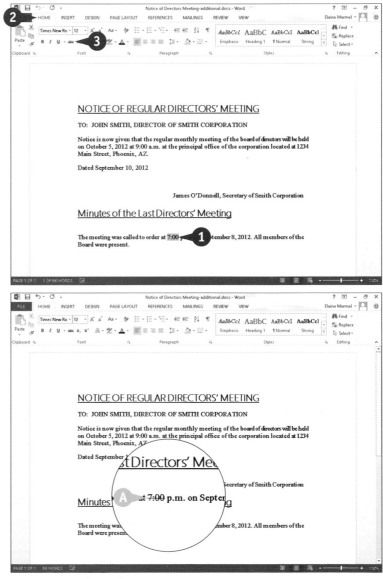

A Word applies strikethrough formatting to the selected text.

You can click anywhere outside the selection to continue working.

You can repeat these steps to remove strikethrough formatting.

Copy Text Formatting

Suppose you have applied a variety of formatting options to a paragraph to create a certain look — for example, you changed the font, the size, the color, and the alignment. If you want to re-create the same look elsewhere in the document, you do not have to repeat the same steps as when you applied the original formatting, again changing the font, size, color, and alignment. Instead, you can use Word's Format Painter feature to "paint" the formatting to the other text.

Copy Text Formatting

1 Select the text containing the formatting that you want to copy.

A If you drag to select, the Mini toolbar appears in the background, and you can use it by moving ▷ toward the Mini toolbar.

2 To use the Ribbon, click the **Home** tab.

3 Click the **Format Painter** button ( ).

The mouse pointer changes to ▲I when you move the mouse over your document.

4 Click and drag over the text to which you want to apply the same formatting.

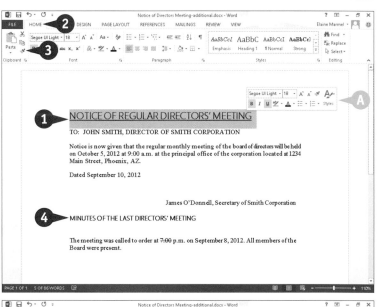

B Word copies the formatting from the original text to the newly selected text.

To copy the same formatting multiple times, you can double-click the **Format Painter** button ( ).

You can press Esc to cancel the Format Painter feature at any time.

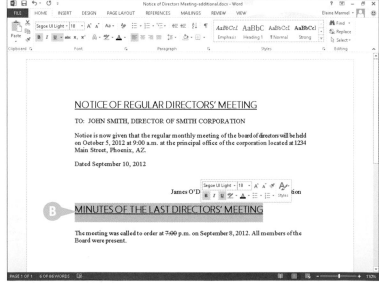

126

Remove Text Formatting

Sometimes, you may find that you have applied too much formatting to your text, making it difficult to read. Instead of undoing all your formatting changes by hand, you can use Word's Clear Formatting command to remove any formatting you have applied to the document text. When you apply the Clear Formatting command, which is located in the Home tab on the Ribbon, Word removes all formatting applied to the text and restores the default settings.

Remove Text Formatting

1 Select the text from which you want to remove formatting.

Note: If you do not select text, Word removes text formatting from the entire document.

2 Click the **Home** tab.

3 Click the **Clear Formatting** button ( ).

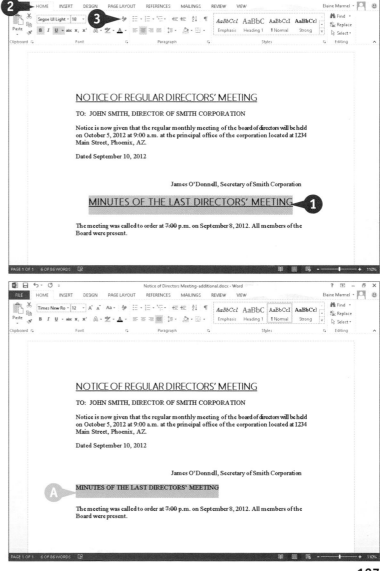

A Word removes all formatting from the selected text.

You can click anywhere outside the selection to continue working.

Set the Default Font for All New Documents

You can change the default font that Word uses for all new documents you create. Word's default font is Calibri, 11 point, a sans serif font. Suppose that most of the documents you create are report-like in nature and you want to use a serif font, such as Cambria or Times New Roman because the serifs on letters will help guide the reader's eye, making reading easier so that the reader can focus on your meaning.

Changing the default font does not affect documents you have already created.

Set the Default Font for All New Documents

1 Click the **Home** tab.

2 Right-click the Normal style.

3 Click **Modify**.

The Modify Style dialog box appears.

4 Click ⮟ to select the font that you want to use for all new documents.

5 Click ⮟ to select the font size that you want to use for all new documents.

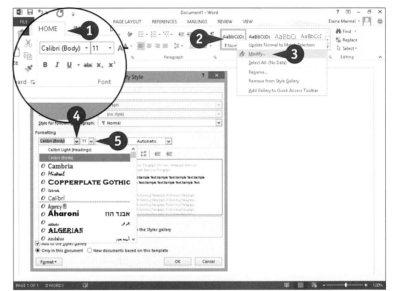

Ⓐ A preview of the new selections appears here.

6 Select **New documents based on this template** (○ changes to ◉).

7 Click **OK**.

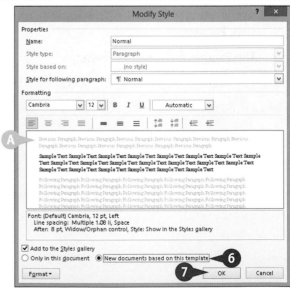

128

B When you open a new document, the default font and font size, if appropriate, are the font and font size you selected.

Note: To open a new document, see Chapter 2.

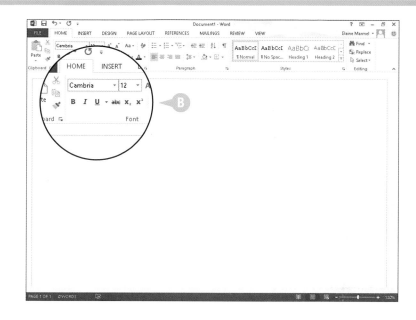

I like the default font, but I want to indent the first line of each paragraph by default. Can I do that?

Yes. Follow these steps:

1 Complete Steps **1** to **3** to open the Modify Style dialog box.

2 Click **Format** and, from the list that appears, click **Paragraph**.

The Paragraph dialog box appears.

3 In the Indentation section, click the **Special** ☑.

4 Click **First line**.

A By default, Word applies a .5" indentation, but you can change the value if you want.

5 Click **OK**.

6 Complete Steps **6** and **7**.

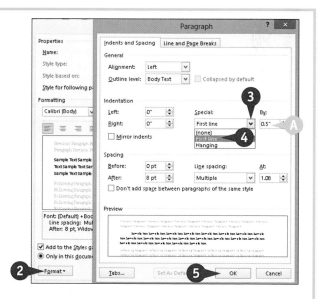

Formatting Paragraphs

Instead of formatting individual words in your document, you can apply changes to entire paragraphs to help certain sections of your text stand out. You can apply formatting such as line spacing, bullets, or borders to the paragraphs in your document to enhance the appearance of the document.

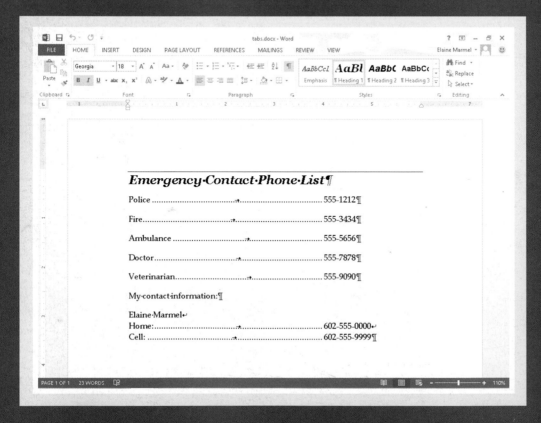

Change Text Alignment

You can use Word's alignment commands to change the way that your text is positioned horizontally on a page. By default, Word left aligns text. You can align text with the left or right margins, center it horizontally between both margins, or justify text between both the left and right margins. You can change the alignment of all the text in your document or change the alignment of individual paragraphs and objects.

To align text vertically, see Chapter 7. The example in this section centers a headline between the left and right margins.

Change Text Alignment

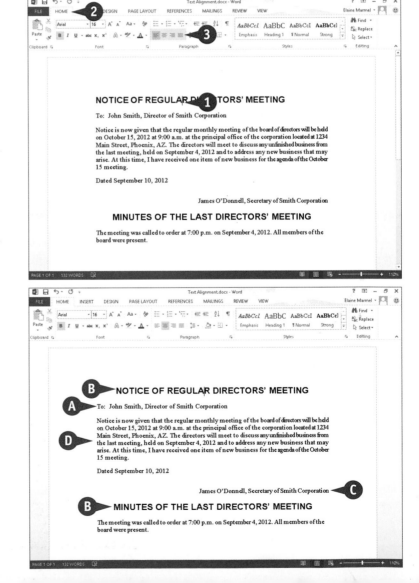

1 Click anywhere in the paragraph that you want to align, or select the paragraphs and objects that you want to align.

2 Click the **Home** tab.

3 Click an alignment button.

The **Align Left** button (☰) aligns text with the left margin, the **Center** button (☰), centers text between the left and right margins, the **Align Right** button (☰) aligns text with the right margin, and the **Justify** button (☰) aligns text between the left and right margins.

Word aligns the text.

Ⓐ This text is aligned with the left margin.

Ⓑ This text is centered between both margins.

Ⓒ This text is aligned with the right margin.

Ⓓ This text is justified between both margins.

Set Line Spacing within a Paragraph

Y ou can change the amount of space Word places between the lines of text within a paragraph. For example, you might set 2.5 spacing to allow for handwritten edits in your printed document, or you may set 1.5 spacing to make paragraphs easier to read. By default, Word assigns single spacing within a paragraph for all new documents that you create.

Word can measure line spacing in inches, but, in keeping with typography tradition, line spacing is most often measured in points, specified as *pts*. Twelve pts equal approximately one line of space.

Set Line Spacing within a Paragraph

1 Click in the paragraph for which you want to change line spacing.

2 Click the **Home** tab.

3 Click the **Line Spacing** button ( ).

Note: As you move the mouse pointer over line spacing options, Word previews the paragraph using each option.

4 Click a number.

A setting of **1** represents single spacing, **1.15** places a small amount of blank space between lines; **1.5** places half a blank line between lines of text; **2** represents double spacing; **2.5** places one and a half blank lines between lines of text; and **3** represents triple spacing.

A Word applies the line spacing you specified to the paragraph containing the insertion point.

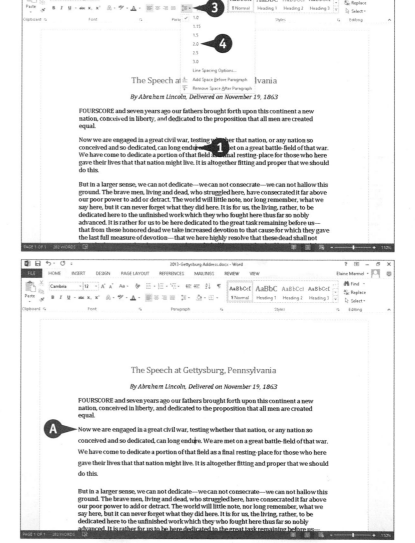

Set Line Spacing between Paragraphs

In addition to changing the spacing between lines within a paragraph, you can change the amount of space Word places between paragraphs of text. For example, you can use this technique to set double spacing between paragraphs while maintaining single spacing within each paragraph.

You can set spacing before a paragraph or after a paragraph. Word measures spacing between paragraphs in points (pts), and one line equals approximately 12 pts. You can create one blank line between paragraphs by adding 6 pts before and 6 pts after the paragraph, or you can simply add 12 pts before or 12 pts after the paragraph.

Set Line Spacing between Paragraphs

1 Select the paragraph or paragraphs for which you want to define spacing.

2 Click the **Home** tab.

3 Click the Paragraph group dialog box launcher (⌐).

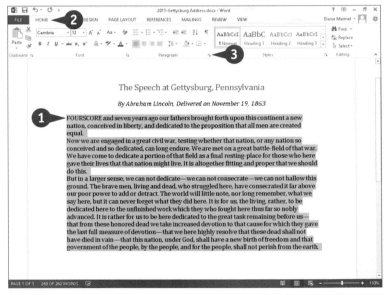

The Paragraph dialog box appears.

4 Click ↕ to increase or decrease the space before the selected paragraph.

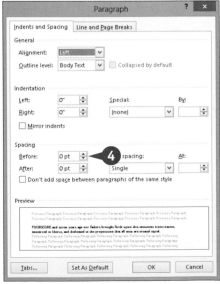

⑤ Click ↕ to increase or decrease the space after the selected paragraph.

⑥ Click **OK**.

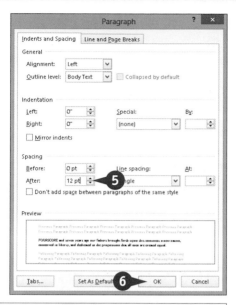

Ⓐ Word applies the spacing before and after the selected paragraph.

You can click anywhere outside the selection to continue working.

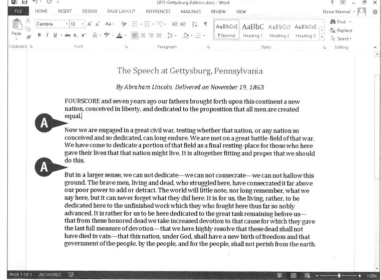

What does the Do Not Add Space between Paragraphs of the Same Style check box do?
As described later in this chapter, you can use styles to assign predefined sets of formatting information, such as font and paragraph information, including line spacing, to paragraphs. By default, Word assigns the Normal style to each paragraph of text. You can select **Do not add space between paragraphs of the same style** (☐ changes to ☑) to use the same spacing both within a paragraph and between paragraphs to which you have assigned the same style.

Create a Bulleted or Numbered List

You can draw attention to lists of information by using bullets or numbers. Bulleted and numbered lists can help you present your information in an organized way. You can create a list as you type it or after you have typed list elements.

A bulleted list adds dots or other similar symbols in front of each list item, whereas a numbered list adds sequential numbers or letters in front of each list item. As a general rule, use bullets when the items in your list do not follow any particular order and use numbers when the items in your list follow a particular order.

Create a Bulleted or Numbered List

Create a List as You Type

1 Type **1.** to create a numbered list or * to create a bulleted list.

2 Press `Spacebar` or `Tab`.

A Word automatically formats the entry as a list item and displays the AutoCorrect Options button ( ) so that you can undo or stop automatic numbering.

3 Type a list item.

4 Press `Enter` to prepare to type another list item.

B Word automatically adds a bullet or number for the next list item.

5 Repeat Steps **3** and **4** for each list item.

To stop entering items in the list, press `Enter` twice.

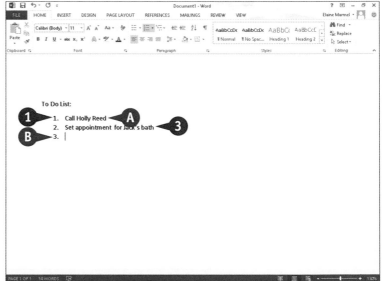

Create a List from Existing Text

1 Select the text to which you want to assign bullets or numbers.

2 Click the **Home** tab.

3 Click the **Numbering** button ( ) or the **Bullets** button ( ).

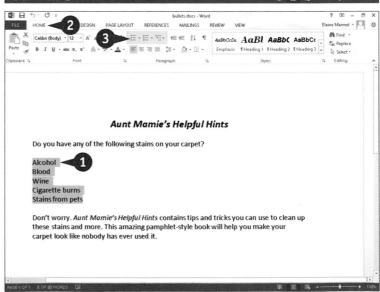

C Word applies numbers or bullets to the selection.

This example uses bullets.

You can click anywhere outside the selection to continue working.

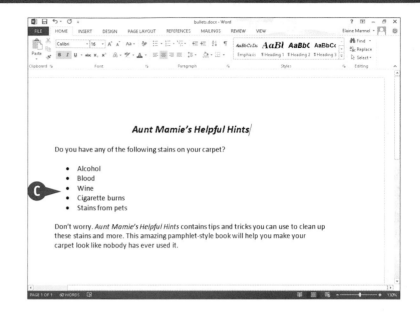

TIP

Can I create a bulleted or numbered list with more than one level, like the type of list you use when creating an outline?

Yes. You can use the Multilevel List button ( ).

1 Click .

2 Click a format.

3 Type your list.

A You can press Enter to enter a new list item at the same list level.

B Each time you press Tab, Word indents a level in the list.

C Each time you press Shift + Tab, Word outdents a level in the list.

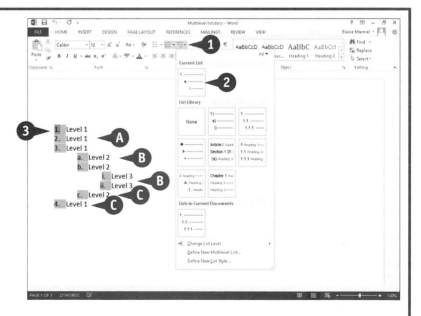

Display Formatting Marks

You can display formatting marks that do not print but help you identify formatting in your document. Displaying formatting marks can often help you identify problems in your documents. For example, if you display formatting marks, you can visibly see the difference between a line break and a paragraph mark. You also can see where spaces were used to attempt to vertically line up text when you should have used tabs, as described in the section "Set Tabs" later in this chapter.

Word can display formatting marks that represent spaces, tabs, paragraphs, line breaks, hidden text, and optional hyphens.

Display Formatting Marks

1 Open any document.

2 Click the **Home** tab.

3 Click the **Show/Hide** button (¶).

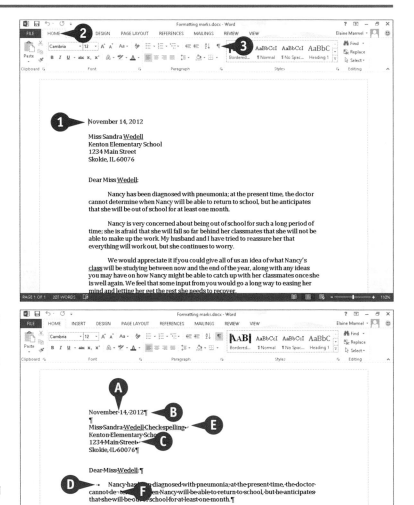

Word displays all formatting marks in your document.

A Single dots (·) represent the spaces you insert each time you press `Spacebar`.

B Paragraph marks (¶) appear each time you press `Enter`.

C Line breaks (↵) appear each time you press `Shift`+`Enter`.

D Arrows (→) appear each time you press `Tab`.

E Hidden text appears underlined with dots.

F Optional hyphens, inserted by pressing `Ctrl`+`-` appear as ¬.

You can click the **Show/Hide** button (¶) again to hide formatting marks.

Hide or Display the Ruler

You can hide or display horizontal and vertical rulers while you work on a Word document in Print Layout, Web Layout, or Draft views. Rulers can help you identify the position of text on the page both horizontally and vertically. You also can use the rulers to align tables and graphic objects.

The horizontal ruler is particularly useful; in addition to helping you align text, tables, and graphic objects vertically on the page, you can use it to indent paragraphs or set tabs in your document, as described in the sections "Indent Paragraphs" and "Set Tabs."

Hide or Display the Ruler

1 Click the **View** tab.

2 Select **Ruler** (☐ changes to ☑).

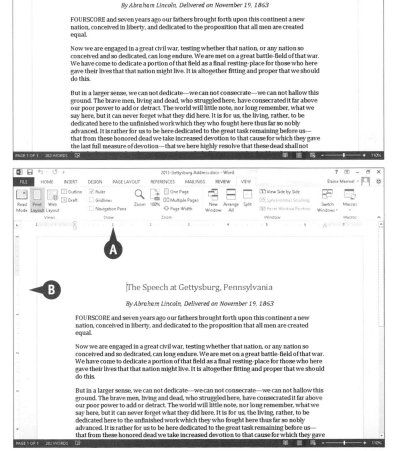

A A ruler appears above your document.

B A ruler appears on the left side of your document.

You can repeat Steps **1** and **2** (☑ changes to ☐) to hide the rulers.

Indent Paragraphs

Y ou can use indents as a way to control the horizontal positioning of text in a document. Indents are simply margins that affect individual lines or paragraphs. You might use an indent to distinguish a particular paragraph on a page — for example, a long quote.

You can indent paragraphs in your document from the left and right margins. You also can indent only the first line of a paragraph or all lines *except* the first line of the paragraph. You can set indents using buttons on the Ribbon, the Paragraph dialog box, and the Word ruler.

Indent Paragraphs

Set Quick Indents

1 Click anywhere in the paragraph you want to indent.

2 Click the **Home** tab on the Ribbon.

3 Click an indent button.

A You can click the **Decrease Indent** button (≡) to decrease the indentation.

B You can click the **Increase Indent** button (≡) to increase the indentation.

C Word applies the indent change.

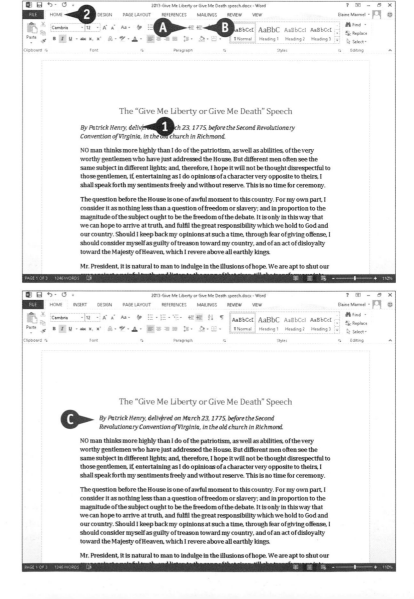

Set Precise Indents

1 Click in the paragraph or select the text you want to indent.

2 Click the **Home** tab.

3 Click the dialog box launcher (⌐) in the Paragraph group.

The Paragraph dialog box appears.

4 Use these boxes to specify the number of inches to indent the left and right edge of the paragraph or selection.

5 Click ☑ to select an indenting option.

First line, shown in this example, indents only the first line of the paragraph, and **Hanging** indents all lines *except* the first line of the paragraph.

6 Click ↕ to set the amount of the first line or hanging indent.

Ⓓ The Preview area shows a sample of the indent.

7 Click **OK**.

Ⓔ Word applies the indent to the paragraph containing the insertion point.

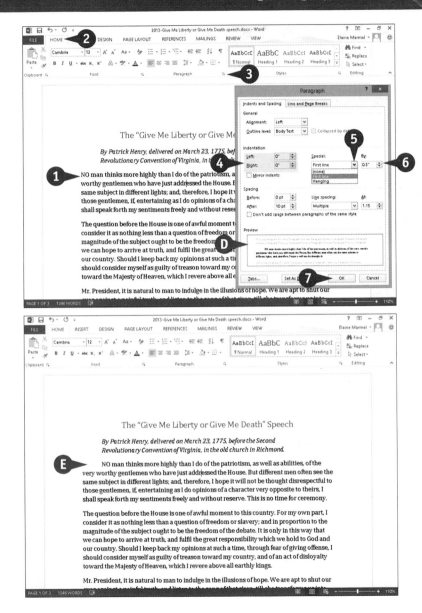

How do I set indents using the Word ruler?

The ruler contains markers for changing the left indent, right indent, first-line indent, and hanging indent. Click the **View** tab, and then click **Ruler** to display the ruler. On the left side of the ruler, drag the **Left Indent** button (▭) to indent all lines from the left margin, drag the **Hanging Indent** button (△) to create a hanging indent, or drag the **First Line Indent** button (▽) to indent the first line only. On the right side of the ruler, drag the **Right Indent** button (△) to indent all lines from the right margin.

Set Tabs

You can use tabs to create vertically aligned columns of text. Using tabs as opposed to spaces ensures that information lines up properly. To insert a tab, press `Tab`; the insertion point moves to the next tab stop on the page.

By default, Word creates tab stops every 0.5 inch across the page and left aligns the text on each tab stop. You can set your own tab stops using the ruler or the Tabs dialog box. You also can use the Tabs dialog box to change the tab alignment and specify an exact measurement between tab stops.

Set Tabs

Add a Tab

1. Click here until the type of tab you want to add appears.

    ⌐ — Left tab, which sets the starting position of text that then appears to the right of the tab.

    ⊥ — Center tab, which aligns text centered around the tab.

    ⌐ — Right tab, which sets the starting position of text that then appears to the left of the tab.

    ⊥ — Decimal tab, which aligns values at the decimal point. Values before the decimal point appear to the left of the tab and values after the decimal point appear to the right of the tab.

    | — Bar tab, which inserts a vertical bar at the tab stop.

2. Select the lines to which you want to add a tab.

3. Click the ruler where you want the tab to appear.

    Word displays the type of tab you selected at the location you clicked on each selected line.

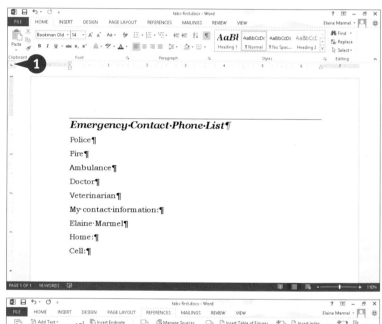

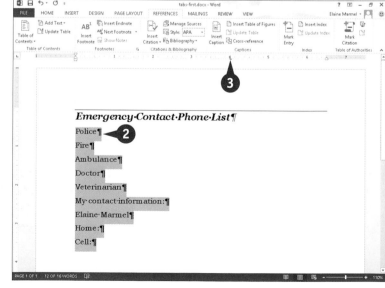

Using a Tab

1 Click to the left of the information you want to appear at the tab; in this example, immediately after the "e" in "Police" to add a tab followed by the phone number.

2 Press **Tab**.

Ⓐ If you display formatting marks, Word displays an arrow representing the tab character.

3 Type your text.

Ⓑ The text appears aligned vertically with the tab.

Move a Tab

1 Click the line using the tab or select the lines of text affected by the tab.

2 Drag the tab to the left or right.

Ⓒ A vertical line marks its position as you drag.

When you click and drag a tab, the text moves to align vertically with the tab.

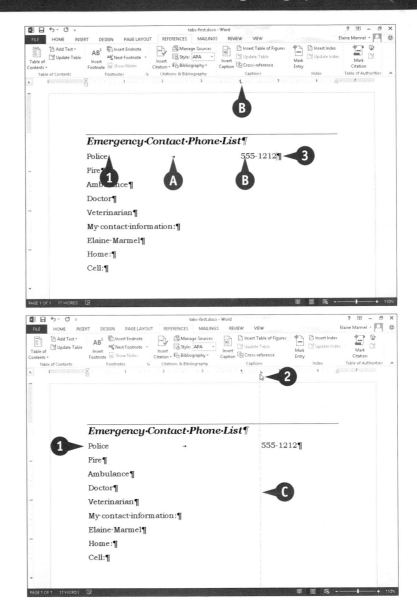

continued ▶

TIP

How can I delete a tab?

Perform the steps that follow. Click in or select the paragraphs containing the tab. Drag the tab off the ruler. When you delete a tab, text aligned at the tab moves to the first preset tab on the line (**Ⓐ**).

Emergency·Contact·

Police → 555-1212¶ ◀Ⓐ

Set Tabs (continued)

Y̶ou can use dot leader tabs to help your reader follow information across a page. Dot leader tabs are often used in tables of contents to help the reader's eye follow the table of content entry across to its associated page number. Dot leader tabs also are helpful when you have a two-column list and the information in the second column is at least three inches away from the information in the first column. Three inches is not a rule, but simply a suggestion. Use your own judgment; if the second column material appears far away from the first column material, use dot leaders.

Set Tabs (continued)

Add Leader Characters to Tabs

1. Follow Steps **1** to **3** in the subsection "Add a Tab" to create a tab stop.

2. Select the text containing the tab to which you want to add dot leaders.

3. Click the **Home** tab.

4. Click the Paragraph group dialog box launcher (⌐).

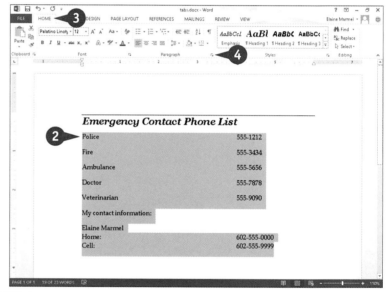

The Paragraph dialog box appears.

5. Click **Tabs**.

The Tabs dialog box appears.

6. Click the tab setting to which you want to add leaders.

7. Select a leader option (○ changes to ●).

8. Click **OK**.

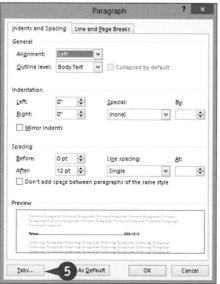

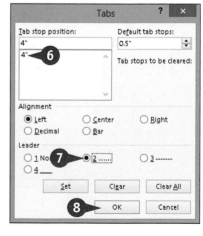

Ⓐ Word adds leading characters from the last character before the tab to the first character at the tab.

You can click anywhere outside the selection to continue working.

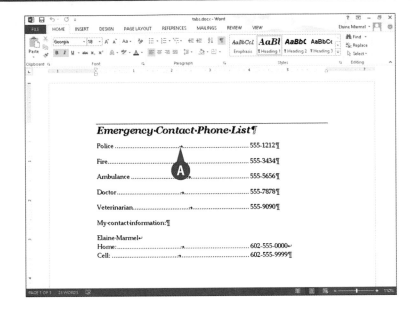

TIP

Can I set tabs using the Tabs dialog box instead of the ruler?

Yes. Follow these steps:

❶ Follow Steps **2** to **5** to display the Tabs dialog box.

❷ Click here and type a tab stop position.

❸ Select a tab alignment option (○ changes to ◉).

❹ Click **Set**.

❺ Repeat Steps **2** to **4** for each tab stop you want to set.

❻ Click **OK** to have the tabs you set appear on the ruler.

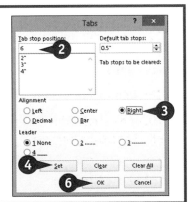

Add a Paragraph Border

The way that you communicate is just as important as the information you want to communicate: You want your important points to come through loud and clear. You can draw attention to a paragraph containing important information by adding a border to it. You can place a border around a paragraph or a page (see Chapter 7 for details on adding a border to a page), and you can control the color, weight, and style of the border. You also can add shading to a paragraph, as described in the section "Add Paragraph Shading" later in this chapter.

Add a Paragraph Border

1 Select the text that you want to surround with a border.

Note: To surround all lines in a paragraph by a border, select both the text and the paragraph mark (¶). To display paragraph marks, click the **Show/Hide** button (¶) on the **Home** tab in the Paragraph group.

2 Click the **Home** tab.

3 Click ▼ beside the Borders button (⊞ ·).

4 Click **Borders and Shading**.

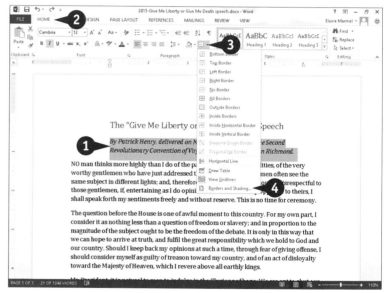

The Borders and Shading dialog box appears.

5 Click the **Borders** tab.

6 Click here to select a type of border.

This example uses Box.

7 Click here to select the style for the border line.

8 Click ☑ and select a color for the border line.

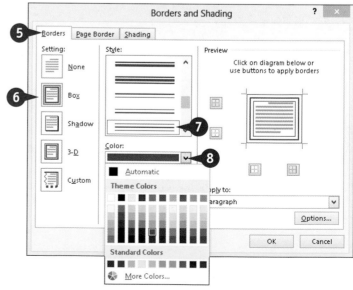

9 Click ⌄ and select a thickness for the border line.

Ⓐ You can use this list to apply the border to an entire paragraph or to selected text.

Ⓑ This area shows the results of the settings you select.

10 Click **OK**.

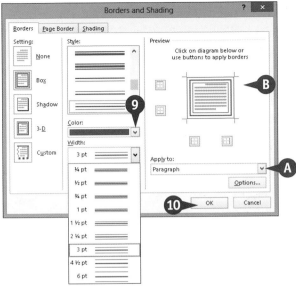

Ⓒ The border appears around the text you selected in Step **1**.

You can click anywhere outside the selection to continue working.

Note: You can apply a border using the same color, style, and thickness you established in these steps to any paragraph by completing Steps **1** to **3** and clicking the type of border you want to apply in Step **4**.

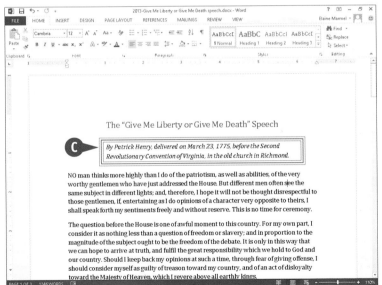

TIP

How do I remove a border?
Perform the steps that follow. Click anywhere in the text surrounded by a border. Click the **Home** tab. Click ▾ beside the Borders button (⊞ ▾). Click **No Border**, and Word removes the border.

Review and Change Formatting

You can review the formatting associated with text in your document to see the details that show the formatting applied to the text. When you reveal formatting for a selection, you can see, simultaneously, all formatting applied to the selected text; you do not need to open individual dialog boxes to view font and paragraph formatting. You also can compare the formatting of two selections to see their differences, as described in the next section, "Compare Formatting."

You also can have Word display wavy blue underlines to mark text you have formatted inconsistently in your document and supply suggestions to correct the formatting inconsistencies.

Review and Change Formatting

1 Select the text containing the formatting you want to review.

2 Click the **Home** tab.

3 Click 🔽 in the Styles group to display the Styles pane.

4 Click the **Style Inspector** button (🔲) to display the Style Inspector pane.

5 Click the **Reveal Formatting** button (🔲) to display the Reveal Formatting pane.

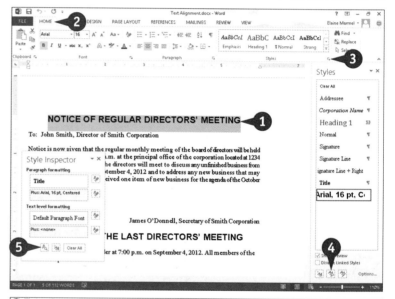

6 Click the **Close** buttons (×) to close the Styles pane and the Style Inspector pane.

Ⓐ A portion of the selected text appears here.

Ⓑ Formatting details for the selected text appear here.

Ⓒ You can click an expand symbol (▷) to display links or a collapse symbol (◀) to hide links.

7 Click the link for the type of change you want to make.

This example uses the Alignment link.

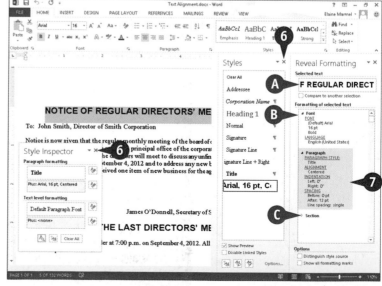

The Indents and Spacing tab of the Paragraph dialog box appears.

8 Select the options you want to change.

9 Click **OK**.

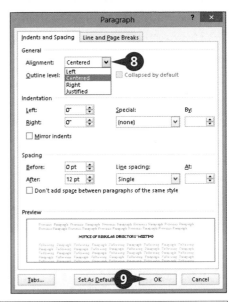

D Word applies the formatting changes.

E The information in the Reveal Formatting pane updates.

F You can click × to close the Reveal Formatting pane.

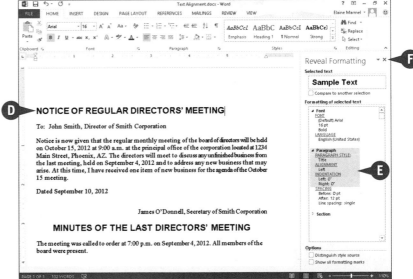

How can I view formatting inconsistencies?
To view wavy blue lines under formatting inconsistencies, click the **File** tab and then click **Options** to display the Word Options dialog box. Click **Advanced** and, in the Editing Options section, select **Keep track of formatting** (☐ changes to ☑) and **Mark formatting inconsistencies** (☐ changes to ☑). Then click **OK**. You can repeat these steps to disable checking for formatting inconsistencies. For suggestions to correct an inconsistency, right-click the underlined word.

Compare Formatting

You can compare the formatting of one selection to another. This feature is useful because it helps you ensure that you apply consistent manual formatting to multiple similar selections. Suppose, for example, that you have a few headings in a document and you do not use heading styles (for more information on using styles, see the next section, "Apply Formatting Using Styles") to format them; by comparing the formatting you apply, you can ensure that you apply formatting consistently. If you find discrepancies, Word can update the second selection so that it matches the first selection.

Compare Formatting

Select Text to Compare

1 Select the first text containing the formatting that you want to compare.

2 Click the **Home** tab.

3 Click ⌐ in the Styles group to display the Styles pane.

A The Styles pane appears.

4 Click the **Style Inspector** button (⧉).

B The Style Inspector pane appears.

5 Click the **Reveal Formatting** button (⧉).

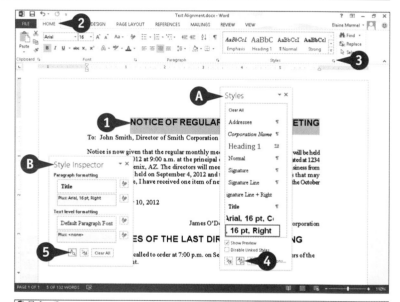

C The Reveal Formatting pane appears.

6 Click × to close the Styles pane and the Style Inspector pane.

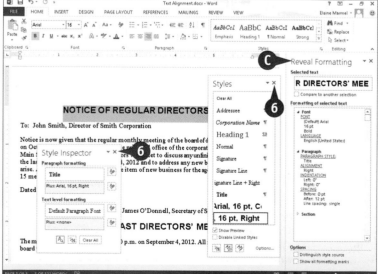

7 Select **Compare to another selection** (☐ changes to ☑).

D A second box for selected text appears.

8 Select the text that you want to compare to the text you selected in Step **1**.

E Formatting differences between the selections appear here.

Match Formatting

1 Slide the mouse pointer over the sample box for the second selection; ▼ appears.

2 Click ▼ .

3 Click **Apply Formatting of Original Selection**.

F Word applies the formatting of the first selection to the second selection.

You can click anywhere to continue working.

G You can click × to close the Reveal Formatting pane.

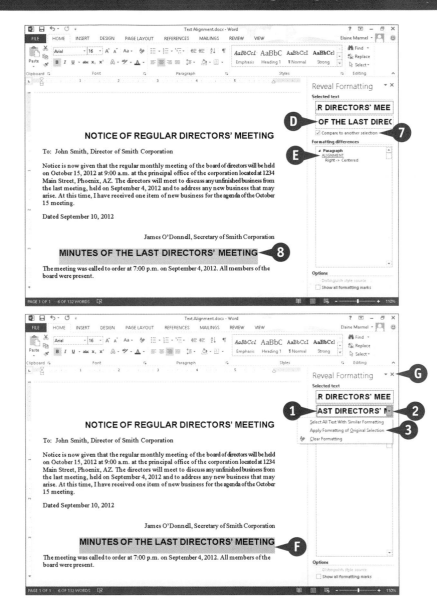

What kind of formatting differences does Word identify in the Reveal Formatting pane?

For any two selections, Word identifies differences in font, paragraph style, alignment, outline level, spacing before and after the paragraphs, line and page breaks, and bullets and numbering. You can make changes to any of these formatting differences by following the steps in the section "Review and Change Formatting."

What happens if I select the Show All Formatting Marks option below the Reveal Formatting pane?

When you select this option, Word displays formatting marks in your document that represent tabs, spaces, paragraphs, line breaks, and so on.

Apply Formatting Using Styles

You can quickly apply formatting and simultaneously maintain formatting consistency to different selections in your document by using styles to format text. *Styles* are predefined sets of formatting that can include font, paragraph, list, and border and shading information. For example, by using heading styles to format headings in your document, you can ensure that all headings use the same formatting and therefore look the same.

You can store styles you use frequently in the Styles Gallery, but you also can easily use styles not stored in the Styles Gallery.

Apply Formatting Using Styles

Using the Styles Gallery

1. Select the text to which you want to apply formatting.

2. Click the **Home** tab.

3. In the Styles group, click ⬆ and ⬇ to scroll through available styles.

4. Click ⬇.

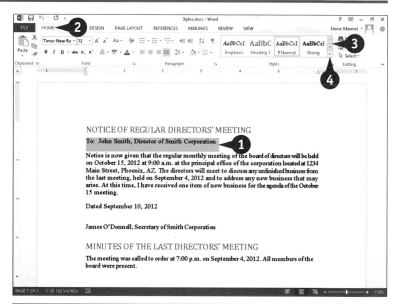

Ⓐ Word displays the Styles Gallery.

Ⓑ The style of the selected text appears highlighted.

Ⓒ As you position the mouse pointer over various styles, Live Preview shows you the way the selected text would look in each style.

You can click a style to apply it to the selected text.

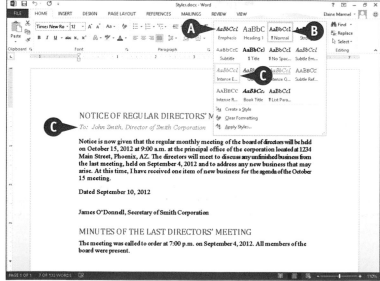

Using Other Styles

1 Select the text to which you want to apply formatting.

2 Click the **Home** tab.

3 In the Styles group, click ⊡ to display the Styles Gallery.

4 Click **Apply Styles**.

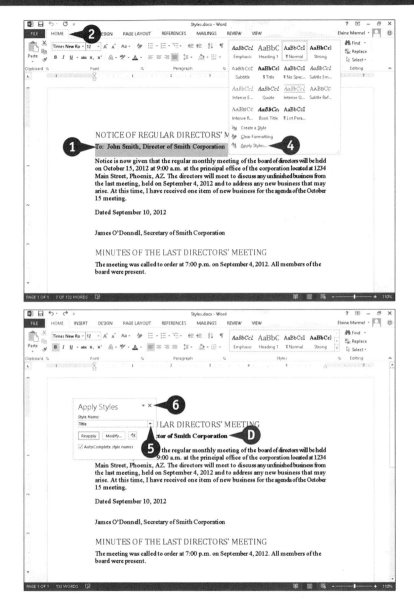

The Apply Styles pane appears.

5 Click ▼ to open the Style Name list, and then select a style.

Ⓓ Word applies the style to the selected text.

6 Click ✕ to close the Apply Styles dialog box.

You can click anywhere to continue working.

TIP

How can I easily view styles as they would appear in my document?

Perform the steps that follow. In the Styles group, click ⌐ to display the Styles pane. In the Styles pane, select **Show Preview** (☐ changes to ☑). Word displays styles using their formatting in the Styles pane.

Switch Styles

You can easily change all text that is formatted in one style to another style. Using this technique can help you maintain formatting consistency in your documents.

For example, suppose that you have been working for a while on a document, and you have been using one particular style for headings. You then decide that you do not like the style you chose to use for headings. Although you could select each heading and change its style, that approach would be tedious and time-consuming — and unnecessary. You can, instead, switch all text in the document formatted in one style to a different style.

Switch Styles

1 Place the insertion point in or select one example of text containing the formatting that you want to change.

2 Click the **Home** tab.

3 Click in the Styles group to display the Styles pane.

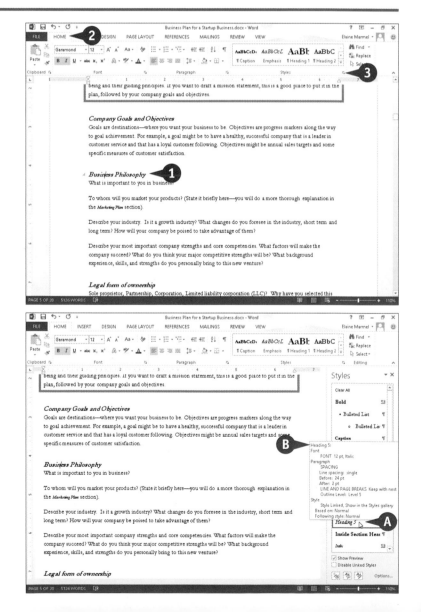

Word displays the Styles pane.

Note: You can dock the pane on-screen if you drag it past the right edge of the screen.

A The style for the selected text appears highlighted.

B You can position over any style to display its formatting information.

④ Position the mouse pointer over a style until ▼ appears.

⑤ Click ▼ to display a list of options.

⑥ Click **Select All Instance(s)**.

ⒸWord selects all text in your document formatted using the style of the text you selected in Step **1**.

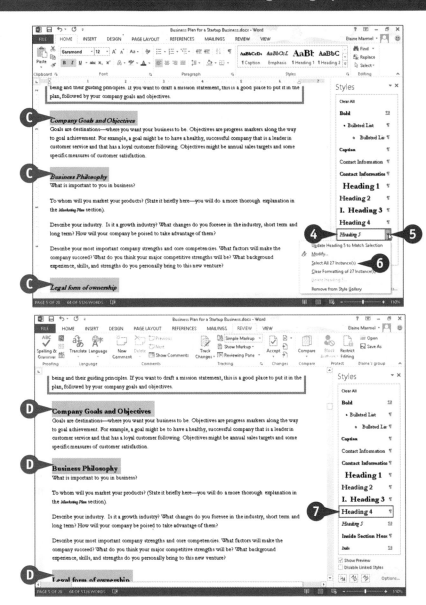

⑦ Click the style you want to apply to all selected text.

ⒹWord changes all selected text to the style you selected in Step **7**.

You can click anywhere to continue working.

TIP

Can I sort styles alphabetically in the Styles pane?
Yes. By default, Word sorts styles using the As Recommended setting, but sorting in alphabetical order is a useful alternative. At the bottom of the Styles pane, click the **Options** link to display the Style Pane Options dialog box. Click the **Select how list is sorted** ☑ and select **Alphabetical**. Then click **OK**.

Save Formatting in a Style

In addition to the styles Word provides for you in the Styles Gallery for headings, normal text, quotes, and more, you can easily create your own styles to store formatting information. Creating your own styles is particularly useful if you cannot find a built-in style that suits your needs.

You can create a new style by formatting text the way you want it to appear when you apply the style. You then use the example text to create the style and store it in the Styles Gallery. You also can modify the style settings at the same time that you create the style.

Save Formatting in a Style

1 Format text in your document using the formatting you want to save in a style.

2 Select the text containing the formatting you want to save.

3 In the Styles group, click ⊡.

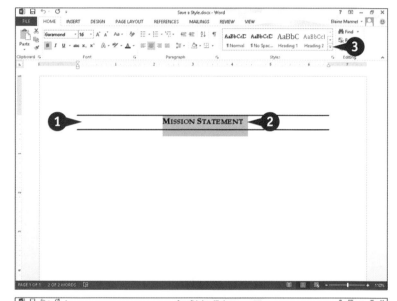

A The Styles Gallery appears.

4 Click **Create a Style.**

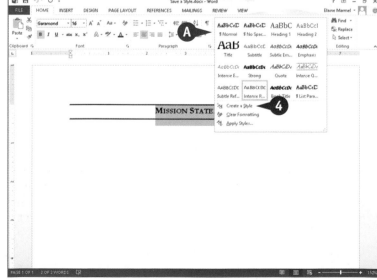

The Create New Style from Formatting dialog box appears.

5 Type a name for the style.

6 Click **Modify**.

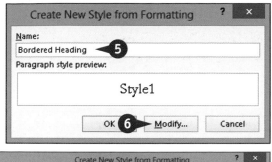

Word displays additional options you can set for the style.

B You can click ☑ and select the style for the following paragraph when you use the style you are creating.

C Use these options to select font formatting for the style.

D Use these options to set paragraph alignment, spacing, and indentation options.

E Select this option to make your style available in new documents (○ changes to ◉).

7 Click **OK**.

Word saves your newly created style.

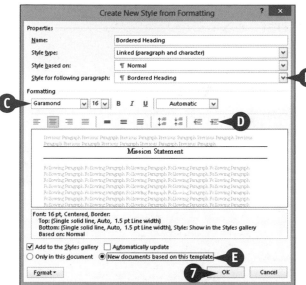

TIPS

What happens if I click Format?
A menu appears that you can use to specify additional formatting. Select the type of formatting, and Word displays a dialog box where you can add more formatting characteristics to the style.

What does the Style Based On option do?
Every style you create is based on a built-in Word style. Changing a built-in style can result in many styles changing. For example, many styles are based on the Normal style. If you change the font of the Normal style, you change the font of all styles based on the Normal style.

Expand or Collapse Document Content

You can hide or display document content by expanding or collapsing headings. Hiding or displaying content can be particularly beneficial if you are working on a long, complicated document. For example, you can hide everything except the portion on which you want to focus your attention. If you send the document to others to review, you can help your reader avoid information overload if you display only the headings and let your reader expand the content of the headings of interest.

To use this feature, you must apply heading styles to text in your document.

Expand or Collapse Document Content

1 In a document, apply heading styles such as Heading 1 or Heading 2.

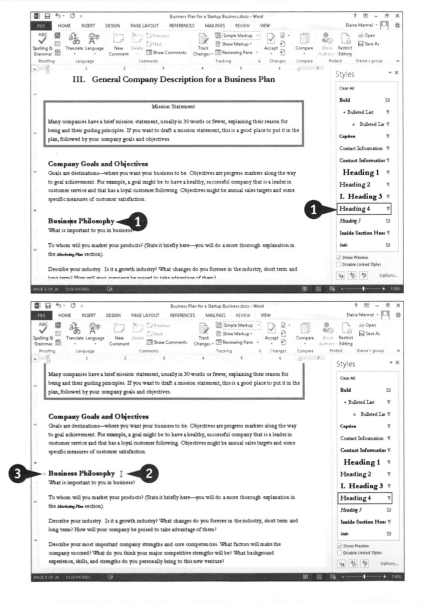

2 Slide the I mouse pointer toward a heading.

A collapse button (◂) appears beside the heading.

3 Click ◂ .

Ⓐ All text following the
heading that is not styled
as a heading disappears
from view.

An expand button (▷)
replaces ◢.

④ Click ▷.

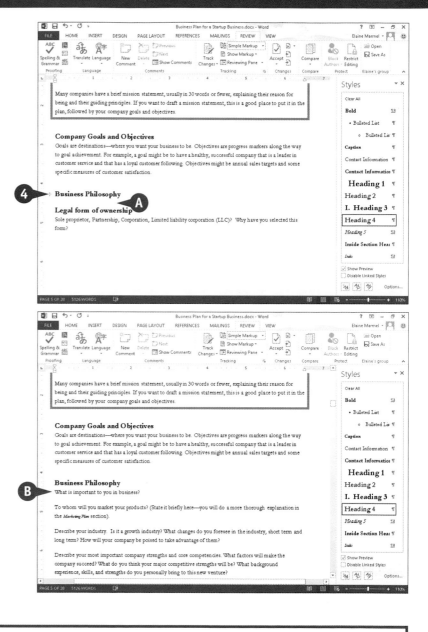

Ⓑ The hidden text reappears.

How can I expand or collapse all headings?
Perform the steps that follow. Right-click any heading. From the menu that
appears, point the mouse at **Expand/Collapse**. Click **Expand All Headings** or
Collapse All Headings (Ⓐ). Collapsing all headings hides all text and headings
except text formatted as Heading 1.

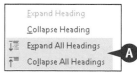

Modify a Style

At some point, you may decide that the formatting of a style is close to but not exactly what you want. For example, you might want to change the size of the font used in a heading style. You do not need to create a new style; you can modify the existing one.

When you change a style, you can add the style to the Styles Gallery, and you can ensure that the style changes appear in new documents you create. You also can have Word update all text in your document that currently uses the style you are modifying.

Modify a Style

1 Open a document containing the style you want to change.

2 Click the **Home** tab.

3 Click ⌐ in the Styles group to display the Styles pane.

4 Right-click the style you want to change.

5 Click **Modify**.

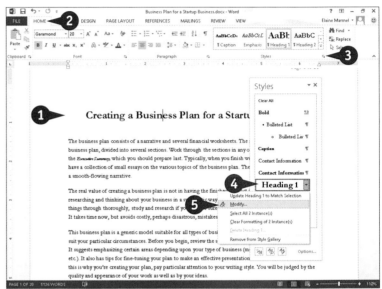

The Modify Style dialog box appears.

6 Make font or paragraph formatting changes.

7 Select the option to make the modified style available in new documents (○ changes to ◉).

8 Select the option to add the style to the Styles Gallery (☐ changes to ☑).

9 Click **OK**.

Word updates all text in the document formatted with the style you changed.

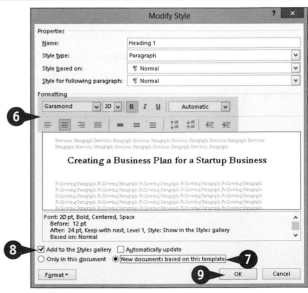

160

Add Paragraph Shading

Shading is another technique you can use to draw your reader's attention. Shading appears on-screen and when you print your document; if you do not use a color printer, paragraph shading will be most effective if you select a shade of gray for your shading.

Add Paragraph Shading

1 Select the paragraph(s) that you want to shade.

2 Click the **Home** tab.

3 Click ▾ beside the Borders button (⊞ ▾).

4 Click **Borders and Shading**.

The Borders and Shading dialog box appears.

5 Click the **Shading** tab.

6 Click ▾.

7 Click a fill color.

8 Click **OK**.

You can click anywhere outside the paragraph(s) you selected in Step **1**.

Ⓐ Word shades the selection you made in Step **1**.

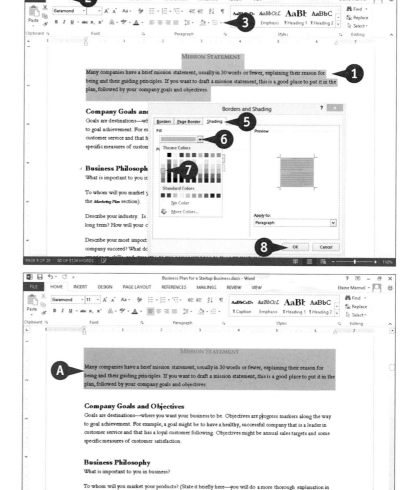

CHAPTER 7

Formatting Pages

In addition to applying formatting to characters and paragraphs, you can apply formatting to pages of your Word document. Find out how to get your page to look its best in this chapter.

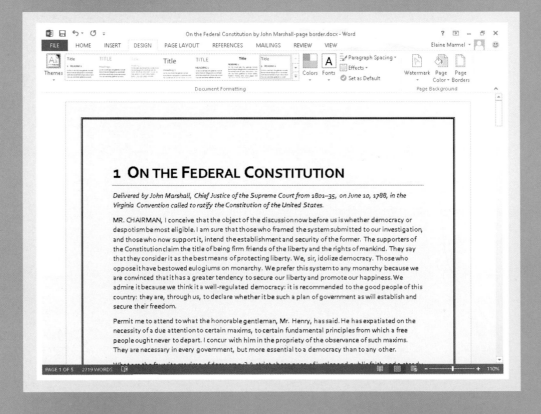

Adjust Margins

By default, Word assigns a 1-inch margin all the way around the page in every new document that you create. You can change these margin settings, however. For example, you can set wider margins to fit more text on a page or set smaller margins to fit less text on a page. You can apply your changes to the current document only or set them as the new default setting, to be applied to all new Word documents you create. When you adjust margins, Word sets the margins from the position of the insertion point to the end of the document.

Adjust Margins

Set Margins Using Page Layout Tools

1. Click anywhere in the document or section where you want to change margins.

2. Click the **Page Layout** tab on the Ribbon.

3. Click **Margins**.

Ⓐ The Margins Gallery appears.

4. Click a margin setting.

Ⓑ Word applies the new settings.

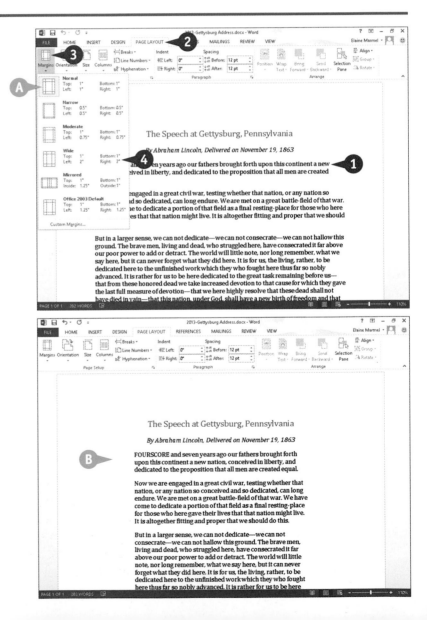

Set a Custom Margin

1 Click the **Page Layout** tab on the Ribbon.

2 Click **Margins**.

C The Margins Gallery appears.

3 Click **Custom Margins**.

The Page Setup dialog box appears, displaying the Margins tab.

4 Type a specific margin in the **Top**, **Bottom**, **Left**, and **Right** boxes.

D You can also click ⬍ to set a margin measurement.

5 Choose a page orientation.

E Preview the margin settings here.

6 Click ⌄, and specify whether the margin should apply to the whole document or from this point forward.

7 Click **OK**.

Word immediately adjusts the margin in the document.

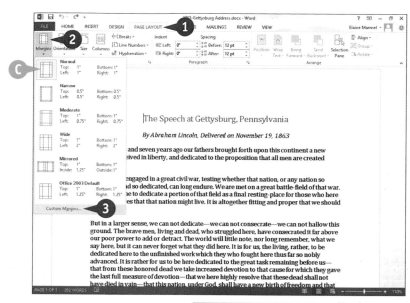

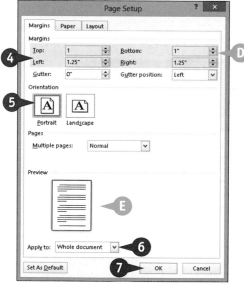

TIPS

How do I set new default margins?
To establish a different set of default margins for every new document that you create, make the desired changes to the Margins tab of the Page Setup dialog box, and click **Set As Default** before clicking **OK**.

Why is my printer ignoring my margin settings?
Some printers have a minimum margin setting, and in most cases, that minimum margin is .25 inches. If you set your margins smaller than your printer's minimum margin setting, you place text in an unprintable area. Be sure to test the margins or check your printer documentation for more information.

Insert a Page Break

Adding page breaks can help you control where text appears. By default, Word automatically starts a new page when the current page becomes filled with text. But you can insert a page break to force Word to start text on a new page, for example, at the end a chapter. You can insert page breaks using the Ribbon or using your keyboard.

You can insert a page break in all views except Read Mode. Page breaks are visible in Print Layout view and, if you display formatting information as described in Chapter 6, page breaks are also visible in Draft, Web Layout, and Outline views.

Insert a Page Break

Using Ribbon Buttons

1. Click in the document where you want to insert a page break.

2. Click the **Insert** tab.

3. Click **Page Break**.

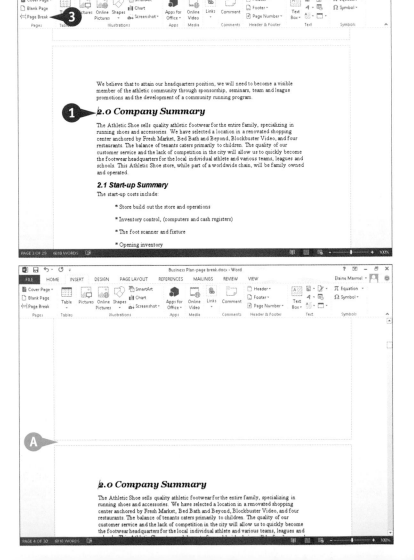

Ⓐ Word inserts a page break and moves all text after the page break onto a new page.

Using the Keyboard

Note: Steps **1** to **3** display formatting information and change your document to Draft view; you can skip these steps and insert a page break in any view except Read Mode.

1 On the Home tab, click the **Show/ Hide** button (¶) to display formatting information.

2 Click the **View** tab.

3 Click **Draft**.

4 Position the insertion point immediately before the text that you want to appear on a new page.

5 Press Ctrl + Enter.

B Word inserts a page break and moves all text after the page break onto a new page.

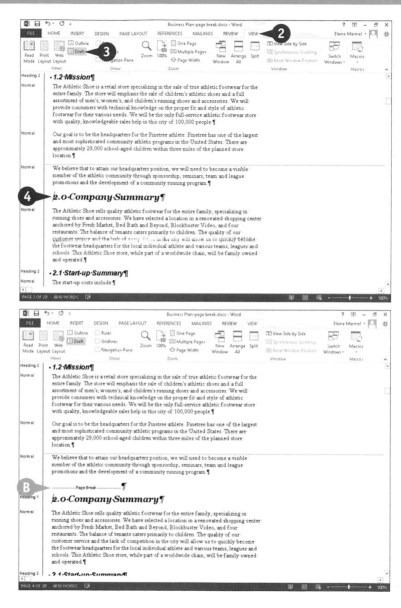

TIP

Can I delete a page break?

Yes. You can delete manually inserted page breaks. With formatting information visible, you can identify these pages breaks in Draft view; they appear as dotted lines containing the words "Page Break." Page breaks that Word inserts automatically also appear as dotted lines but do not contain the words "Page Break." Perform Steps **1** to **3** in the subsection "Using the Keyboard." Click anywhere on a manually inserted page break line and press Delete.

Control Text Flow and Pagination

Although you cannot delete automatic page breaks that Word inserts when you fill a page with text, you can control the placement of page breaks in a number of ways to help your reader more easily understand the document's content.

You can eliminate widows and orphans. You can keep selected lines of a paragraph together on the same page; similarly, you can keep selected paragraphs together, forcing the paragraphs to appear on the same page. You also can force Word to insert a page break before a selected paragraph. The benefits of these controls appear most obviously in Draft view (see Chapter 6).

Control Text Flow and Pagination

Note: To switch to Draft view, click **View** and then click **Draft**.

1. Select the text whose flow you want to affect.

Note: To control widows and orphans, you do not need to select any text.

2. Click **Home**.

3. Click the Paragraph group dialog box launcher (🔾).

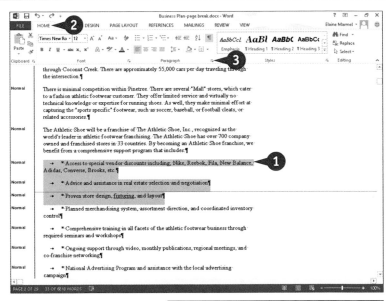

The Paragraph dialog box appears.

4. Click the **Line and Page Breaks** tab.

Ⓐ This area contains the options you can use to control text flow and automatic pagination.

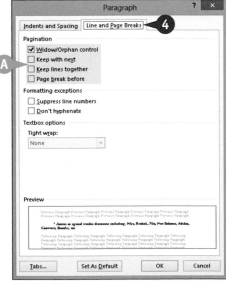

5 Select an option (☐ changes to ☑).

Note: This example keeps lines together on a page.

6 Repeat Step **5** as needed.

7 Click **OK**.

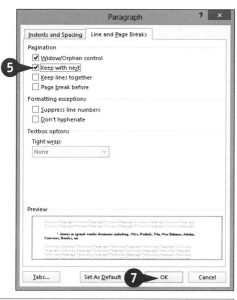

B Word groups the selected text in the manner you specified; in this example, Word inserts a page break before the selected text to keep it together on a page.

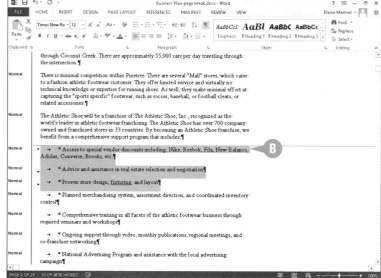

TIPS

What is a widow?

Widow is the term used to describe text grouped so that the first line of a paragraph appears at the bottom of a page and subsequent lines appear on the following page. Widows are distracting to reading comprehension.

What is an orphan?

Orphan is the term used to describe text grouped so that the last line of a paragraph appears at the top of a new page and all preceding lines appear at the bottom of the previous page. Like widows, orphans are distracting to reading comprehension.

Align Text Vertically on the Page

You can align text between the top and bottom margins of a page if the text does not fill the page. For example, you might want to center text vertically on short business letters or report cover pages to improve their appearance.

By default, Word applies vertical alignment to your entire document, but you can limit the alignment if you first divide the document into sections. You will need to use this technique to vertically align the cover page of a report; otherwise, you will align all pages of the report vertically. See the section "Insert a Section Break" for more information.

Align Text Vertically on the Page

Note: To align a report cover page, insert a Next Page section break after the cover page and click anywhere on the cover page.

1. In the document you want to align, click the **Page Layout** tab.

2. Click the Page Setup group dialog box launcher (⌐).

   The Page Setup dialog box appears.

3. Click the **Layout** tab.

4. Click the **Vertical alignment** ∨, and select a vertical alignment choice.

   Ⓐ To align a cover page, click the **Apply to** ∨ and select **This section**.

5. Click **OK**.

   Ⓑ Word applies vertical alignment.

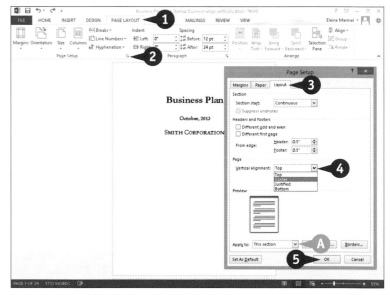

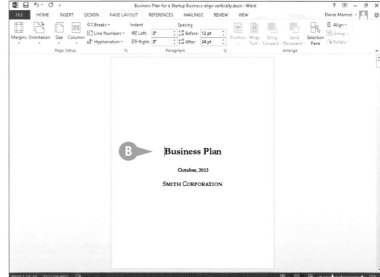

Change Page Orientation

You can change the direction that text prints from the standard portrait orientation of 8 1/2 inches x 11 inches to the landscape orientation of 11 inches x 8 1/2 inches. Changing orientation is particularly helpful on pages containing tables with many columns; using a landscape orientation might help you fit all columns on a single page.

Change Page Orientation

Note: To change the page orientation of a single page in a multi-page document, first insert a Next Page section break before and after the page and click anywhere on the page.

1 Click anywhere in the document or on the page whose orientation you want to change.

2 Click the **Page Layout** tab.

3 Click **Orientation**.

A The current orientation appears highlighted.

4 Click an option.

B Word changes the orientation.

Note: The document in this example appears zoomed out to show orientation changes more clearly.

Note: By default, Word changes the orientation for the entire document. To limit orientation changes, divide the document into sections. See the section "Insert a Section Break."

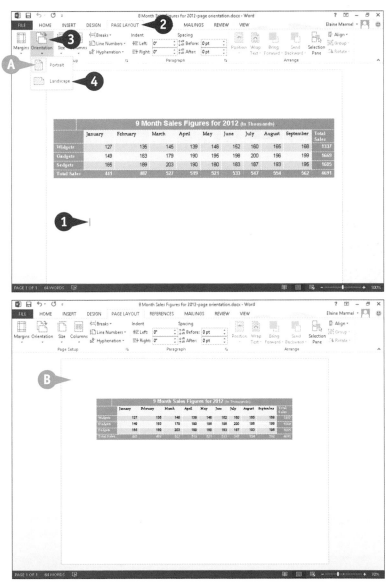

171

Insert a Section Break

You can use section breaks in a document to establish separate margins, headers, footers, vertical page alignment, and other page formatting settings within a single document.

You can start a new section on a new page or anywhere on a page. For example, to establish separate page numbers for chapters, your break should start a new page. But suppose that your document includes a table that will fit on a portrait-oriented page if you can establish narrower margins to accommodate the table; in this case, you can insert continuous section breaks before and after the table and establish margins for the table between the breaks.

Insert a Section Break

1 Click in the location where you want to start a new section in your document.

2 Click the **Page Layout** tab.

3 Click **Breaks**.

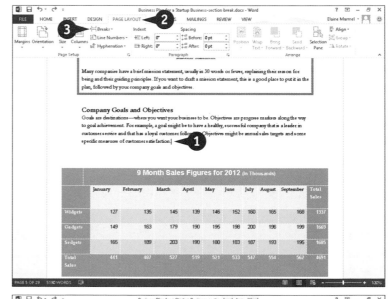

Ⓐ The Breaks Gallery appears.

4 Click an option to select the type of section break you want to insert.

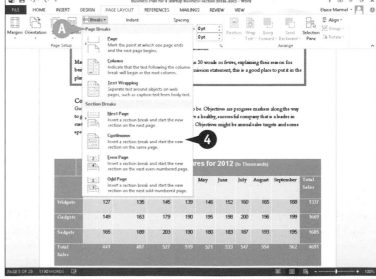

Word inserts the type of break you selected.

5 Click the **View** tab.

6 Click **Draft** to display the document in Draft view.

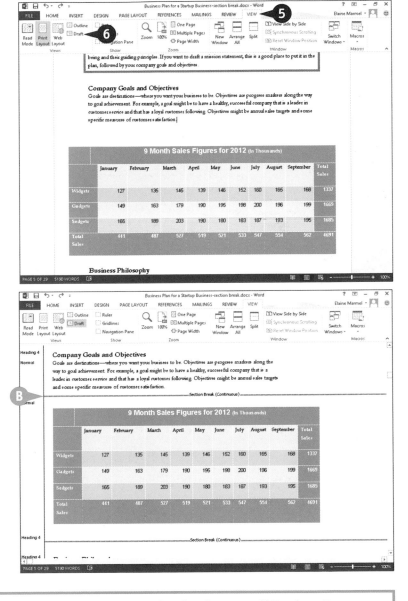

B A section break line appears.

You can remove the section break by clicking the section break line and pressing Delete.

How does Word handle printing when I insert a section break?
Section breaks are formatting marks that do not print; instead, the effects of the section break are apparent when you print. If you insert a Next Page section break, Word starts the text that immediately follows the section break on a new page. But if you insert a Continuous section break as shown in this section, text flows continuously.

What happens if I select Even Page or Odd Page?
Word starts the next section of your document on the next even or odd page. If you insert an Even Page section break on an odd page, Word leaves the odd page blank.

Add Page Numbers to a Document

You can add page numbers to make your documents more manageable. You can choose to add page numbers to the header or footer area at the top or bottom of a page or in the page margins, or you can add a single page number at the current position of the insertion point.

Page numbers in headers and footers appear on-screen only in Print Layout view. A single page number at the current position of the insertion point also appears in Read Mode view. As you edit your document to add or remove text, Word adjusts the document and the page numbers accordingly.

Add Page Numbers to a Document

Note: To place a single page number at a specific location in the document, click that location.

1. Click the **Insert** tab.

2. Click **Page Number**.

A. Page number placement options appear.

3. Click a placement option.

Note: If you choose **Current Position**, Word inserts a page number only at the current location of the insertion point — and nowhere else in the document.

B. A gallery of page number alignment and formatting options appears.

4. Click an option.

C. The page number appears in the location and using formatting you selected.

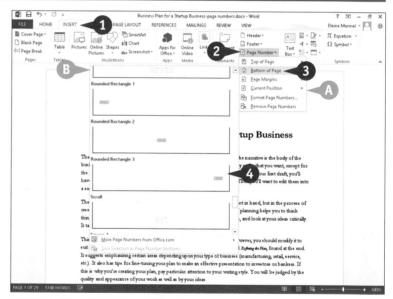

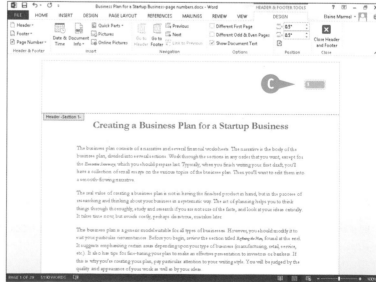

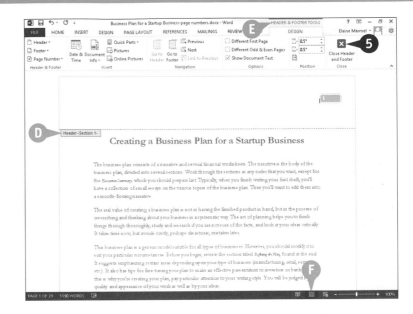

Ⓓ For page numbers placed anywhere *except* at the current position of the insertion point, Word opens the header or footer pane.

Ⓔ Header & Footer Tools appear on the Ribbon.

Ⓕ If you do not see the page number, click the **Print Layout** button (▣) on the status bar to display the document in Print Layout.

5 Click **Close Header and Footer** to continue working in your document.

Note: In Print Layout view, all page numbers *except* those placed at the current position of the insertion point appear gray and unavailable for editing. To work with these page numbers, you must open the header or footer pane. See the section "Add a Header or Footer" later in this chapter.

TIP

How can I start each section of my document with page 1?
You can break the document into sections as described in the section "Insert a Section Break" and then use these steps to start each section on page 1:

1 Complete the steps in this section to insert page numbers in your document.

2 Place the insertion point in the second section of your document, and repeat Steps **1** to **3**, selecting **Format Page Numbers** in Step **3**.

3 In the Page Numbering section, select **Start at** (○ changes to ●) and type **1** in the box.

4 Click **OK**.

5 Repeat these steps for each subsequent section of your document.

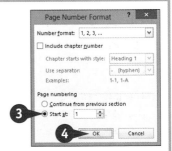

Add Line Numbers to a Document

You can add numbers to the left edge of every line of your document. Line numbers are particularly useful for proofreading; proofreaders can refer to locations in the document by their line numbers. You can number lines in your document continuously, or you can have numbering restart on each page or at each new section. And you can suppress line numbers for selected paragraphs. Line numbers appear on-screen only in Print Layout view.

By default, line numbers appear beside every line in your document, but using line numbering options, you can display lines at intervals you establish.

Add Line Numbers to a Document

Add Line Numbers

1. Click ▦ to display the document in Print Layout view.

2. Click the **Page Layout** tab.

3. Click **Line Numbers**.

4. Click a line numbering option.

   This example shows Continuous.

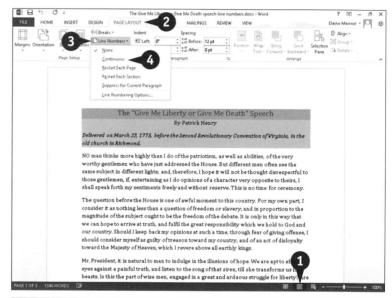

A Word assigns line numbers to each line of your document.

Note: To remove line numbers, complete Steps **1** to **4**, clicking **None** in Step **4**.

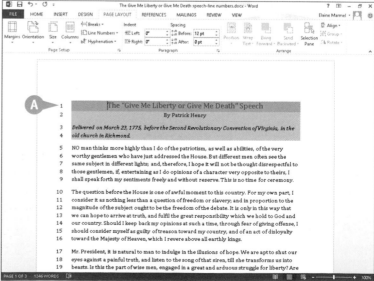

176

Number in Unusual Increments

1 Repeat Steps **1** to **3**, selecting **Line Numbering Options** in Step **3**.

The Layout tab of the Page Setup dialog box appears.

2 Click **Line Numbers** to display the Line Numbers dialog box.

3 Click the **Count by** ↕ to specify an increment for line numbers.

4 Click **OK** to close the Line Numbers dialog box.

5 Click **OK** to close the Page Setup dialog box.

B Line numbers in the increment you selected appear on-screen.

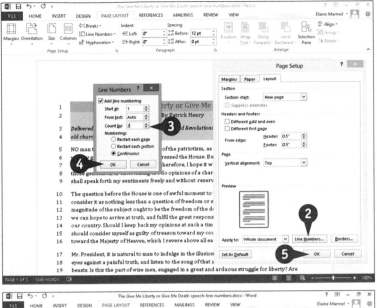

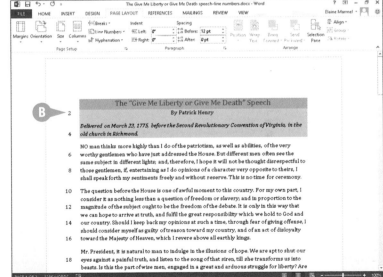

How can I skip numbering certain lines?

To skip numbering certain lines, such as a page title or introductory text, follow Steps **1** to **4** in the subsection "Add Line Numbers." Then perform the steps that follow. Select the paragraphs for which you do not want to display line numbers. Click the **Page Layout** tab and click **Line Numbers**. In the Line Numbers dialog box, click **Suppress for Current Paragraph**. Word removes line numbers from the selected paragraph and renumbers subsequent lines.

Using the Building Blocks Organizer

Building blocks are preformatted text and graphics that you can use to quickly and easily add a splash of elegance and pizzazz to your documents. Some building blocks appear by default as gallery options in Word. And some building blocks provide placeholder text that you replace to customize the building block in your document.

Word organizes building blocks into different galleries, such as cover pages, headers, footers, tables, and text boxes, so that you can sort the building blocks by gallery to easily find something to suit your needs. This section adds a header building block to a document.

Using the Building Blocks Organizer

① Open a document to which you want to add a building block.

Note: Depending on the type of building block you intend to use, you may need to position the insertion point where you want the building block to appear.

② Click the **Insert** tab.

③ Click the **Quick Parts** button (▣ ▾).

④ Click **Building Blocks Organizer**.

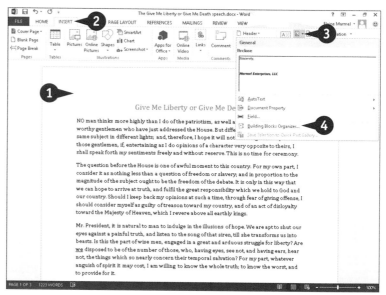

The Building Blocks Organizer window appears.

Ⓐ Building blocks appear here.

Ⓑ You can preview a building block here.

⑤ Click a column heading to sort building blocks by that heading.

Sorting by Gallery is most useful to find a building block for a specific purpose.

⑥ Click a building block.

⑦ Click **Insert**.

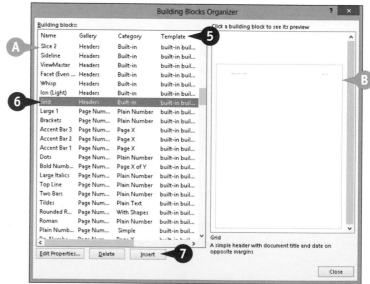

C The building block appears in your document.

This example incorporates a place for a title and date in the header.

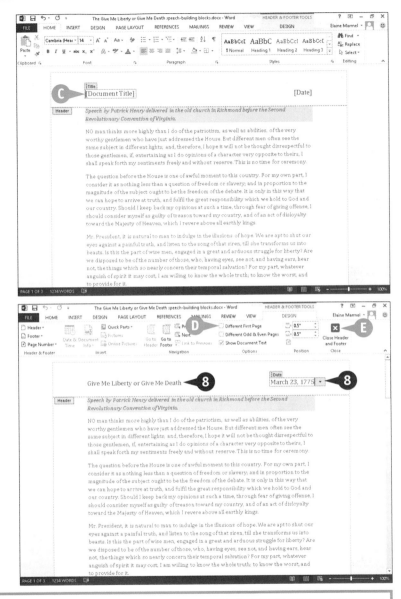

8 Click in the building block, and fill in any required information.

D For headers and footers, you can make the building block appear on all pages of your document if you do not select **Different First Page**.

E You can click **Close Header and Footer** to continue working in your document.

TIP

How do I know where in my document Word will insert a building block?

Word places a building block in your document based on the building block's properties. Complete Steps **1** to **4** in this section to display the Building Blocks Organizer window. Click a building block and click **Edit Properties** to display the Modify Building Block dialog box. Click the **Options** ☑ to determine where a particular building block will appear in your document, in its own paragraph or in its own page (**A**).

Modify Building Block	? ×
Name:	Automatic Table 2
Gallery:	Table of Contents
Category:	Built-In
Description:	Automatic table contents (labeled "Table of Contents") that includes all text formatted with the Heading 1-3 styles
Save in:	built-in building blocks.dotx
Options:	Insert content in its own paragraph
	Insert content only
	Insert content in its own paragraph
	Insert content in its own page

Add a Header or Footer

I f you want to include text at the top or bottom of every page, such as the title of your document, your name, or the date, you can use headers and footers. Header text appears at the top of the page above the margin; footer text appears at the bottom of the page below the margin.

To view header or footer text, you must display the document in Print Layout view. To switch to this view, click the **View** tab and click the **Print Layout** button. Then double-click the top or bottom of the page, respectively, to view the header or footer.

Add a Header or Footer

1 Click the **Insert** tab.

2 Click the **Header** button to add a header, or click the **Footer** button to add a footer.

This example adds a footer.

A The header or footer gallery appears.

3 Click a header or footer style.

Word adds the header or footer and displays the Header & Footer Tools tab.

B The text in your document appears dimmed.

C The insertion point appears in the Footer area.

D Header & Footer Tools appear on the Ribbon.

E Some footers contain information prompts.

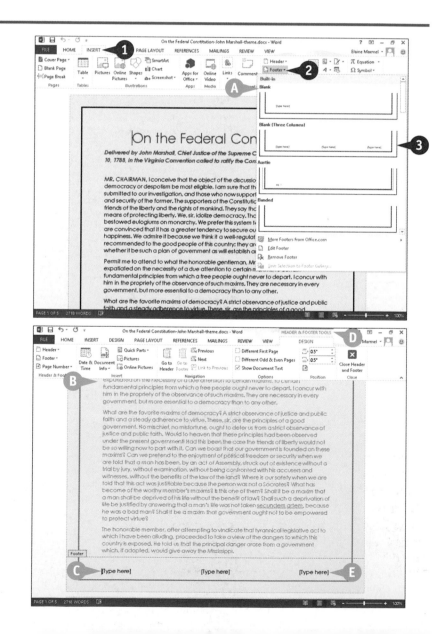

4 Click or select an information prompt.

5 Type footer information.

6 Click **Close Header and Footer**.

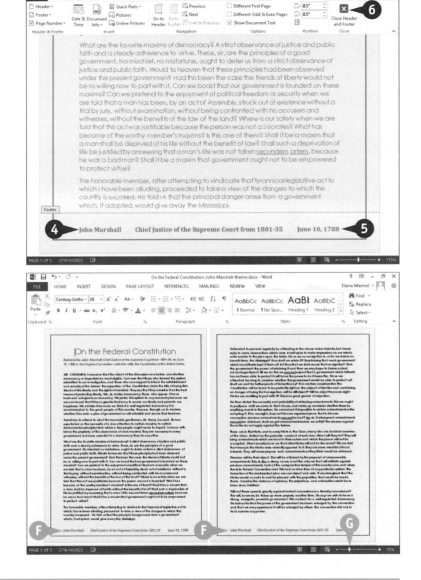

F Word closes the Header & Footer Tools tab and displays the header or footer on the document page.

G You can zoom out to view the header or footer on multiple pages of your document.

Note: To edit a header or footer, click the **Insert** tab on the Ribbon, click the **Header** or **Footer** button, and click **Edit Header** or **Edit Footer** to redisplay the Header & Footer Tools tab.

TIPS

Can I format text in a header or footer?

Yes. You can apply boldface, italics, underlining, and other character formatting the same way that you apply them in the body of a document. And the header area and footer area each contain two predefined tabs so that you can center or right-align text you type.

How do I remove a header or footer?

Click the **Insert** tab, click the **Header** or **Footer** button, and click the **Remove Header** or **Remove Footer** command. Word removes the header or footer from your document.

Using Different Headers or Footers within a Document

You can use different headers or footers in different portions of your document. For example, suppose that you are preparing a business plan and you intend to divide it into chapters. You could create separate headers or footers for each chapter. If you plan to use more than one header or footer in your document, insert section breaks before you begin. See the section "Insert a Section Break" for details.

This section shows how to create different headers in your document, but you can use the steps to create different footers by substituting "footer" wherever "header" appears.

Using Different Headers or Footers within a Document

1 Click in the first section for which you want to create a header.

2 Click the **Insert** tab.

3 Click **Header**.

The Header Gallery appears.

4 Click a header.

Ⓐ Word inserts the header.

Ⓑ The text in your document appears dimmed.

Ⓒ The insertion point appears in the First Page Header-Section 1 box.

Ⓓ To make all headers for a section the same, you can deselect **Different First Page** (☑ changes to ☐).

Note: This example uses different first page headers.

5 Type any necessary text in the header.

6 Click **Next** to move the insertion point to the next page of the first section, Header-Section 1.

7 Click **Next** again.

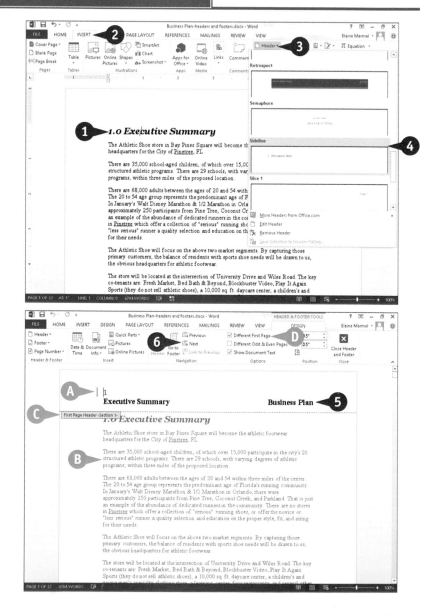

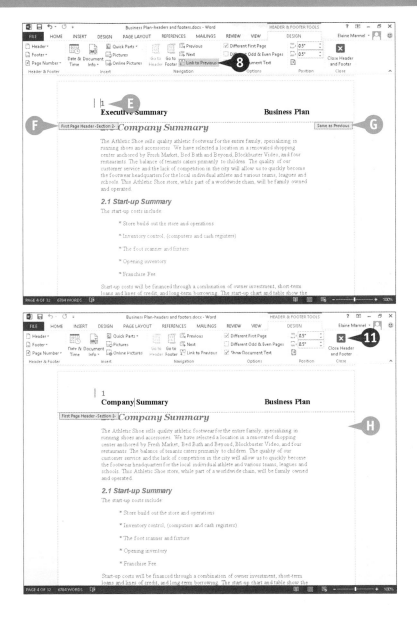

E Word moves the insertion point into the header for Section 2.

F The First Page Header-Section 2 box appears.

G Word identifies the header or footer as "Same as Previous."

8 Click **Link to Previous** to deselect it and unlink the headers of the two sections.

H Word removes the "Same as Previous" marking from the right side of the header box.

9 Repeat Steps **2** to **5** to insert a new header in the second section.

This example displays new text on the left side of the header.

10 Repeat Steps **6** to **9** for each section for which you want a different header.

11 Click **Close Header and Footer**.

TIP

Can I create different headers or footers for odd or even pages?

Yes, and you do not need to insert section breaks. Complete Steps **2** to **5**. Then, on the Design tab of the Header & Footer Tools, click **Different Odd & Even Pages**. Each header or footer box is renamed to Odd Page or Even Page. Click **Next** to switch to the Even Page Header box or the Even Page Footer box and type text.

Add a Footnote

You can include footnotes in your document to identify sources or references to other materials or to add explanatory information. When you add a footnote, a small number appears alongside the associated text, and footnote text appears at the bottom of a page. As you add, delete, and move text in your document, Word also adds, deletes, moves, or renumbers associated footnotes.

Footnotes appear within your document in Print Layout view and Read Mode view. Footnote references appear in the body of your document in all views.

Add a Footnote

1 Click where you want to insert the footnote reference.

2 Click the **References** tab.

3 Click **Insert Footnote**.

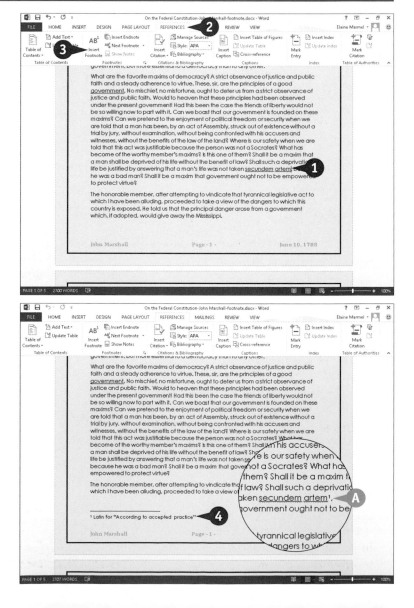

A Word displays the footnote number in the body of the document and in the note at the bottom of the current page.

4 Type the footnote text.

You can double-click the footnote number or press **Shift** + **F5** to return the insertion point to the place in your document where you inserted the footnote.

184

Add an Endnote

You can include endnotes in your document to identify sources or references to other materials or to add explanatory information. Endnotes are numbered i, ii, iii, and so on and their content appears at the end of your document in Print Layout view and Read Mode view. Endnote references appear in the body of your document in all views.

Word automatically numbers endnotes for you. As you add, delete, and move text in your document, Word adds, deletes, moves, or renumbers any associated endnotes.

Add an Endnote

① Click where you want to insert the endnote reference.

Ⓐ In this example, the endnote number appears on page 1.

② Click the **References** tab.

③ Click **Insert Endnote**.

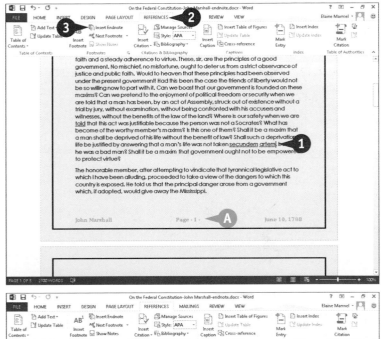

Word inserts the endnote number in the body of your document.

Ⓑ Word inserts the endnote number at the end of your document and displays the insertion point in the endnote area at the bottom of the last page of the document.

④ Type your endnote text.

You can double-click the endnote number or press Shift + F5 to return the insertion point to the place in your document where you inserted the endnote.

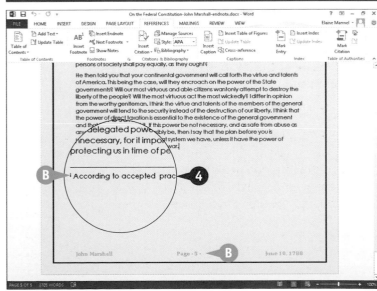

Find, Edit, or Delete Footnotes or Endnotes

As you work, you might find that you need to edit or delete the content of a footnote or an endnote. To make changes to a footnote or an endnote, you must first find the footnote or endnote reference and the associated footnote or endnote text.

You can work in any view to find, edit, or delete a footnote or an endnote. Remember that you do not need to worry about renumbering or moving footnotes or endnotes because Word handles those functions for you automatically. Although you can include both footnotes and endnotes, people typically use only one type of note.

Find, Edit, or Delete Footnotes or Endnotes

Find Footnotes or Endnotes

1 Press **Ctrl**+**Home** to move the insertion point to the top of the document.

2 Click **References**.

3 Click ▼ beside Next Footnote.

4 Click an option to find the next or previous footnote or endnote.

Word moves the insertion point to the reference number of the next or previous footnote or endnote.

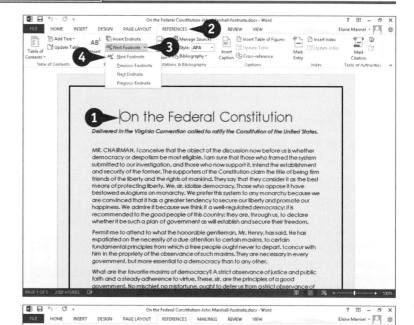

Edit Footnotes or Endnotes

1 Select the footnote or endnote reference number in your document.

2 Double-click the selection.

Note: To easily edit endnotes, press **Ctrl**+**End** to move the insertion point to the end of the document.

A In Print Layout view, Word moves the insertion point into the footnote or endnote.

Ⓑ In Draft view, Word displays footnotes in the Footnotes pane.

③ Edit the text of the note as needed.

④ In Draft view, click the **Close** button (×) when you finish editing.

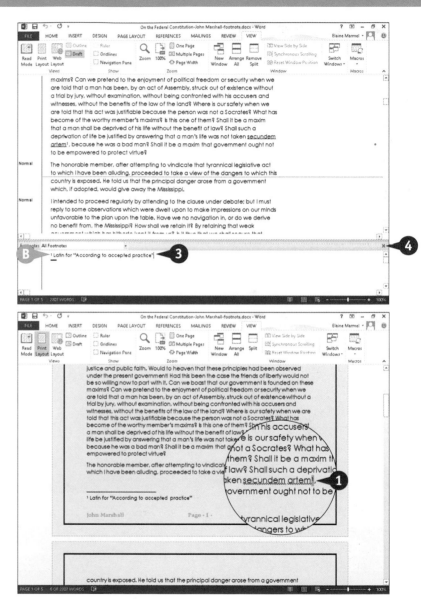

Delete a Footnote or Endnote

① Select the reference number of the footnote or endnote you want to delete.

② Press Delete.

Word removes the footnote or endnote number and related information from the document and automatically renumbers subsequent footnotes or endnotes.

TIP

Can I print endnotes on a separate page?
Yes. Perform the steps that follow. Click in your document before the first endnote. Click the **Insert** tab and click **Page Break**. Word inserts a page break immediately before the endnotes, placing them on a separate page at the end of your document.

Convert Footnotes to Endnotes

You can convert endnotes to footnotes or footnotes to endnotes. Converting footnotes to endnotes or endnotes to footnotes gives you the flexibility to try one type of note and then decide that you prefer the other type of note. Converting notes also helps if you accidentally enter one type of note when you meant to enter the other type. You do not need to delete existing notes of one type and then re-enter them as the other type of note. Instead, you can save time by converting footnotes or endnotes.

Although you can include both footnotes and endnotes, people typically use only one type of note.

Convert Footnotes to Endnotes

1 Click the **References** tab.

2 Click the Footnotes group dialog box launcher (⌐).

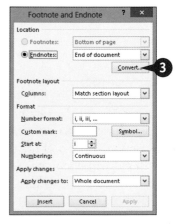

The Footnote and Endnote dialog box appears.

3 Click **Convert**.

The Convert Notes dialog box appears.

4 Select the option that describes what you want to do (⊙ changes to ⊙).

5 Click **OK** to redisplay the Footnote and Endnote dialog box.

In the Footnote and Endnote dialog box, **Cancel** changes to **Close**.

6 Click **Close**.

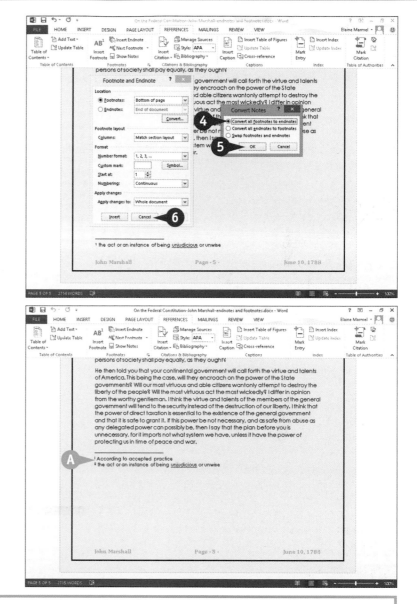

A Word makes the conversion and renumbers footnotes and endnotes appropriately.

What does the Show Notes button in the Footnotes group do?
If your document contains only footnotes or only endnotes, Word jumps to the footnote section on the current page or the endnote section at the end of the document. If your document contains both footnotes and endnotes, Word displays this dialog box so that you can select an option to view.

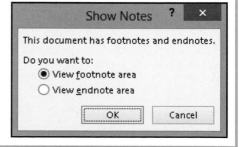

Generate a Table of Contents

You can use Word to generate a table of contents (TOC) for your document that automatically updates as you change your document. You select from Word's gallery of TOC styles to establish the TOC's look and feel. You can most easily create a TOC if you apply heading styles — Heading 1, Heading 2, and Heading 3 — to text that should appear in the TOC. Word searches for text that you format using a heading style and includes that text in the TOC.

You can create a table of contents at any time, continue working, and update the table of contents automatically with new information whenever you want.

Generate a Table of Contents

Insert a Table of Contents

1 Place the insertion point in your document where you want the table of contents to appear.

A This example places the table of contents on a blank page after the cover page of a report.

2 Click the **References** tab.

3 Click **Table of Contents**.

The Table of Contents Gallery appears.

4 Click a table of contents layout.

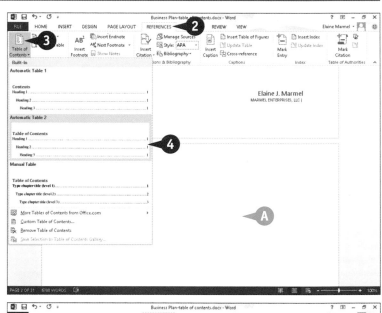

B Word inserts a table of contents at the location of the insertion point.

The information in the table of contents comes from text to which Heading styles 1, 2, and 3 are applied.

You can continue working in your document, adding new text styled with heading styles.

Note: Do not type directly in the table of contents; make corrections in the document.

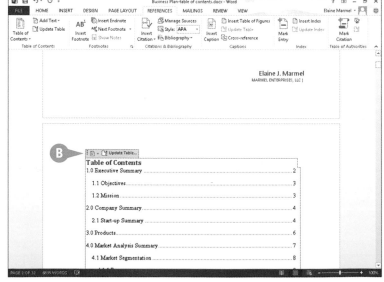

Update the Table of Contents

1. Add or change text styled with heading styles or remove heading styles from text in your document.

2. Click anywhere in the table of contents.

3. Click **Update Table**.

   The Update Table of Contents dialog box appears.

4. Select **Update entire table** (○ changes to ◉).

5. Click **OK**.

C. Word updates the table of contents to reflect your changes.

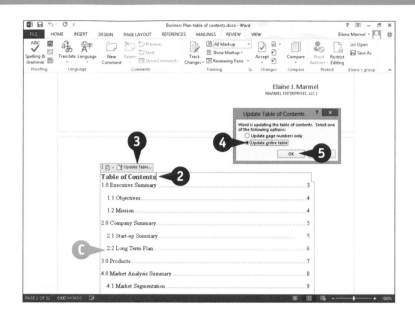

Can I include additional heading styles, such as Heading 4, in the table of contents?

Yes. Simply follow these steps:

1. Complete Steps **2** to **4** in the subsection "Insert a Table of Contents," selecting **Custom Table of Contents** in Step **4** to display the Table of Contents dialog box.

2. Click the **Show levels** ‡ to change the number of heading styles included in the table of contents.

3. Click **OK**.

   Word prompts you to replace the current table of contents.

4. Click **Yes** to update the table of contents.

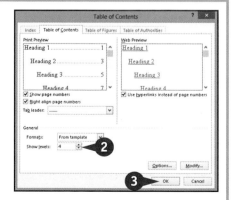

Add a Watermark

You can add a watermark to your document to add interest or convey a message. A watermark is faint text that appears behind information in a document. For example, you can place a watermark on a document that marks it confidential or urgent. Or you can place a watermark on a document to mark it as the original or as a copy. Using a "Draft" watermark can help distinguish a final copy from a review copy. And for material that should not be reproduced, you can apply a "Do Not Copy" watermark.

Watermarks are visible in Print Layout view and when you print your document.

Add a Watermark

1 Click 🔳 to display your document in Print Layout view.

2 Click the **Design** tab.

3 Click **Watermark**.

Ⓐ If you see the watermark you want to use in the Watermark Gallery, you can click it and skip the rest of the steps in this section.

4 Click **Custom Watermark**.

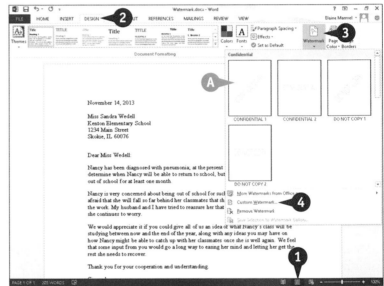

The Printed Watermark dialog box appears.

5 Select **Text watermark** (○ changes to ⦿).

6 Click ⌄, and select the text to use as a watermark or type your own text.

Ⓑ You can use these options to control the font, size, color, intensity, and layout of the watermark.

7 Click **OK**.

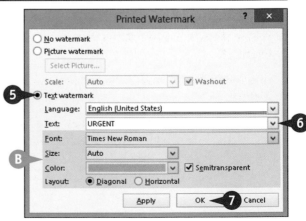

C Word displays the watermark on each page of your document.

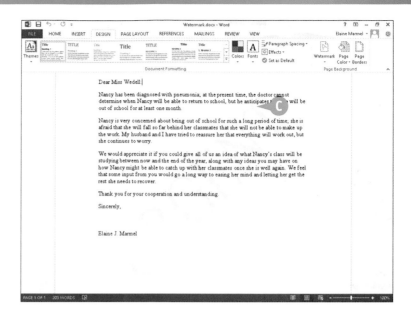

TIP

What happens if I select the Picture Watermark option in the Printed Watermark dialog box?

Word enables you to select a picture stored on your hard drive or to search an online source to select a picture as the watermark in your document. Follow these steps:

1 Follow Steps **1** to **5**, selecting **Picture watermark** in Step **5**.

2 In the Printed Watermark dialog box, click **Select Picture**.

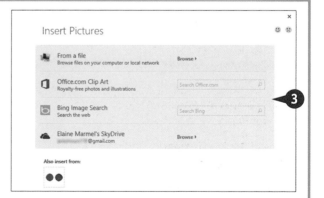

3 In the Insert Picture dialog box, navigate to and insert the picture you want to use as a watermark.

4 Click **OK** in the Printed Watermark dialog box to add the picture watermark to your document.

Add a Page Border

You can add a border around each page of your document to add interest or make the document aesthetically appealing. You also can add borders around a single or multiple paragraphs, as described in Chapter 6, but be careful not to use too many effects; you risk making your document difficult to read. For example, do not use both paragraph and page borders.

You can apply one of Word's predesigned borders to your document, or you can create your own custom border — for example, bordering only the top and bottom of each page.

Add a Page Border

1 Click ▣ to display your document in Print Layout view.

2 Click the **Design** tab.

3 Click **Page Borders**.

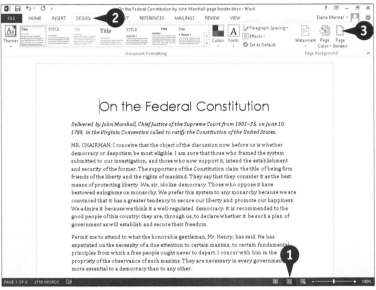

The Borders and Shading dialog box appears, displaying the Page Border tab.

4 Click the type of border you want to add to your document.

5 Click a style for the border line.

Ⓐ This area shows a preview of the border.

Ⓑ You can click ⌄ to select a color for the border from the palette that appears.

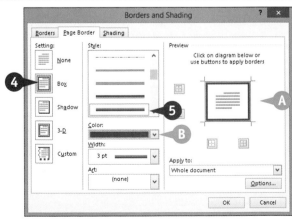

C You can click ☑ to select a width for the border.

6 Click ☑ to specify the pages on which the border should appear.

7 Click **OK**.

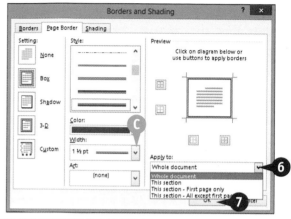

D Word applies the border you specified.

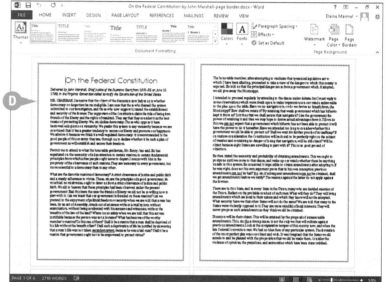

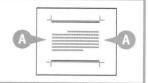

Apply Document Formatting

You can give a professional look to a document using document formatting. You can apply a document theme, which consists of a set of theme colors that affect fonts, lines, and fill effects. Applying a theme to a document is a quick way to add polish to it. And once you apply a theme, you also can apply style sets, which vary the fonts.

The effect of applying a theme is more obvious if you have assigned styles such as headings to your document. The effects of themes are even more pronounced when you assign a background color to a page.

Apply Document Formatting

Apply a Theme

1 Open a document.

The document uses current colors and styles for its fonts, lines, page color, and fill effects.

2 Click the **Design** tab.

3 Click **Themes**.

Note: You can point at a theme, and Live Preview will show you how the document would look using that theme.

4 Click a theme.

Your document appears using the theme you selected.

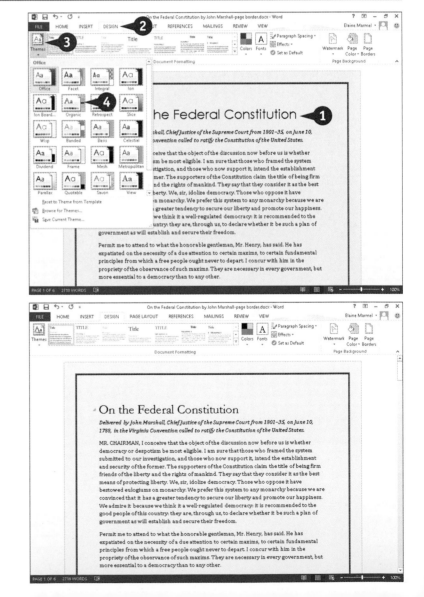

Apply a Style Set

1 Complete Steps **1** to **4** in the previous subsection.

2 Click the **Design** tab.

3 Point the mouse at various style sets.

Note: Live Preview shows you how the document would look using that style set.

4 Click a style set.

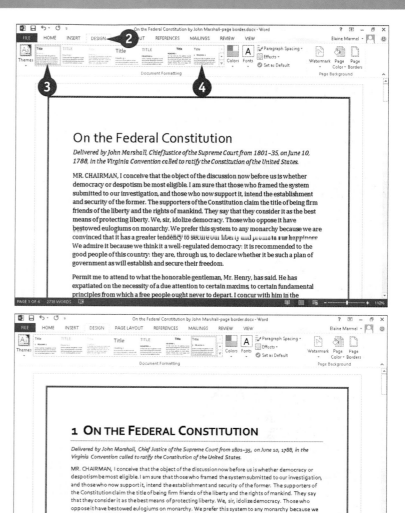

Your document appears using the style set you selected.

How can I make the effects of my theme more obvious?
The effects of applying a theme become more obvious if you have applied heading styles and a background color to your document. To apply a background color, click the **Design** tab, click the **Page Color** button (**A**), and click a color in the palette (**B**); Word applies the color you selected to the background of the page. For help applying a style, see Chapter 6.

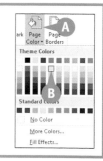

Create Newspaper Columns

You can create columns in Word to present your text in a format similar to a newspaper or magazine, where columnar information runs from the bottom of one column to the top of the next column. For example, if you are creating a brochure or newsletter, you can use columns to make text flow from one block to the next.

If you simply want to create a document with two or three columns, you can use one of Word's preset columns. Alternatively, you can create custom columns, choosing the number of columns you want to create in your document, indicating the width of each column, and more.

Create Newspaper Columns

Create Quick Columns

Note: If you want to apply columns to only a portion of your text, select that text.

1. Click the **Page Layout** tab.

2. Click the **Columns** button.

3. Click the number of columns that you want to assign.

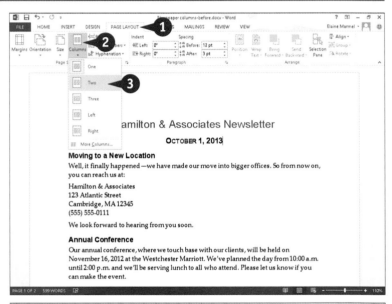

Word displays your document in the number of columns that you specify.

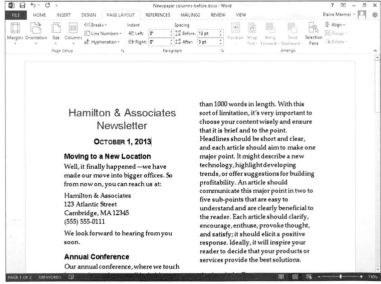

Create Custom Columns

Note: If you want to apply columns to only a portion of your text, select that text.

1 Click the **Page Layout** tab.

2 Click the **Columns** button.

3 Click **More Columns**.

The Columns dialog box appears.

4 Click a preset for the type of column style that you want to apply.

A You can select this option (☐ changes to ☑) to include a vertical line separating the columns.

5 Deselect this option to set exact widths for each column (☑ changes to ☐).

6 Set an exact column width and spacing here.

B You can specify whether the columns apply to the selected text or the entire document.

7 Click **OK**.

Word applies the column format to the selected text.

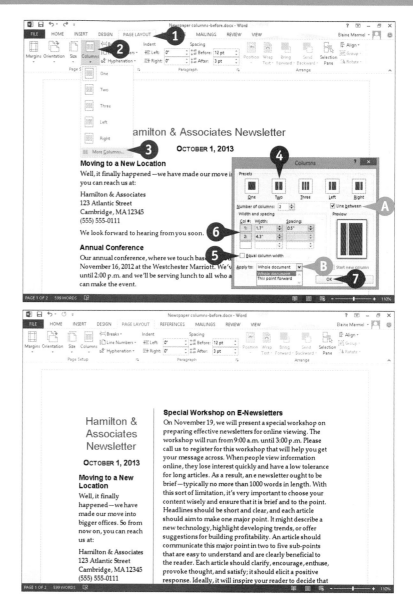

TIPS

How do I wrap column text around a picture or other object?

Click the picture or other object that you want to wrap, click the **Format** tab, click the **Wrap Text** button, and then click the type of wrapping that you want to apply.

Can I create a break within a column?

Yes. To add a column break, click where you want the break to occur and then press **Ctrl**+**Shift**+**Enter**. To remove a break, select it and press **Delete**. To return to a one-column format, click the **Columns** button on the Page Layout tab, and then select the single-column format.

CHAPTER 8

Printing Documents

After your document looks the way you want it to look, you are ready to distribute it. In this chapter, you learn how to preview and print documents, print envelopes, and print labels.

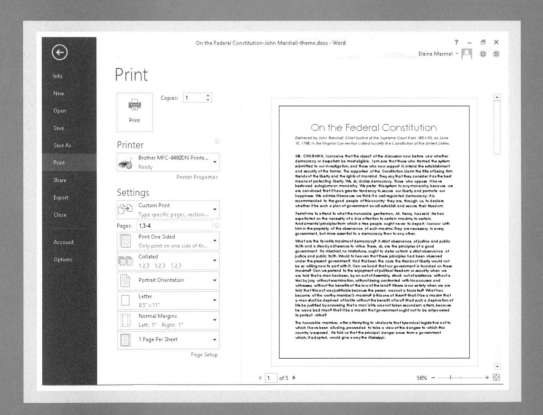

Preview and Print a Document

If a printer is connected to your computer, you can print your Word documents. For example, you might print a document to look for layout errors and other possible formatting inconsistencies or to distribute it as a handout in a meeting.

When you print a document, you have two options. You can send a document directly to the printer using the default settings, or you can change these settings. For example, you might opt to print just a portion of the document or print using a different printer. You can preview your document before you print it.

Preview and Print a Document

1 Open the document you want to print.

Note: To print only selected text, select that text.

2 Click the **File** tab.

Backstage view appears.

3 Click **Print**.

Ⓐ A preview of your document appears here.

4 Click these arrows to page through your document.

5 To magnify the page, drag the Zoom slider.

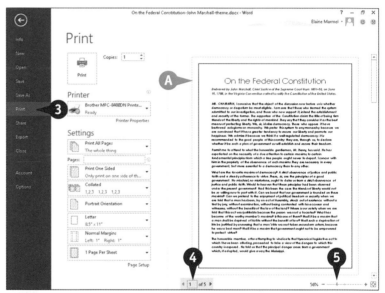

6 Click ▼ to select a printer.

7 To print more than one copy, type the number of copies to print here or click ⬍.

8 Click ▼ to select what to print.

Ⓑ You can print the entire document, text you selected, or only the current page.

Ⓒ You can click ▲ and ▼ to select document elements to print, such as document properties or a list of styles used in the document.

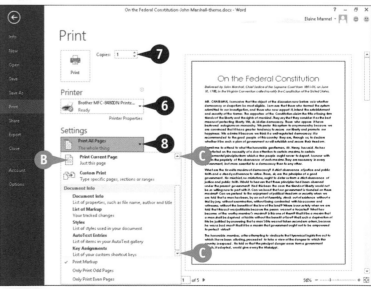

9 To print noncontiguous pages, type the pages you want to print, such as **1,5,6–9** or **1,3-4** in the Pages box.

10 To print the document, click the **Print** button.

D If you change your mind and do not want to print, click ⊙ to return to the document window.

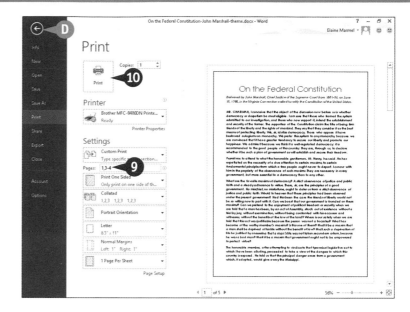

What other print options can I set?
In the Settings section, click buttons to select options:

Option	Purpose
Print One Sided — Only print on one sid...	Determine whether to print on one or both sides of the paper.
Collated 1,2,3 1,2,3 1,2,3	When printing multiple copies, specify whether to collate the copies or print multiple copies of each page at the same time.
Portrait Orientation	Choose to print in Portrait or Landscape orientation.
Letter 8.5" x 11"	Select a paper size.
Normal Margins Left: 1" Right: 1"	Select page margins.
1 Page Per Sheet	Specify the number of pages to print on a single sheet of paper.

Print on Different Paper Sizes

You can print one part of your document on one size of paper and another part on a different size of paper. For example, you may want to print one portion of your document on legal-sized paper to accommodate a particularly long table and then print the rest of the document on letter-sized paper.

You must insert section breaks in your document for each portion of the document that you want to print on different paper sizes. To learn how to insert section breaks, see Chapter 7.

Print on Different Paper Sizes

1 After dividing your document into sections, place the insertion point in the section that you want to print on a different paper size.

2 Click the **Page Layout** tab.

3 Click the Page Setup group dialog box launcher (⌐).

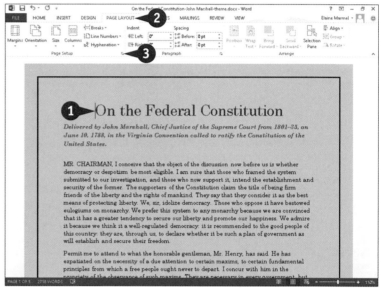

The Page Setup dialog box appears, displaying the Margins tab.

4 Click the **Paper** tab.

5 Click ⌄, and select the paper size you want to use.

Ⓐ The width and height of the paper size you select appear here.

Ⓑ A preview of your selection appears here.

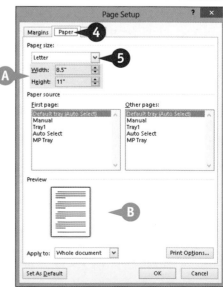

6 Click here to select a paper tray for the first page in the section.

7 Click here to select a paper tray for the rest of the section.

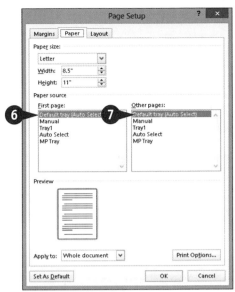

8 Click the **Apply to** ⌄.

9 Click **This section**.

10 Repeat these steps for other sections of the document.

11 Click **OK** to save your changes.

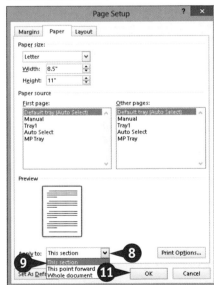

What happens when I click Print Options in the Page Setup dialog box?
The Display tab of the Word Options dialog box appears. In the Printing Options section, you can select check boxes to control the printing of various Word elements.

Printing options

☑ Print drawings created in Word ⓘ

☐ Print background colors and images

☐ Print document properties

☐ Print hidden text

☐ Update fields before printing

☐ Update linked data before printing

Print an Envelope

If your printer supports printing envelopes, Word can print a delivery and return address on an envelope for you. You also can have Word automatically fill in the recipient's name and address. Word checks the currently open document for information that appears to be an address; if Word finds an address, Word fills in the address automatically. To save yourself time and typing, open the letter you intend to mail before you follow the steps in this section to print the envelope.

Consult your printer manual to determine whether your printer supports printing envelopes.

Print an Envelope

1 Click the **Mailings** tab.

2 Click **Envelopes**.

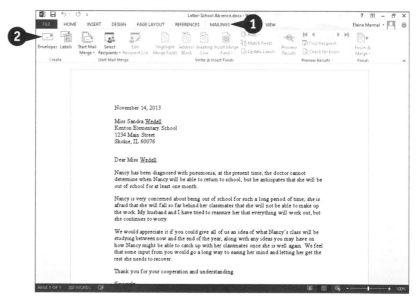

The Envelopes and Labels dialog box appears.

3 Click the **Envelopes** tab.

Note: If Word finds an address near the top of your document, it displays and selects that address in the Delivery address box.

4 You can type a delivery address.

You can remove an existing address by pressing Delete.

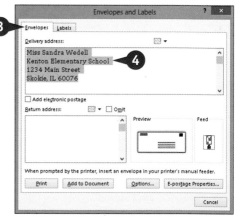

By default, Word displays no return address in the Return address box.

⑤ Click here to type a return address.

⑥ Click **Print**.

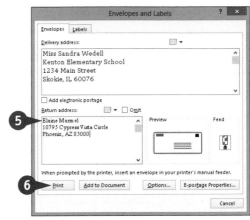

A dialog box appears if you supplied a return address.

Note: If you save the return address, Word displays it each time you print an envelope and does not display this dialog box.

⑦ Click **Yes**.

Word saves the return address as the default return address and prints the envelope.

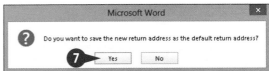

TIP

What happens if I click Options in the Envelopes and Labels dialog box?
Word displays the Envelope Options dialog box. On the Envelope Options tab, you can set the envelope size, include a delivery bar code, and set fonts for the delivery and return addresses. On the Printing Options tab, you can set the feed method and tray for your printer.

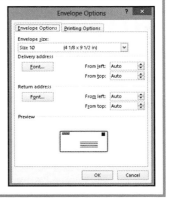

Set Up Labels to Print

You can format a Word document so that you can use it to type and print labels using an assortment of standard labels from a variety of vendors, including Avery, 3M, Microsoft, Office Depot, and Staples, to name just a few. Printing address labels is useful when you need to mail packages or envelopes that are not letter-size. You also are not limited to printing address labels; you also can create name tag and file folder labels, for example.

This section demonstrates how to create a blank page of address labels onto which you can type address label information.

Set Up Labels to Print

1 Click the **Mailings** tab.

2 Click **Labels**.

The Envelopes and Labels dialog box appears.

3 Click the **Labels** tab.

Ⓐ This area shows the label currently selected.

4 Click **Options**.

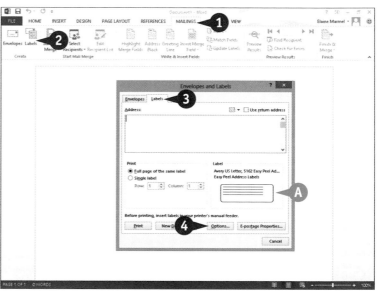

The Label Options dialog box appears.

5 In this area, select the type of printer and printer tray to print labels (○ changes to ◉).

6 Click ∨ to select the vendor that makes your labels.

7 Click the product number of your labels.

8 Click **OK**.

9 Click **New Document** in the Envelopes and Labels dialog box.

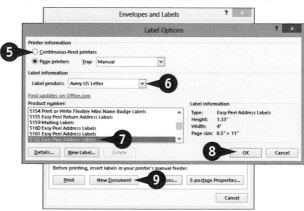

Word displays a blank document, set up for label information.

10 If you do not see gridlines separating labels, click the **Layout** tab.

11 Click **View Gridlines**.

12 Type a label.

13 Press **Tab** to move to the next label and type an address.

Note: To print labels, see the section "Preview and Print a Document" earlier in this chapter.

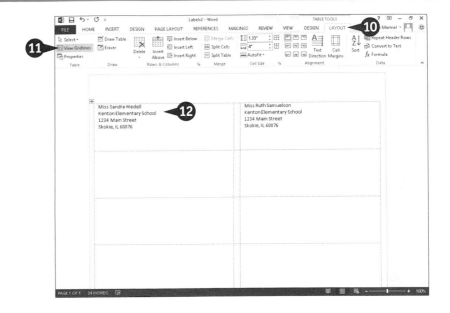

TIP

Can I print a single label?

1 Complete Steps **1** to **3** in this section to open the Envelopes and Labels dialog box.

2 Select **Single label** (○ changes to ◉).

3 Type the row and column of the label on the label sheet that you want to use.

4 Click here to display the Label Options dialog box and select the label you use (refer to Steps **5** to **8**).

5 Type the label information here.

6 Click **Print**, and Word prints the single label.

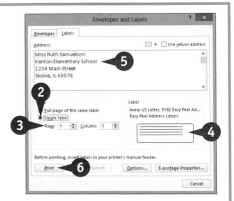

CHAPTER 9

Working with Tables and Charts

Do you want to keep the information in your Word document easy to read? The answer may very well be to add a table to contain your data. In this chapter, you learn how to create and work with tables in Word.

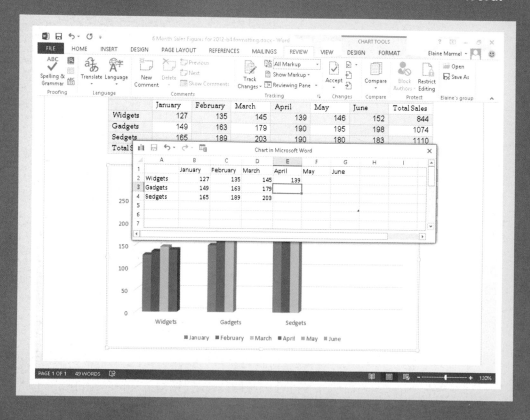

Create a Table

You can use tables to present data in an organized fashion. For example, you might add a table to your document to display a list of items or a roster of classes. Tables contain columns and rows, which intersect to form *cells*. You can insert all types of data in cells, including text and graphics.

To enter text in cells, click in the cell and then type your data. As you type, Word wraps the text to fit in the cell. Press `Tab` to move from one cell to another. You can select table cells, rows, and columns to perform editing tasks and apply formatting.

Create a Table

Insert a Table

1 Click in the document where you want to insert a table.

2 Click the **Insert** tab.

3 Click the **Table** button.

A Word displays a table grid.

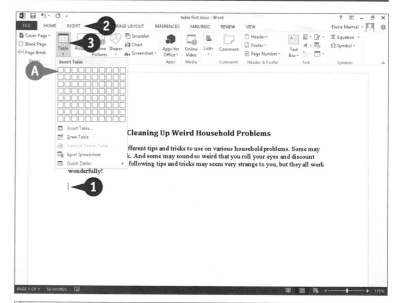

4 Slide the mouse pointer across the squares that represent the number of rows and columns you want in your table.

B Word previews the table as you drag over cells.

5 Click the square representing the lower-right corner of your table.

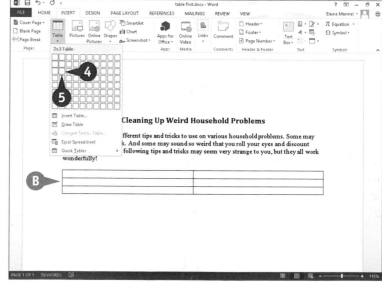

The table appears in your document.

C Table Tools appear on the Ribbon.

6 Click in a table cell, and type information.

D If necessary, Word expands the row height to accommodate the text.

You can press **Tab** to move the insertion point to the next cell.

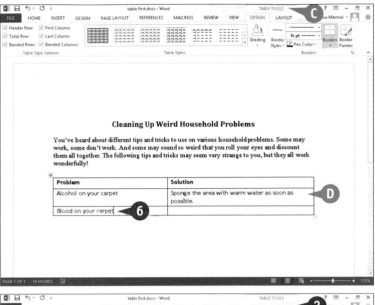

Delete a Table

1 Click anywhere in the table you want to delete.

2 Click the **Layout** tab.

3 Click **Delete**.

4 Click **Delete Table**.

Word removes the table and its contents from your document.

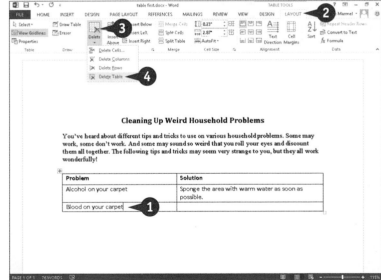

TIPS

Can I add rows to a table?

Yes. To add a row to the bottom of the table, place the insertion point in the last cell and press **Tab**. To add a row anywhere else, use the buttons in the Rows & Columns section of the Layout tab.

What, exactly, is a table cell?

Cell refers to the intersection of a row and a column. In spreadsheet programs, columns are named with letters, rows are named with numbers, and cells are named using the column letter and row number. For example, the cell at the intersection of Column A and Row 2 is called A2.

Change the Row Height or Column Width

You can change the height of rows or the width of columns to accommodate your table information. Be aware that Word changes row height automatically to accommodate information but leaves column width unchanged unless you take action to change a column's width. Most people change row height or column width to improve the appearance of their table.

You cannot change either row height or column width unless you work in Print Layout view or Web Layout view, so use the buttons on the status bar to switch to one of these views before you try to change row height or column width.

Change the Row Height or Column Width

Change the Row Height

1 Click the **Print Layout** button (▣) or the **Web Layout** button (▣).

2 Position the mouse pointer over the bottom of the row you want to change (I changes to ↕).

3 Drag the row edge up to shorten or down to lengthen the row height.

A A dotted line marks the proposed bottom of the row.

4 When the row height suits you, release the mouse button.

B Word adjusts the row height.

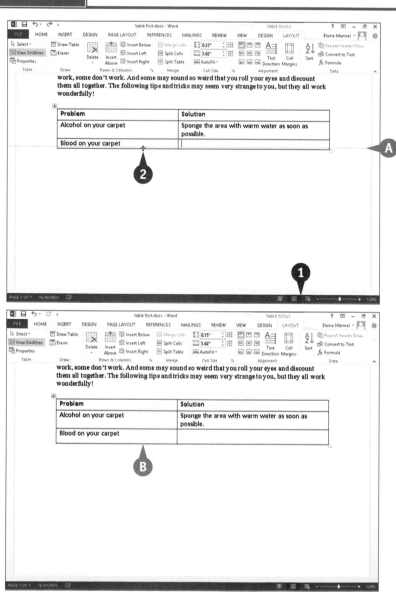

214

Change the Column Width

1 Position the mouse pointer over the right side of the column you want to change (I changes to +‖+).

2 Drag the column edge right to widen or left to narrow the column width.

C A dotted line marks the proposed right side of the column.

3 Release the mouse.

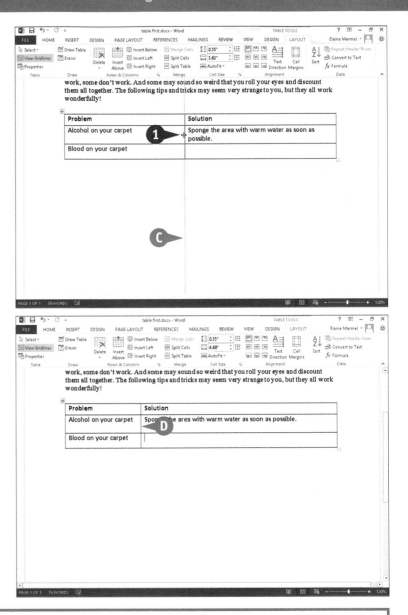

D Word adjusts the column width.

Note: For any column except the rightmost column, changing a column's width also changes the width of the column to its right, but the overall table size remains constant. When you change the width of the rightmost column, you change the width of the entire table.

I tried to change the row height, but the mouse pointer did not change, and I could not drag the row. What did I do wrong?

You can change row height only when displaying your document in either Print Layout view or Web Layout view. Make sure you select one of those views by clicking ▦ or ▥. See Chapter 3 for more on understanding document views and switching between them.

Can I easily make a column the size that accommodates the longest item in it?

Yes. Double-click the right edge of the column. Word widens or narrows the column based on the longest entry in the column and adjusts the overall table size.

Move a Table

You can move a table to a different location in your document. You might discover, for example, that you inserted a table prematurely in your document and, as you continue to work, you decide that the table would better help you make your point if you move it to a location further down in your document. You do not need to reinsert the table and re-enter its information; instead, move it.

Make sure that you are working from Print Layout or Web Layout view; you can use the buttons on the status bar or on the View tab to switch views if necessary.

Move a Table

1. Click the **Print Layout** button (▤) or the **Web Layout** button (▥).

2. Position the mouse pointer over the table.

   A table selection handle (⊞) appears in the upper-left corner of the table.

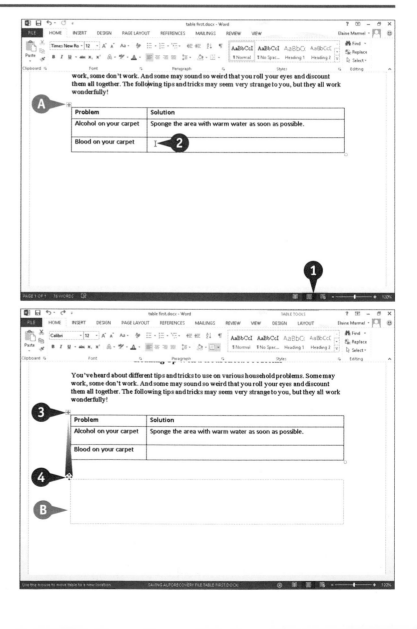

3. Position the mouse pointer over ⊞ (I changes to ⬉).

4. Drag the table to a new location (⬉ changes to ✛).

   B A dashed line represents the proposed table position.

5. Release the mouse button.

   The table appears in the new location.

   To copy the table, perform these steps but press and hold Ctrl in Step **3**.

Resize a Table

If you find that your table dimensions do not suit your purpose, you can resize the table from Print Layout view or Web Layout view. For example, you may want to resize a table to make it longer and narrower, especially if your table is small; in that case, you could reduce the space occupied by the table and wrap text in your document around it using the Table Properties box.

Make sure that you are working from Print Layout or Web Layout view; you can use the buttons on the status bar to switch views if necessary.

Resize a Table

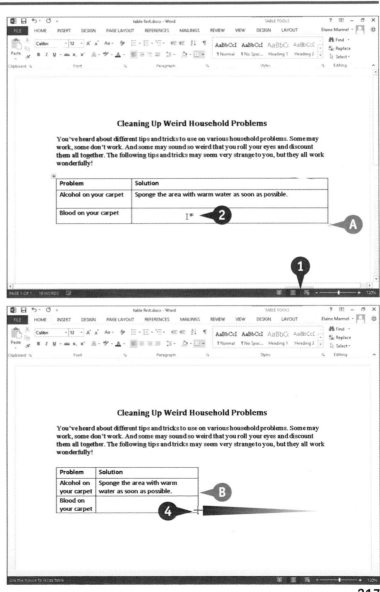

① Click the **Print Layout** button (▣) or the **Web Layout** button (▣).

② Position the mouse pointer over the table.

Ⓐ A handle (▫) appears in the lower-right corner of the table.

③ Position the mouse pointer over the handle (I changes to ↖).

④ Drag up, down, left, or right to adjust the table's size (↖ changes to +).

Note: You can also drag diagonally to simultaneously change both the width and height of the table.

Ⓑ The table outline displays the proposed table size.

⑤ Release the mouse button to change the table's size.

Note: On the Table Tools Layout tab, you can click **Properties** to control how text wraps around the outside of your table.

217

Add or Delete a Row

You can easily add rows to accommodate more information or remove rows of information you do not need. Word automatically adds rows to the bottom of a table if you place the insertion point in the last table cell and press **Tab**. If you accidentally insert an extra row at the bottom of the table, you can delete it. If you need additional rows in the middle of your table to accommodate additional information, you can insert extra rows.

To add a new first row to your table, see the first tip at the end of this section.

Add or Delete a Row

Add a Row

1 Slide I outside the left edge of the row below where you want a new row to appear.

A I changes to ⬦ and a plus sign (⊕) attached to a pair of horizontal lines that span the width of the table appears.

2 Click ⊕.

B Word inserts a row above the row you identified in Step **1** and selects it.

When you slide the mouse away from the row, ⊕ disappears. You can click in the row to add information to the table.

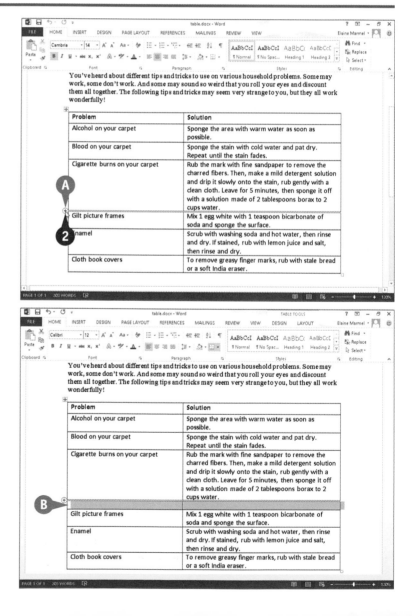

Delete a Row

1 Click anywhere in the row you want to delete.

2 Click the **Layout** tab.

3 Click **Delete**.

4 Click **Delete Rows**.

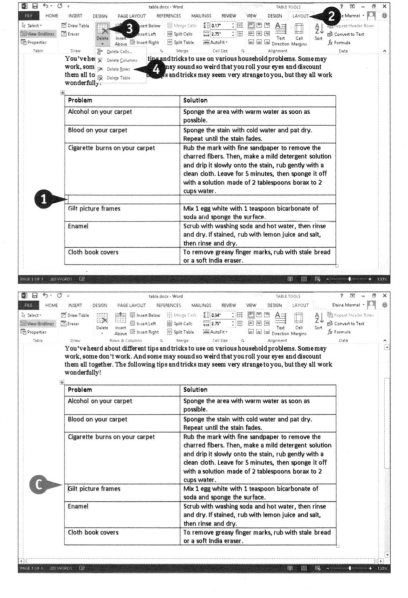

C Word removes the row and any text it contained from the table.

How can I insert a new first row in my table?

Place the insertion point anywhere in the first table row. Click the **Layout** tab and then click **Insert Above**.

Can I delete more than one row at a time?

Yes. Select the rows you want to delete and perform Steps **2** to **4** in the subsection "Delete a Row." To select the rows, position 🗗 outside the left side of the table. Drag to select the rows you want to delete. The same approach works for inserting rows; select the number of rows you want to insert before you begin.

Add or Delete a Column

You can add or delete columns to change the structure of a table to accommodate more or less information. If you need additional columns in the middle of your table, you can insert extra columns. If you insert too many extra columns, you can delete those columns, too. When you add columns, Word decreases the size of the other columns to accommodate the new column but retains the overall size of the table.

Add or Delete a Column

Add a Column

Note: If you need to add a column to the left side of your table, click anywhere in the first column and, on the Layout tab, click the **Insert Left** button.

1 Slide I outside the top edge of the column to the left of the column you want to add.

A I changes to ⮕ and a plus sign (⊕) attached to a pair of vertical lines that span the height of the table appears.

2 Click ⊕.

B Word inserts a new column in the table to the right of the column you identified in Step **1** and selects the new column.

Note: Word maintains the table's overall width.

You can click in the column to add text to it.

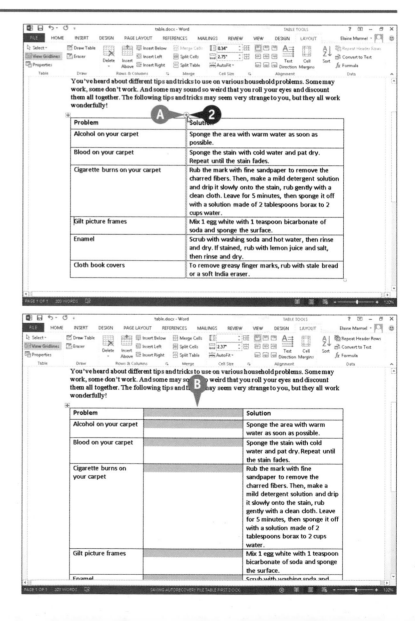

Delete a Column

1. Click anywhere in the column you want to delete.

2. Click the **Layout** tab.

3. Click **Delete**.

4. Click **Delete Columns**.

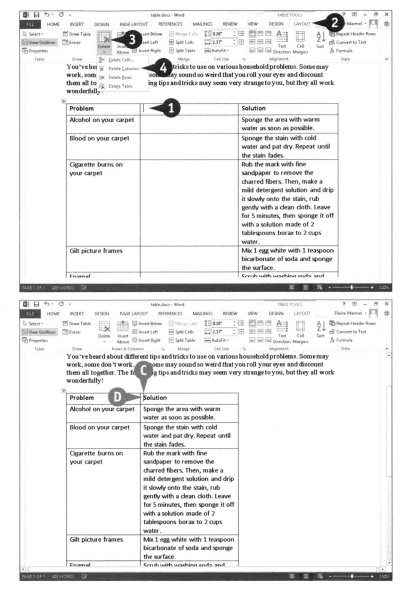

Ⓒ Word removes the column and any text it contained from the table.

Ⓓ The insertion point appears in the column to the right of the one you deleted.

Word does not resize existing columns to use the space previously occupied by the deleted column.

TIP

Is there a way I can easily enlarge a table to fill up the space between the left and right margins after deleting a column?

Yes. Perform the steps that follow. Click anywhere in the table. Then click the **Layout** tab. Click **AutoFit** in the Cell Size group and then click **AutoFit Window** (Ⓐ). The table content and columns readjust to fill the space.

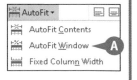

Set Cell Margins

You can set margins in table cells to make table information more legible. For example, you might want to use the top and bottom margins of table cells to add space above and below text in the cells of your table. When you increase top and bottom cell margins, you create more space between rows of the table, making table information easier to read. You also can adjust left and right cell margins to add more space vertically between cells, again creating an easier-to-read table. When you adjust cell margins, you can have Word automatically adjust the cell contents within the margins.

Set Cell Margins

1 Click anywhere in the table.

2 Click the **Layout** tab.

3 Click **Cell Margins**.

The Table Options dialog box appears.

4 Type margin settings here.

5 Click **OK**.

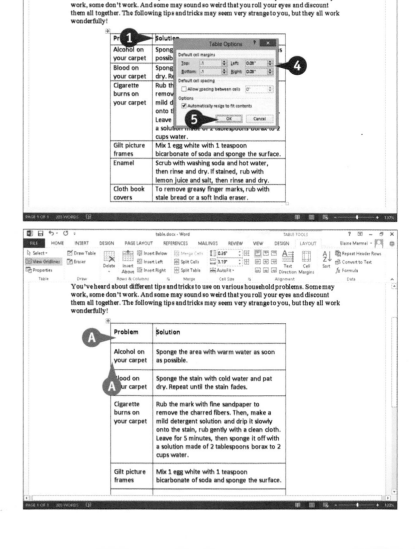

A Word applies cell margin settings.

Add Space between Cells

You can set spacing between table cells. For example, additional spacing between cells can make table information easier to read. When you allow additional spacing between cells, Word applies the spacing both horizontally and vertically; you cannot allow additional space in only one direction. To adjust space in only one direction, adjust cell margins as described in the previous section, "Set Cell Margins." When you adjust cell margins, you can have Word automatically adjust the cell contents within the margins.

Add Space between Cells

1 Click anywhere in the table.

2 Click the **Layout** tab.

3 Click **Cell Margins**.

The Table Options dialog box appears.

4 Select **Allow spacing between cells** (☐ changes to ☑), and type a setting for space between cells.

5 Click **OK**.

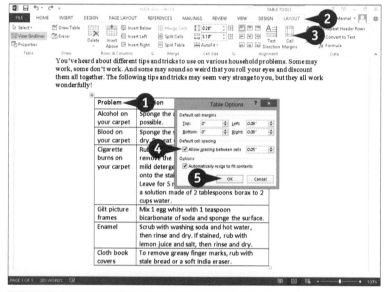

A Word adds space between cells.

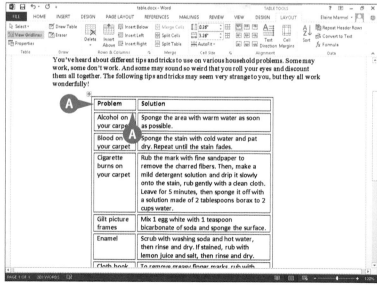

Combine Cells

You can combine two or more cells to create one large cell in which you can store, for example, a table title. Word uses the term *merge* for this function.

You cannot add a single cell to a table; you must add either a row or a column. To create a single cell that stores a table title, insert a table row as described in the section "Add or Delete a Row" earlier in this chapter. Then use the steps in this section to combine the cells of that row into a row that contains one cell that spans the width of the table.

Combine Cells

1 Slide the mouse pointer inside and at the left edge of the first cell you want to merge (I changes to ↗).

2 Drag ↗ across the cells you want to merge to select them.

3 Click the **Layout** tab.

4 Click **Merge Cells**.

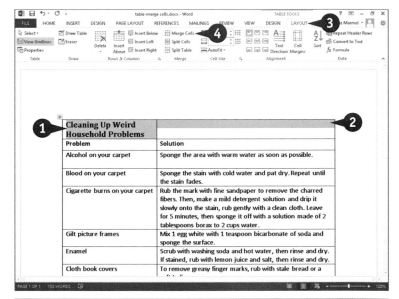

Ⓐ Word combines the cells into one cell and selects that cell.

To center a table title, see the section "Align Text in Cells," later in this chapter.

5 Click anywhere to cancel the selection.

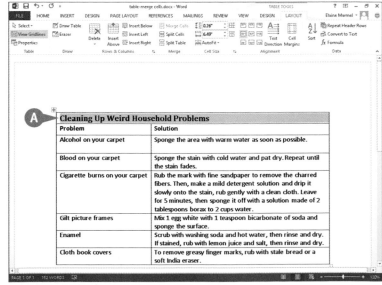

Split Cells

Y ou can split one cell into two or more cells. Splitting a cell can be advantageous if you find that you have more information in one cell than you want. By splitting the cell, you can make room for additional information.

You can split any cell; you are not limited to splitting a cell that you previously merged. When you split a cell, the new cells that you create can span one row or multiple rows. The new cell can also span one column or multiple columns. The new cell can also span both rows and columns.

Split Cells

1 Click anywhere in the cell you want to split.

2 Click the **Layout** tab.

3 Click **Split Cells**.

The Split Cells dialog box appears.

4 Type the number of columns and rows into which you want to split the cell here.

5 Click **OK**.

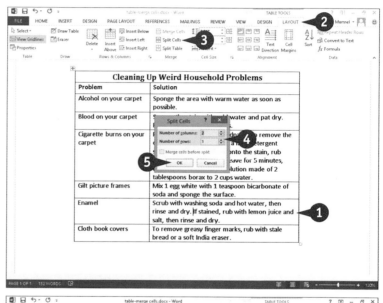

A Word splits and selects the cell.

Split a Table

You can split one table into two. This feature is useful if you discover, after entering information in a table, that you should have created separate tables.

Suppose, for example, that you are putting together a table of methods one can use to clean up common household stains. Initially, you create one table for all the stains, but after working awhile, you realize that the information might be more useful if you create one table that covers cleaning up liquid stains and another table that addresses cleaning up dry stains. You can split the table.

Split a Table

① Position the insertion point anywhere in the row that should appear as the first row of the new table.

② Click the **Layout** tab.

③ Click **Split Table**.

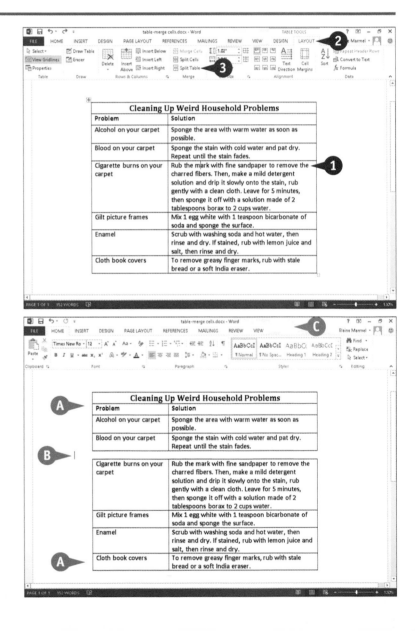

Ⓐ Word separates the table into two tables.

Ⓑ The insertion point appears between the tables.

Ⓒ Because the insertion point is not resting in a table cell, Table Tools no longer appear on the Ribbon.

Add a Formula to a Table

You can place a formula in a cell and let Word automatically do the math for you. Word generally suggests the correct formula for the situation and can calculate a variety of values. For example, Word can sum or average values, identify a maximum or minimum value, and count the number of values in a selected range, among other functions.

You can accept the suggested formula, or you can modify the formula as necessary. For example, Word sums the values of a selected cell, when you might need to sum values beside a selected cell.

Add a Formula to a Table

1 In a table containing numbers, click in a cell that should contain the sum of a row or a column.

2 Click the **Layout** tab.

3 Click **Formula**.

The Formula dialog box appears, suggesting a formula.

A You can click ⌄ to select a number format.

B You can click ⌄ to select a different formula.

4 Click **OK**.

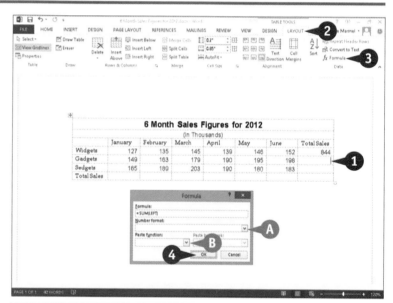

C Word places the formula in the cell containing the insertion point and displays the calculated result of the formula.

If you change any of the values in the row or column that the formula calculates, you can click in the cell containing the formula and press **F9** to update the formula result.

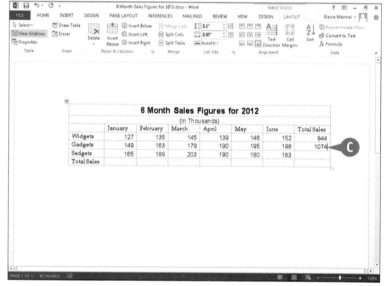

Align Text in Cells

To make your text look more uniform, you can align text or numbers with the top, bottom, left, right, or center of cells. By default, Word aligns table entries at the top-left edge of each cell. But, in some cases, Word's default alignment is not appropriate for the data you are presenting.

For example, many people prefer to center the title of a table in its cell. And most people want values to align along the right side of the cell, especially if the total of the values appears in the table.

Align Text in Cells

1 Click in the cell you want to align.

You can position the mouse pointer over the left edge of the cell whose alignment you want to change ($\mathcal{I}$ changes to ➘) and drag to select multiple cells.

2 Click the **Layout** tab.

3 Click an alignment button.

This example uses the Align Center button (🗐) to align a title vertically and horizontally in a cell.

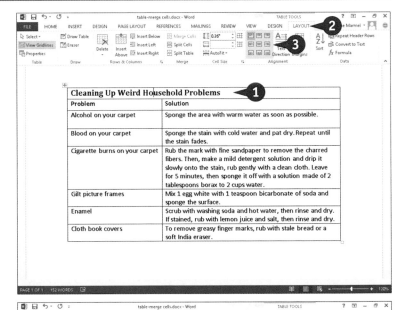

A Word selects the text and aligns it accordingly in the cell.

4 Click anywhere to cancel the selection.

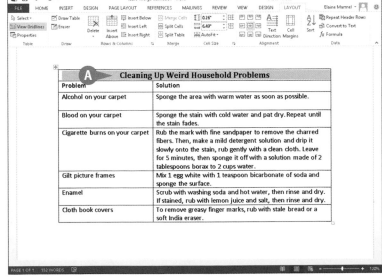

Add Shading to Cells

You can add shading to cells to call attention to them. Shading adds depth to drawings, and it can improve the appearance of a table if you apply it properly. For example, you might want to shade a table title or table column or row headings, or both title and headings. By shading these particular cells, you subtly draw your reader's eye to them to help ensure that the reader will notice them, which helps the reader understand the table content.

Be careful not to apply too much shading or too dark a shade, which can make text unreadable.

Add Shading to Cells

1 Click anywhere in the cell to which you want to add shading.

A You can position the mouse pointer over the left edge of any cell (I changes to ↗) and drag to select multiple cells.

2 Click the **Design** tab.

3 Click the bottom half of **Shading**.

B The Shading Gallery appears.

You can position the mouse pointer over a color, and Live Preview displays a sample of the selected cells shaded in the proposed color.

4 Click a color.

C Word applies the shading to the selected cells.

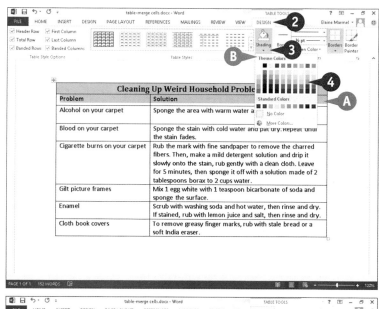

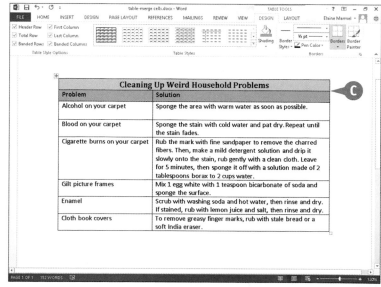

Change Cell Borders

You can change the appearance of cell borders. By default, Word displays the borders that separate each cell to help you enter information into a table and to help your reader read the table's information. You might want to change the appearance of the borders surrounding selected cells to call attention to them.

You can select a border style, which applies a predetermined line style, weight, and color, or you can manually select these characteristics. And you can apply your selection to individual borders using the Border Painter tool or to an entire cell using the Borders tool.

Change Cell Borders

Paint a Border Style

1 Click the **Design** tab.

2 Click the bottom half of **Border Styles**.

A The Theme Borders Gallery appears.

3 Click a color and style.

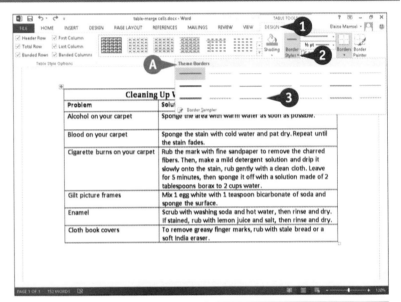

4 Slide ▷ into the document area (▷ changes to ✐).

5 Click a border to which you want to apply the border style you chose in Step **3**.

B Word applies the selected border style.

6 Repeat Step **5** for each border you want to change.

C You can click **Border Painter** to stop applying the border.

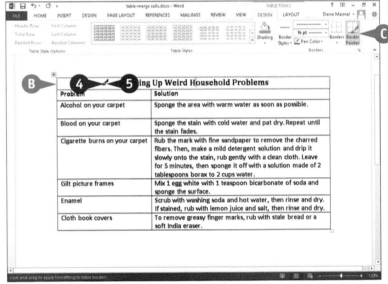

Manually Change Cell Borders

1 Click in the cell whose borders you want to change.

2 Click the **Design** tab.

3 Click the **Line Style** ▼ to display the Line Style Gallery, and click the line style you want to apply.

D You can repeat Step **3** for the **Line Weight** ▼ and the **Pen Color** ▼ to select the weight and color of the border line.

4 Click the bottom half of **Borders** to display the Borders Gallery.

5 Click the type of border to apply.

This example uses Outside Borders.

E Word applies the border using the selected line style, weight, and pen color to the selected cells.

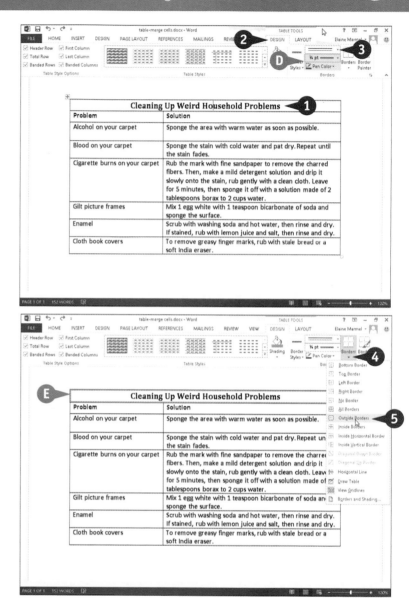

TIP

How can I remove borders from table cells?
Perform the steps that follow. Click in the cell whose borders you want to remove. Click the **Design** tab. Click the bottom half of **Borders** and then click **No Border**. Word removes the borders from the table cells and replaces them with dotted gridlines, which do not print.

Format a Table

You can easily apply formatting to your tables by using the table styles found in the Table Styles Gallery on the Design tab. Earlier sections in this chapter showed you how to apply shading and borders to your table. Each table style in the Table Styles Gallery contains its own unique set of formatting characteristics, and when you apply a table style you simultaneously apply shading, color, borders, and fonts to your table. You also can set table style options that add a header row or a total row, emphasize the table's first column, and more.

Format a Table

1. Click anywhere in the table.

2. Click the **Design** tab.

3. Click ▼ in the Table Styles group.

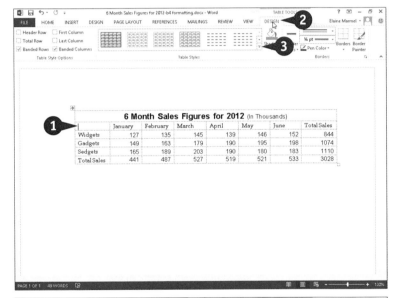

Ⓐ The Table Styles Gallery appears.

4. Position the mouse pointer over a table style.

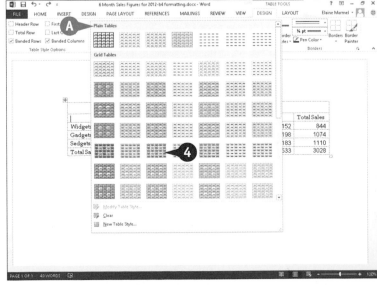

B Live Preview displays the table in the proposed table style, using the style's fonts, colors, and shading.

5 Repeat Step **4** until you find the table style you want to use.

6 Click the table style you want to use.

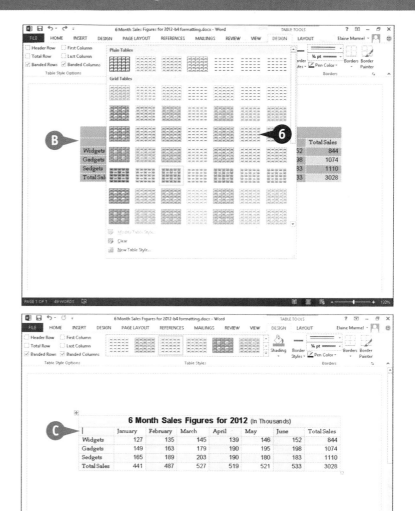

C Word displays the table in the style you selected.

How can I remove a table formatting design?

You have a few options. If you just applied the formatting, you can click the **Undo** button (↶). However, if you performed other actions since applying the table formatting design, perform Steps **1** to **3** in this section and then click **Clear**.

Add a Chart

You can chart data stored in a Microsoft Word 2013 document using Microsoft Excel 2013. When you create a chart in a Word document, you supply all data for the chart in Excel. Although you might have a table containing the information in Word, you do not use the information in that table to create the chart.

If your Word document contains a table and you choose to chart that data, remember that the chart you create is completely independent of the table. You could easily delete either the chart or the table and the other element remains unaffected.

Add a Chart

1 Click in the document where you want a chart to appear.

2 Click the **Insert** tab.

3 Click **Chart**.

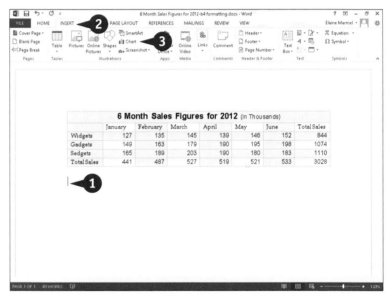

The Insert Chart dialog box appears.

A Chart types appear here.

4 Click a chart type.

B You can click a variation within a given chart type.

5 Click **OK**.

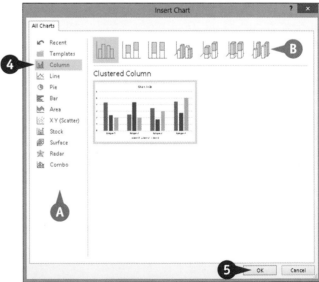

C Microsoft Excel opens, displaying sample data.

D A sample chart of the data appears in Word.

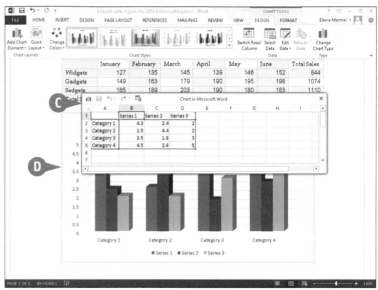

6 Change the data in Excel.

E The chart in Word updates to reflect the changes in Excel.

7 You can close Excel without saving by clicking the **Close** button (×).

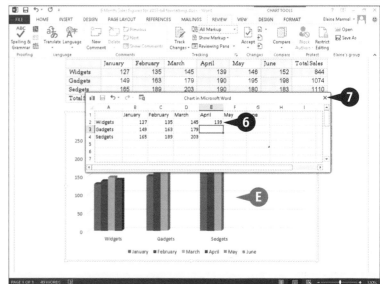

Can I format the chart in Word?

Yes. When you select the chart, Word displays Chart Tools on the Ribbon and, beside the chart, formatting buttons: the **Layout Options** button ( ), the **Chart Elements** button (+), the **Chart Styles** button ( ), and the **Chart Filters** button ( ). Using either Ribbon tools or formatting buttons, you can select a layout and style, add and format shape styles and WordArt styles, set up chart and axis titles, add data labels and a data table, and modify the legend. You also can control how text wraps around your chart, change the color and style of your chart, and filter data from your chart to highlight select values.

Chart Concepts

When creating a chart, you have a wide variety of choices. You can create column charts, line charts, pie charts, bar charts, area charts, XY charts, stock charts, surface charts, doughnut charts, bubble charts, and radar charts. Each chart type serves a different purpose and communicates information in a different way to the reader. The type of chart you use depends on the information you are trying to convey to your reader. In addition, you are not limited to the first chart type you select; if you discover that you have not selected the optimal chart type, try a different one.

Column Charts

A column chart shows data changes over a period of time and can compare different sets of data. A column chart contains vertically oriented bars.

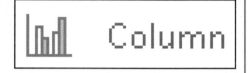

Line Charts

Line charts help you see trends. A line chart connects many related data points; by connecting the points with a line, you see a general trend.

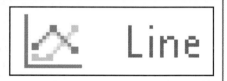

Pie Charts

Pie charts demonstrate the relationship of a part to the whole. Pie charts are effective when you are trying to show, for example, the percentage of total sales for which the Midwest region is responsible.

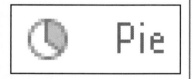

Bar Charts

Bar charts typically compare different sets of data and can also show data changes over time. A bar chart closely resembles a column chart, but the bars are horizontally oriented.

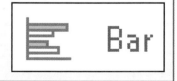

Area Charts

Area charts show data over time, but an area chart helps you see data as broad trends, rather than individual data points.

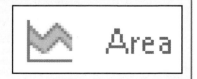

XY (Scatter) Charts

Statisticians often use an XY chart, also called a scatter chart, to determine whether a correlation exists between two variables. Both axes on a scatter chart are numeric, and the axes can be linear or logarithmic.

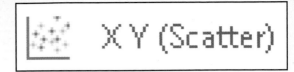

Stock Charts

Also called High-Low, Open-Close charts, stock charts are used for stock market reports. This chart type is very effective for displaying data that fluctuates over time.

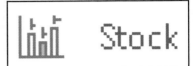

Surface Charts

Topographic maps are surface charts, using colors and patterns to identify areas in the same range of values. A surface chart is useful when you want to find the best-possible combination between two sets of data.

Radar Charts

You can use a radar chart to compare data series that consist of several variables. Each data series on a radar chart has its own axis that "radiates" from the center of the chart — hence the name radar chart. A line connects each point in the series.

Combo

You can use a combination of charts to help make your point. Word provides three predefined combination charts: a clustered column–line chart, a clustered column–line on a secondary axis chart, and a stacked area–clustered column chart. If none of these meets your needs, you can create your own custom combination chart.

CHAPTER 10

Working with Graphics

You can spruce up documents by inserting a variety of graphics; the technique to insert graphics varies, depending on the type of graphic. You can edit graphics in a variety of ways using the tools that appear when you select the graphic. In this chapter, you learn how to edit a picture, clip art image, screenshot, WordArt drawing, shape, and text box.

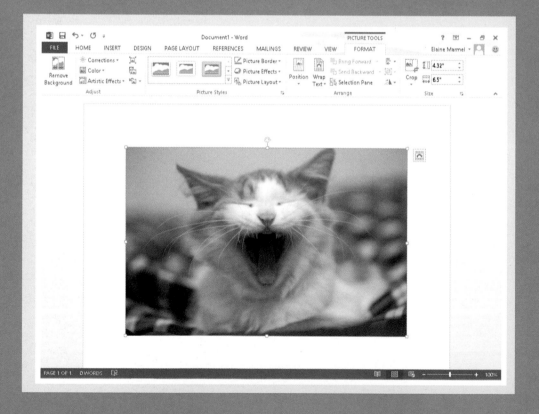

Add WordArt

WordArt is decorative text that you can add to a document as an eye-catching visual effect. You can create text graphics that bend and twist or display a subtle shading of color. You find the various WordArt options on the Insert tab of the Ribbon.

You can create WordArt text at the same time that you create a WordArt graphic, or you can apply a WordArt style to existing text. After you convert text into a WordArt object, you can resize, move, or modify the graphic in the ways described in the section "Understanding Graphics Modification Techniques," later in this chapter.

Add WordArt

1 Click in the document where you want to add WordArt or select existing text and apply WordArt to it.

2 Click the **Insert** tab.

3 Click the **WordArt** button ($4 \cdot$).

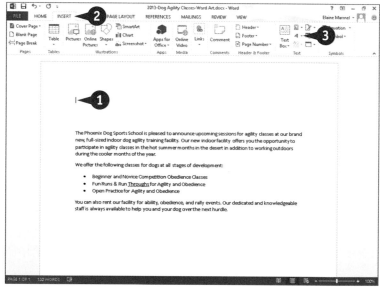

A The WordArt Gallery appears.

4 Click the WordArt style you want to apply.

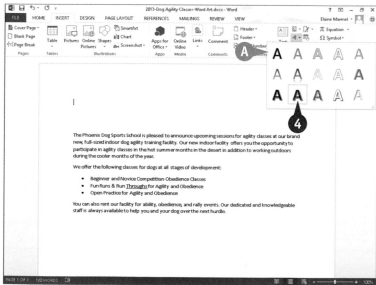

B If you selected text in Step **1**, your text appears selected in the WordArt style you applied; otherwise, the words "Your Text Here" appear selected in the upper-left corner of your document.

C Handles (⊡) surround the WordArt graphic.

D Drag ⟳ to rotate the graphic.

E ⬚ controls text flow as described in "Wrap Text around a Graphic."

F Drawing Tools appear on the Ribbon; you can use these tools to format WordArt.

5 If necessary, type text.

G Word converts the text to a WordArt graphic.

You can click anywhere outside the WordArt to continue working.

Note: You can move, resize, or rotate the WordArt; see the section "Move or Resize a Graphic."

Note: You can change the size of the WordArt font by selecting the WordArt text and, on the Home tab, selecting a different font size from the Font list in the Font group.

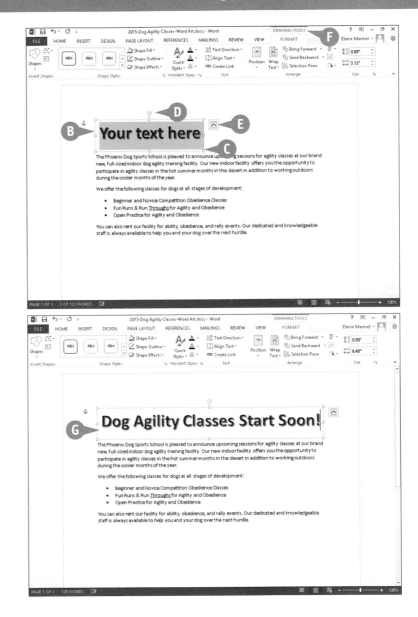

TIPS

Can I edit the WordArt drawing?
Yes. Click inside the WordArt drawing. Handles (⊡ and ⟳) appear around the WordArt. Edit the text the way you would edit any text, deleting and changing as needed. Use ⟳ to rotate the WordArt drawing.

Can I delete a WordArt drawing?
Yes, but be aware that deleting the drawing also deletes the text. Click near the edge of the drawing or if you click inside the drawing, click any handle (⊡) to select the drawing. Then press Delete.

Add a Picture

You can include a picture stored on your computer to add punch to your Word document. For example, if you have a photo or graphic file that relates to the subject matter in your document, you can insert it into the document to help the reader understand your subject. After you insert a picture, you can resize, move, or modify the graphic in a variety of ways. The section "Understanding Graphics Modification Techniques," later in this chapter, describes the many ways you can edit an image or add effects to an image.

Add a Picture

1 Click in your document where you want to add a picture.

2 Click the **Insert** tab.

3 Click **Pictures**.

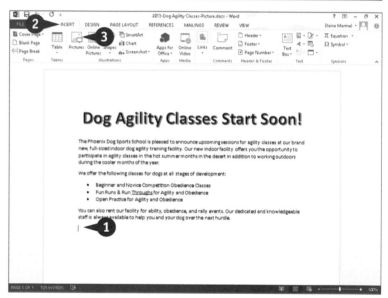

The Insert Picture dialog box appears.

Ⓐ The folder you are viewing appears here.

Ⓑ You can click here to navigate to commonly used locations where pictures may be stored.

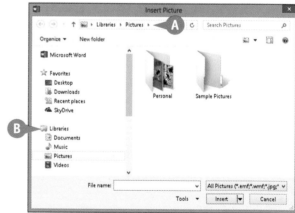

4 Navigate to the folder containing the picture you want to add.

5 Click the picture you want to add to your document.

6 Click **Insert**.

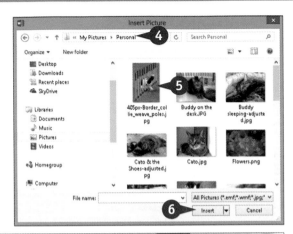

C The picture appears in your document, selected and surrounded by handles (⬚).

D Drag ↻ to rotate the picture.

E 🔲 controls text flow around the picture as described in "Wrap Text around a Graphic."

F Picture Tools appear on the Ribbon; you can use these tools to format pictures.

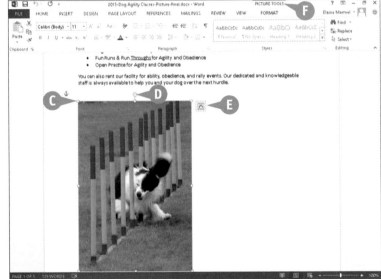

TIP

How can I delete a picture?

1 Move the mouse pointer over the picture.

A The pointer changes to ⇖.

2 Click the picture to select it.

3 Press Delete.

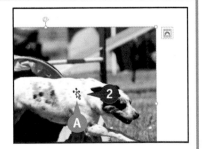

Insert an Online Picture

In addition to pictures stored on your computer's hard drive, you can insert a picture from an online source into a Word document. Exercise care in choosing online pictures, and make sure that they fall into the public domain or that you have written permission to use the picture.

The clip art found at Office.com is all public domain art, and you can freely use any images available at Office.com. Word 2013 does not come with any preinstalled clip art as previous versions did; instead, use the clip art available at Office.com.

Insert an Online Picture

1 Click in your document where you want to add a picture.

2 Click the **Insert** tab.

3 Click **Online Pictures**.

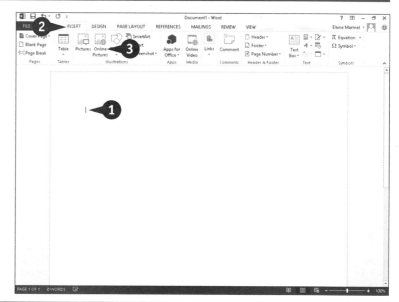

The Insert Picture window appears.

4 Click here and type a description of the type of image you want.

5 Click the Search button (🔍).

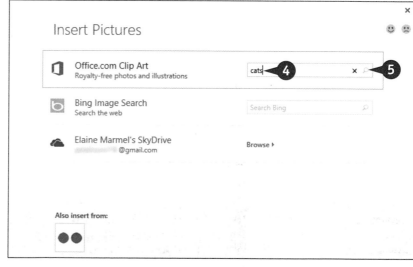

The results of your search appear.

A You can click here (∧ and ∨) to navigate through the search results.

B You can click here to return to the Insert Picture window and search for a different image.

6 Click the picture you want to add to your document.

7 Click **Insert**.

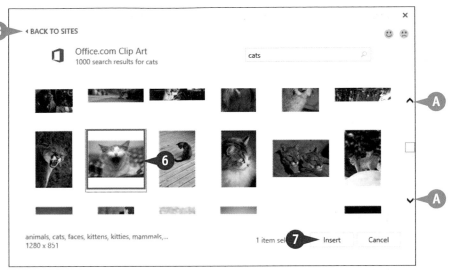

C The picture appears in your document, selected and surrounded by handles (▱).

D Drag ⟳ to rotate the picture.

E 🖼 controls text flow around the picture as described in "Wrap Text around a Graphic."

F Picture Tools appear on the Ribbon; you can use these tools to format the picture.

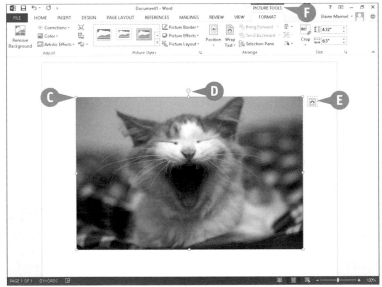

TIPS

Why must I make sure that the image I choose falls into the public domain?

Images that are privately owned are often available for use only if you agree to pay a fee and/or give credit to the owner of the image. To use a public domain image, you do not need to pay a royalty or get permission from an image owner to use the image.

What happens when I search using Bing?

A Bing search results window appears in your default browser, and you can navigate to the listed sites to look for pictures. Be aware that the Bing search does not exclude pictures outside the public domain, and you need to determine if an image is royalty-free and available for use without permission.

Insert an Online Video

Y ou can insert a video available on the Internet into a Word document. After you have inserted the video, you can play it directly from the Word document.

You can insert videos you find using Bing Search or videos available on YouTube, or you can insert a video embed code — an HTML code that uses the `src` attribute to define the video file you want to embed. Most videos posted on the Internet are public domain, but if you are unsure, do some research to determine if you can use the video freely.

Insert an Online Video

1 Click in your document where you want to add a video.

2 Click the **Insert** tab.

3 Click **Online Video**.

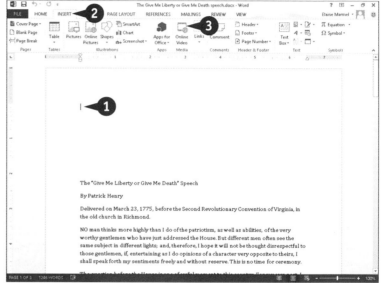

The Insert Video window appears.

4 In one of the search boxes, type a description of the video you want to insert.

Note: This example searches YouTube. To search YouTube, click the YouTube button at the bottom of the window; Word redisplays the window with a search box.

5 Click the Search button (🔎).

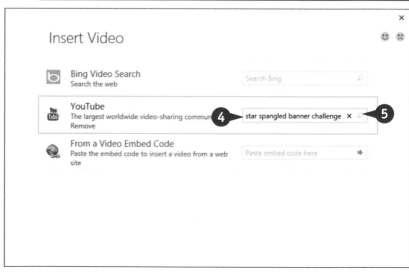

The results of your search appear.

A You can click here (∧ and ∨) to navigate through the search results.

B You can click here to return to the Insert Video window and search for a different video.

6 Click the video you want to add to your document.

7 Click **Insert**.

C The video appears in your document, selected and surrounded by handles (⊡).

D Drag ⬇ to rotate the video.

E ⊠ controls text flow around the video as described in "Wrap Text around a Graphic."

F Picture Tools appear on the Ribbon; you can use these tools to format the appearance of the video in your document.

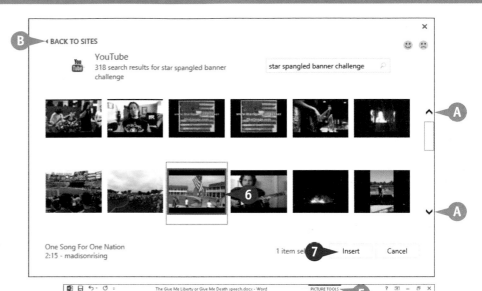

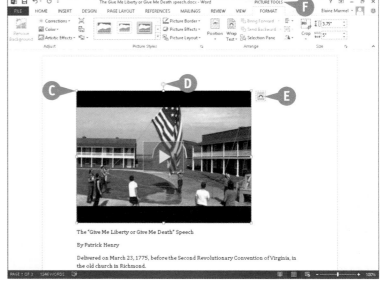

TIP

How do I play an inserted video?

From Print Layout view or Read Mode view, click the video Play button (▶). The video appears in its own window. Click the Play button again to start the video. To stop the video and return to the document, click outside the video anywhere on the document.

Add a Screenshot

You can insert into a Word document an image called a *screenshot*. You can capture a screenshot of another document open in Word or of a document open in another program.

Screenshots are exact pictures of the open document at the moment you take the screenshot. In addition to including a screenshot in a Word document, if you are having a problem on your computer, you can use a screenshot to help capture the problem so that you can provide accurate and detailed information to the technical support person who helps you.

Add a Screenshot

1 Open the document you want to capture.

Ⓐ This example shows a chart in Excel.

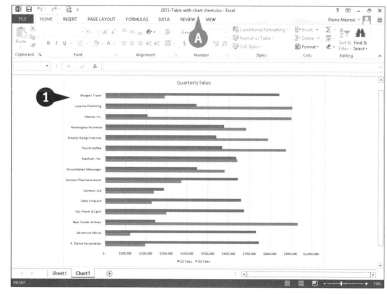

2 Open the Word document in which you want to insert a screenshot of the document you opened in Step **1**.

3 Position the insertion point where you want the screenshot to appear.

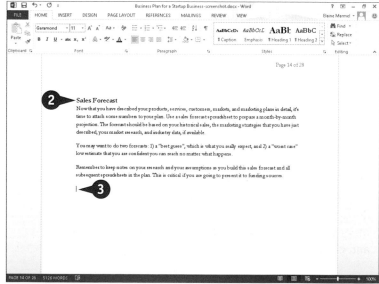

4 Click **Insert**.

5 Click **Screenshot**.

B The Screenshot Gallery shows open programs and available screenshots of those programs.

Note: You can open as many programs and documents as your computer permits. In this example, in addition to the chart in Excel and Word, another Excel workbook is also open.

6 Click the screenshot you want to insert in your Word document.

C The screenshot appears in your Word document, selected and surrounded by handles ( ).

D Drag to rotate the screenshot.

E controls text flow around the screenshot as described in "Wrap Text around a Graphic."

F Picture Tools appear on the Ribbon; you can use these tools to format the screenshot.

You can click anywhere outside the screenshot to continue working.

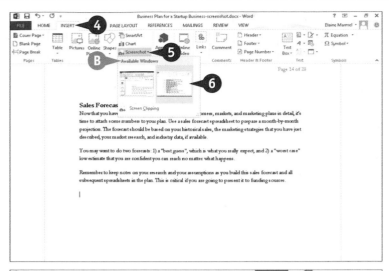

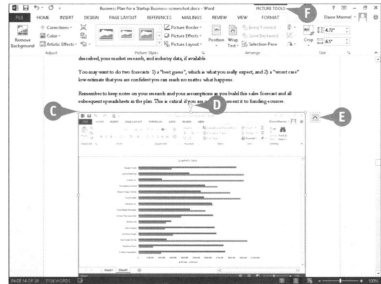

TIPS

Can I use the Screenshot feature to insert a screenshot of the current Word document into the same document?

No, but here is a workaround. Open the document in which you want to insert a screenshot, and then open a second, blank document. From the blank document, shoot a screen of the first document. The screen appears in the blank document, already selected. Click **Copy** ( ), switch to the other document, click where the screenshot should appear, and click **Paste**.

Can I use the Screenshot feature to take a picture of my desktop?

No, but use this workaround: While viewing your desktop, press `Print scrn`. Then switch to Word, and position the insertion point where you want the screenshot to appear. Press `Ctrl`+`V` to paste the image into your Word document.

Add a Shape

To give your Word document pizzazz, you can add graphic shapes such as lines, arrows, stars, and banners. Suppose, for example, that you are part of a barbershop quartet that wants to sell and deliver singing telegrams for Valentine's Day — the perfect fun way to raise money to support your hobby. You can create a flyer that advertises your unique gift offering, suitable not only for lovers, but for anyone who occupies a special place in the life of the sender — a grandparent, parent, child, or long-time friend.

Shapes are visible in Print Layout, Web Layout, and Reading Layout views.

Add a Shape

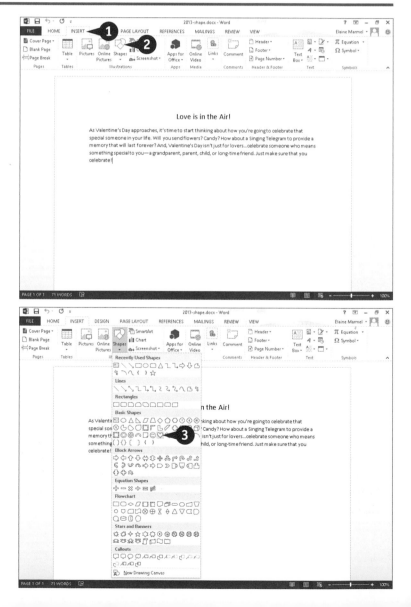

1 Click the **Insert** tab.

2 Click **Shapes**.

The Shapes Gallery appears.

3 Click a shape.

The Shapes Gallery closes and the mouse pointer (I⁼) changes to +.

4 Position the mouse pointer at the upper-left corner of the place where you want the shape to appear.

5 Drag the mouse pointer (+) down and to the right until the shape is the size you want.

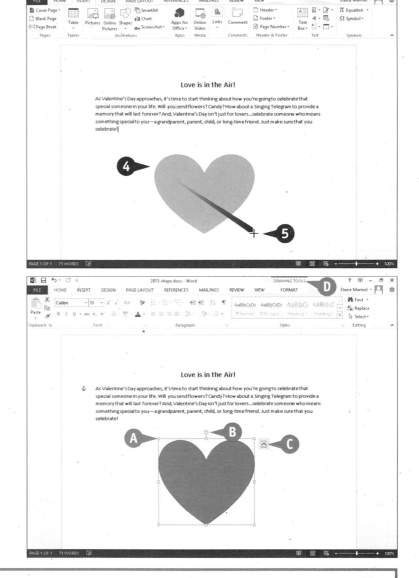

A When you release the mouse button, the shape appears in your document, selected and surrounded by handles (□).

B Drag ⟳ to rotate the shape.

C ▧ controls text flow around the shape as described in the section "Wrap Text around a Graphic."

D Drawing Tools appear on the Ribbon.

You can press **Esc** or click anywhere to continue working in your document.

TIP

Can I change the color of a shape?

Yes, you can change the color inside a shape as well as the shape's outline color. Click the shape to select it. On the Ribbon, in the Shape Styles group, click the **Shape Fill** button (**A**) to display the color gallery. Move the mouse pointer over the color gallery; Live Preview displays the outline of the shape in the proposed color. Click a color (**B**). Repeat these steps, selecting **Shape Outline** in Step **2**.

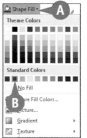

Add a Text Box

You can add a text box to your document to control the placement and appearance of the text that appears in the box. Text boxes are graphics that are designed specifically to help you work with text. You can use text boxes to help you draw attention to specific text or to easily move text around within a document. You also can use a text box to display text vertically instead of horizontally.

Word inserts your text box near the insertion point, but you can move the text box the same way you move any graphic element; see the next section for details. Text boxes are visible only in Print Layout, Web Layout, and Read Mode views.

Add a Text Box

1 Click near the location where you want the text box to appear.

2 Click the **Insert** tab.

3 Click **Text Box**.

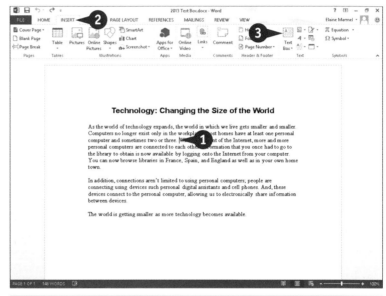

The Text Box Gallery appears.

4 Click a text box style.

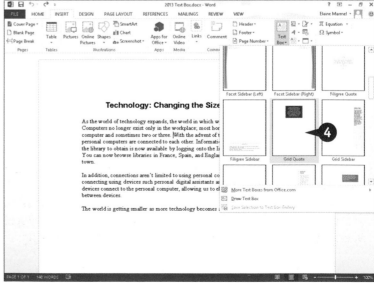

Ⓐ The Text Box Gallery closes and Word places a text box in your document.

Sample text appears inside a text box, and Word selects the sample text.

Ⓑ Existing text flows around the box.

Ⓒ Drag to rotate the text box as described in "Wrap Text around a Graphic."

Ⓓ Drawing Tools appear on the Ribbon; you can use these tools to format the text box.

5 To replace the sample text, start typing.

6 Click outside the text box.

Your text appears in the box.

Note: You can format the text using the techniques described in Chapter 5.

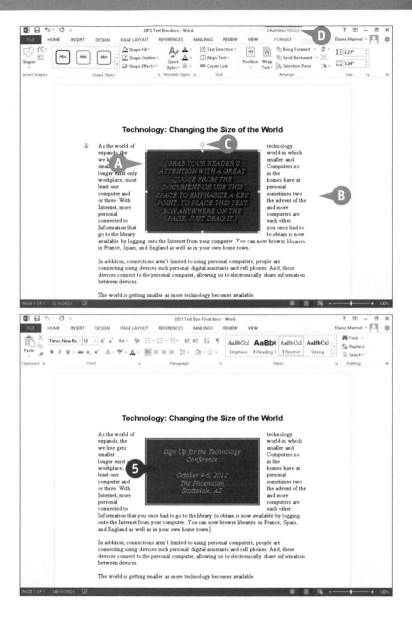

TIP

What should I do if I do not like any of the predefined text box formats?
You can examine additional styles on Office.com, or you can draw your own text box and format it. Perform the steps that follow. Complete Steps **1** to **3** in this section. Click **More Text Boxes from Office.com** to view some additional text box styles. If you still do not see a style you like, click **Draw Text Box** (I⁼ changes to ⌖). Drag the mouse pointer (⌖) from the upper-left to the lower-right corner of the place where you want the text box to appear; the text box appears.

Move or Resize a Graphic

If you find that a graphic — a picture, clip art image, shape, text box, or WordArt graphic — is not positioned where you want it or it is too large or too small, you can move or resize it. Alignment guides — green lines — appear as you move a graphic to help you determine where to place the graphic. After you have picked the spot for the graphic, the alignment guides disappear. Text automatically reflows around a graphic wherever you place it or however you size it; see "Wrap Text around a Graphic," later in this chapter, to control the way text flows.

Move or Resize a Graphic

Move a Graphic

1 Click the graphic.

Ⓐ Handles ( ) surround the graphic.

2 Position the mouse pointer over the WordArt image, picture, video, or shape, or over the edge of the text box (changes to).

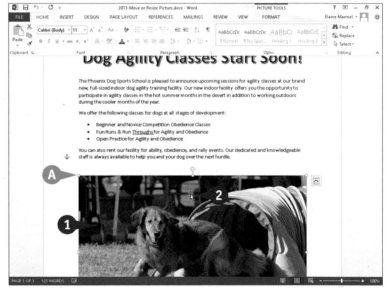

3 Drag the graphic to a new location.

Ⓑ Green alignment guides help you position the graphic.

4 Release the mouse button.

The graphic appears in the new location, and the alignment guides disappear.

5 Click outside the graphic to cancel its selection.

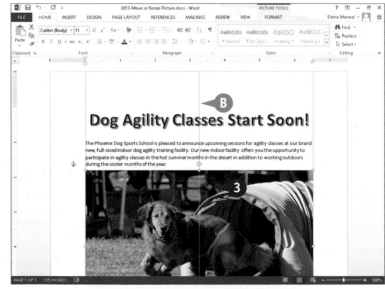

Resize a Graphic

1 Click the graphic.

C Handles (⌷) surround the graphic.

2 Position the mouse pointer over one of the handles ($I^=$ changes to ⬀, ↕, ⬈, or ⬌).

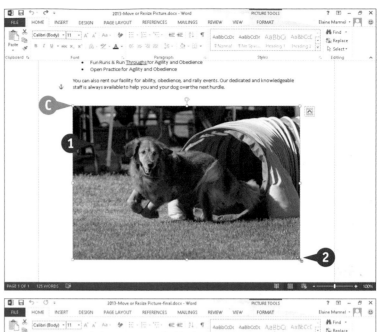

3 Drag the handle inward or outward until the graphic is the appropriate size (⬀, ↕, ⬈, or ⬌ changes to +).

4 Release the mouse button.

The graphic appears in the new size.

5 Click outside the graphic to cancel its selection.

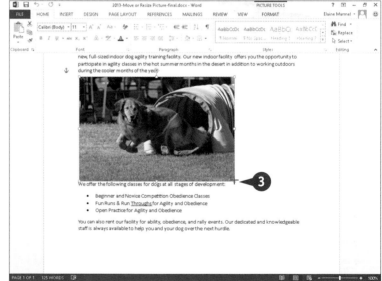

TIPS

The green alignment guides do not appear when I drag a graphic. Why not?

The new Alignment Guide feature works only on documents created in or converted to Word 2013 format. You cannot work in Compatibility Mode. See Chapter 2 for details on converting older Word documents to Word 2013 format.

Does it matter which handle I use to resize a graphic?

If you click and drag any of the corner handles, you maintain the proportion of the graphic as you resize it. The handles on the sides, top, or bottom of the graphic resize the width or the height only of the graphic, so using one of them can make your graphic look distorted, especially if you resize a picture, video, or screenshot using any handle except a corner handle.

Understanding Graphics Modification Techniques

In addition to moving or resizing graphics, you can modify their appearance using a variety of Ribbon buttons. When you select a graphic, Word displays additional tabs specific to the graphic you select. These tabs contain the buttons you can use to modify the appearance of the selected image.

You can adjust the size, brightness or contrast, and color of a picture. You can rotate a graphic or make it three-dimensional. You also can add a shadow or apply a color outline or style to a graphic. And you can change the color of a graphic.

Crop a Picture

You can use the Crop tool to create a better fit, to omit a portion of the image, or to focus the viewer on an important area of the image. You can crop a picture, screenshot, or clip art image. When you crop an object, you remove vertical and/or horizontal edges from the object. The Crop tool is located on the Format tab on the Ribbon, which appears when you click the object you want to crop.

Rotate or Flip a Graphic

After you insert an object such as a piece of clip art or a photo from your hard drive into a Word document, you may find that the object appears upside down or inverted. Or maybe you want to rotate or flip pictures, clip art images, and some shapes for dramatic effect. For example, you might flip a clip art image to face another direction or rotate an arrow object to point elsewhere on the page. You cannot rotate text boxes.

Correct Images

You can change the brightness and contrast of a picture, clip art image, or screenshot to improve its appearance, and you can sharpen or soften an image. Suppose the image object you have inserted in your Word file is slightly blurry or lacks contrast. You find the image-correction tools on the Picture Tools Format tab on the Ribbon, which appears when you click to select the object to which you want to apply the effect.

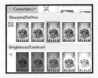

Make Color Adjustments

You can adjust the color of a picture, screenshot, or clip art image by increasing or decreasing color saturation or color tone. You also can recolor a picture, screenshot, or clip art image to create an interesting effect.

Color saturation controls the amount of red and green in a photo, while color tone controls the amount of blue and yellow.

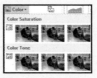

Remove the Background of an Image

You can remove the background of a picture, screenshot, or clip art image. Suppose that you inserted a screenshot of an Excel chart in a Word document; the screenshot would, by default, include the Excel Ribbon. You can use the Remove Background tool in the Adjust group on the Picture Tools Format tab to remove the Excel Ribbon and focus the reader's attention on the chart.

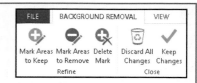

Add a Picture or Shape Effect

You can use tools to assign unique and interesting special effects to objects. For example, you can apply a shadow effect, create a mirrored reflection, apply a glow effect, soften the object's edges, make a bevel effect, or generate a 3D rotation effect. You can find these tools on the Format tab of the Ribbon, which appears when you click to select the object to which you want to apply the effect.

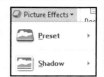

Apply a Style to a Graphic

You can apply a predefined style to a shape, text box, WordArt graphic, picture, or clip art image. Styles contain predefined colors and effects and help you quickly add interest to a graphic. Applying a style removes other effects that you may have applied, such as shadow or bevel effects. Sample styles appear on the Picture Tools Format or Drawing Tools Format tab when you click ⊡ in the Picture Styles or Shape Styles group.

Add a Picture Border or Drawing Outline

You can add a border to a picture, shape, text box, WordArt graphic, clip art image, or screenshot. Using the Picture Border or Shape Outline tool, which appears on the Picture Tools Format or Drawing Tools Format tab, you can control the thickness of the border, set a style for the border (a solid line or dashed line), and change the color of the border.

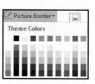

Apply Artistic Effects

You can apply artistic effects to pictures, screenshots, and clip art images in order to liven them up. For example, you can make an image appear as though it was rendered in marker, pencil, chalk, or paint. Other artistic effects might remind you of mosaics, film grain, or glass. You find the Artistic Effects button on the Picture Tools Format tab, which appears when you click to select the object to which you want to apply the effect.

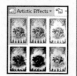

Understanding Text Wrapping and Graphics

When you insert graphics into a Word document, you can control the way text wraps around the graphic. For example, you can wrap text around a graphic, force text to skip a graphic and leave its left and right sides blank, or place a graphic on top of text or underneath text. By default, most graphics have a relatively square boundary, even if the graphic is not a square, and most text wrapping options relate to that relatively square boundary.

By editing a graphic's wrap points, you can change the square boundary to more closely match the graphic's shape and wrap text more closely around the shape.

Button	Function
In Line with Text	Text does not wrap around the graphic. Word positions the graphic exactly where you placed it. The graphic moves to accommodate added or deleted text, but no text appears on the graphic's right or left.
Square	This option wraps text in a square around your graphic regardless of its shape. You can control the amount of space between text and all your graphic's sides.
Tight	This option wraps text around the graphic's outside edge. The difference between this option and Square becomes apparent with a nonsquare shape; with Tight, you can control the space between the text and the graphic's right and left sides. Word leaves no space between text and the graphic's top and bottom sides.
Through	With this option, if you edit a graphic's wrap points by dragging them to match the shape of the graphic, you can wrap text to follow the graphic's shape.
Top and Bottom	Wraps text around the graphic's top and bottom but leaves the space on either side of a graphic blank.
Behind Text	With this option, the text runs over the graphic, as if the graphic were not there.
In Front of Text	With this option, the graphic appears to block the text underneath the graphic's location.
Edit Wrap Points	Displays handles that represent an image's wrap points. You can drag the handles to change the position of the wrap points. Changing a wrap point does not change the image's appearance but affects the way text wraps around the image.
✓ Move with Text / Fix Position on Page	Choose one of these options to determine the way Word positions an image. It can move as you add text or it can remain on the page exactly where you placed it.

Wrap Text around a Graphic

You can control the way that Word wraps text around a graphic image in your document. Controlling the way text wraps around a graphic becomes very important when you want to place graphics in a document where space is at a premium, such as a two-columned newsletter. You can, for example, wrap text around all sides of a graphic or only around the top and bottom of a graphic. See the previous section for details on text wrapping methods. The information in this section shows text wrapping for a picture but applies to text wrapping for any kind of graphic.

Wrap Text around a Graphic

1 Click a graphic.

A Handles (□) appear around the image.

2 Click **Format**.

3 Click **Wrap Text**.

4 Point the mouse at each wrapping style to see how it affects the text and the image.

Note: You can click 🖾 to display text layout options, but these buttons do not provide a live preview.

5 Click the wrapping style you want to apply.

Word wraps text around the graphic using the text wrapping option you selected.

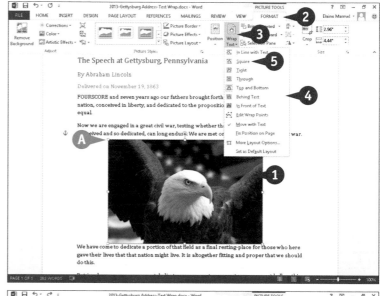

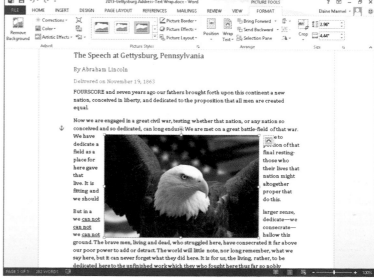

Work with Diagrams

You can use the SmartArt feature to create all kinds of diagrams to illustrate concepts and processes. For example, you might insert a diagram in a document to show the hierarchy in your company or to show the workflow in your department. SmartArt offers predefined diagram types, including list, process, cycle, hierarchy, relationship, matrix, pyramid, and picture. In addition, you can choose from several diagram styles within each type. For example, if you choose to create a hierarchy diagram, you can choose from several different styles of hierarchy diagrams.

The example in this section demonstrates adding an organizational chart.

Work with Diagrams

Add a Diagram

1 Click in your document where you want the diagram to appear.

2 Click the **Insert** tab.

3 Click **SmartArt**.

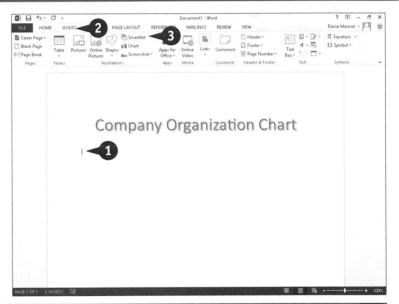

The Choose a SmartArt Graphic dialog box appears.

4 Click a diagram category.

5 Click the type of diagram you want to add.

Ⓐ A description of the selected diagram appears here.

6 Click **OK**.

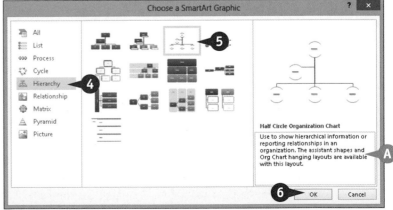

Word adds the diagram.

B The graphic border surrounding the diagram indicates that the diagram is selected; the border will not print.

C SmartArt Tools appear.

Note: You might also see the text pane, described in the next subsection.

Each object within the diagram is called a *shape*.

Add Text to the Diagram

1 On the Design tab of SmartArt Tools, click **Text Pane**.

D The text pane appears. Each bullet in the text pane matches the selected text block in the diagram.

2 Type the text you want to add.

3 Click the next item in the text pane.

Note: You do not need to use the text pane; you can click and type directly in a shape.

4 Repeat Steps **2** and **3** for each shape in the diagram. When you finish, click × to close the text pane and click a blank spot on the diagram.

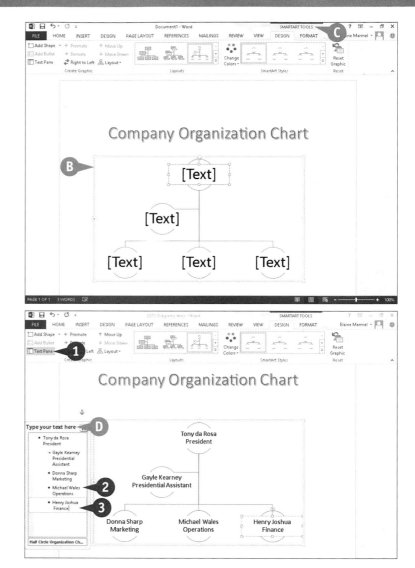

TIPS

How can I add two lines of text to a shape?

After you type the first line of the text in the text pane, press Shift+Enter. Then type the second line. Word adjusts the font size of the text to fit the shape, and for consistency, Word adjusts the font size of all text in the diagram to match.

Can I control the size and position of the diagram on the page?

Yes. You can size the diagram using its handles, or you can click the **Format** tab, click **Size**, and then click the spinner arrows (⬍) to change the height and width. Word sets the default position on the diagram in line with your text. You can position the diagram by dragging it, or you can use the Position Gallery to place the diagram in one of nine predetermined positions on the page. On the Format tab, click **Arrange** and then click **Position** to display the Position Gallery.

continued ▶ **261**

No SmartArt diagram comes with all the shapes you need to create your diagram, but you can easily add shapes at any place in the diagram to accommodate your needs. And when circumstances change, you can easily revise a diagram by adding or deleting shapes as appropriate.

To keep your diagrams interesting, you can apply styles to diagrams. Styles enhance the appearance of a diagram, providing a professional look and adding dimension and depth to the diagram. These style enhancements draw a reader's attention to a diagram and help you get your point across.

Work with Diagrams (continued)

Add or Delete Shapes

1 Click the **Design** tab.

2 Click the shape above or beside which you want to add a shape.

A Handles ( ) surround the shape.

3 Click ▼ beside Add Shape, and select the option that describes where the shape should appear.

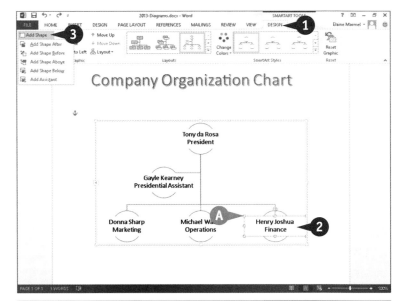

B The new shape appears.

You can add text to the new shape by following the steps in the subsection "Add Text to the Diagram" on the previous page.

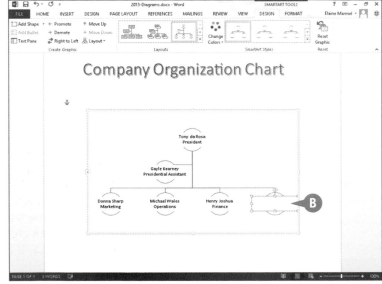

Apply a Diagram Style

1 Click the **Design** tab.

2 Click ⊡ in the SmartArt Styles group to display the Quick Styles Gallery.

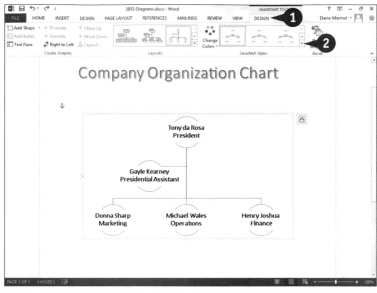

The SmartArt Styles Gallery appears.

You can slide the mouse pointer over an option in the gallery, and Live Preview displays the appearance of the diagram using that style.

3 Click a style.

C Word applies the selected style to the diagram.

You can click anywhere outside the diagram to continue working.

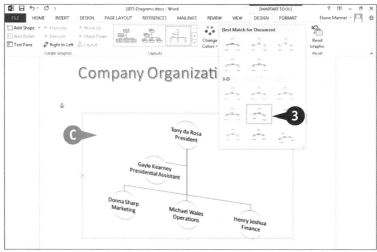

TIPS

How can I delete a shape?
Click the outside border of the shape; handles (⬚) appear around the shape. Press Delete to remove the selected shape from the diagram.

Can I change the layout of an organization chart diagram after I insert it?
Yes. Click the border of the organization chart to select it. Then click the **SmartArt Tools Design** tab and, in the Layouts group, click ⊡ to display the Layouts Gallery for the type of diagram you chose when you inserted the diagram. Select a different organization chart structure, and Word applies the new layout to the diagram. To select a different type of diagram, you can click **More Layouts** at the bottom of the Layouts Gallery to reopen the Choose a SmartArt Graphic dialog box.

CHAPTER 11

Customizing Word

Do you like the default Word settings? If not, you can easily customize portions of the Word program to make it perform more in line with the way you work.

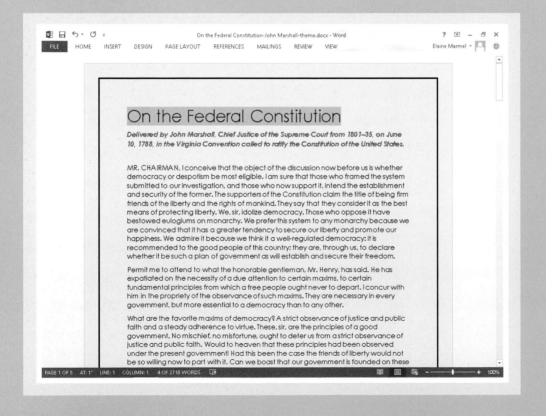

Control the Display of Formatting Marks

As described in Chapter 6, you can view the formatting marks that Word automatically inserts as you type. These formatting marks help you understand why your document looks the way that it looks — for example, why paragraphs seem farther apart than you expect. Formatting marks are always in documents, but they are hidden from you unless you display them.

Using the Show/Hide button displays all formatting marks. But you also can limit the formatting marks that Word displays to view just the ones that interest you.

Control the Display of Formatting Marks

1. Click the **Show/Hide** button (¶) on the Home tab to display formatting marks.

2. Click the **File** tab.

   Backstage view appears.

3. Click **Options**.

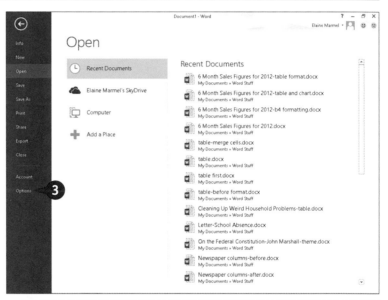

The Word Options dialog box appears.

4. Click **Display**.

Ⓐ You can select **Show all formatting marks** (☐ changes to ☑) to display all formatting marks.

5. Select the formatting marks you want to display (☐ changes to ☑).

6. Click **OK**.

   Word displays only the selected formatting marks in your document.

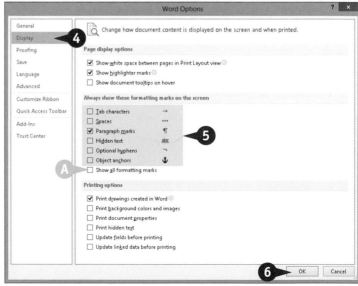

Customize the Status Bar

You can customize the status bar to display information you want visible while you work. By default, Word displays some information on the status bar, such as the page number and number of pages and words in your document, the shortcuts to the Read Mode, Print Layout, and Web Layout views, and the zoom slider and zoom indicator. You can add a wide variety of information, such as the position of the insertion point by line and column number or by vertical page position. You also can display indicators of spelling and grammar errors and typing mode — insert or overtype.

Customize the Status Bar

1 Right-click the status bar to display the Customize Status Bar menu.

2 Click the option you want to display on the status bar.

3 Repeat Step **2** for each option you want to display.

A Word displays the option(s) you selected on the status bar.

You can click anywhere outside the menu to close it.

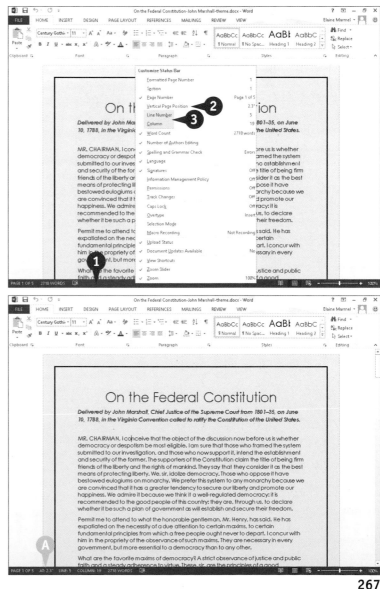

Hide or Display Ribbon Buttons

By default, Word pins the Ribbon on-screen, but you can unpin the Ribbon to hide it while you work and then redisplay it when you need it. Unpinning the Ribbon can make your screen appear less crowded and less distracting, enabling you to concentrate on your document as opposed to the controls you use as you prepare it.

When you unpin and hide the Ribbon, you hide the buttons on each tab, but the tab names continue to appear. When you click a tab name, the Ribbon reappears. Note that unpinning the Ribbon has no effect on the Quick Access Toolbar.

Hide or Display Ribbon Buttons

Ⓐ By default, Word displays the Ribbon.

① Click the **Unpin the Ribbon** button (⌃).

Ⓑ Word unpins the Ribbon, hiding the buttons but continuing to display the tabs.

② Work in your document as usual.

③ When you need a Ribbon button, click that Ribbon tab.

Note: You can click any Ribbon tab, but you will save time if you click the tab containing the button you need.

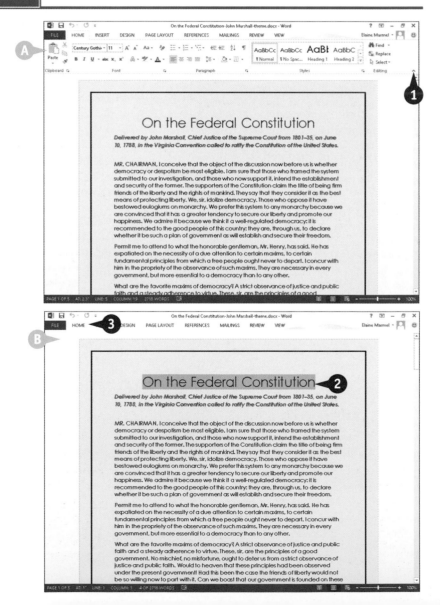

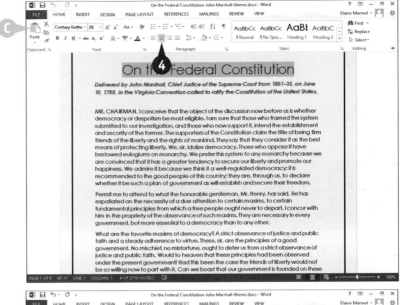

C Word redisplays the Ribbon buttons.

④ Click the button you need.

D Word performs the button's action.

⑦ Click anywhere outside the Ribbon.

E Word hides the Ribbon buttons again.

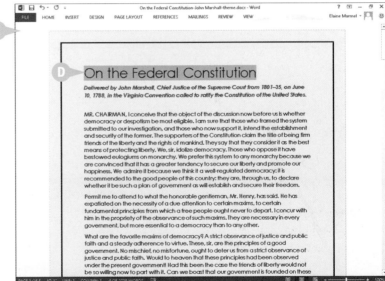

How can I redisplay the Ribbon buttons permanently?
Click any Ribbon tab to display the Ribbon. Then click the **Pin the Ribbon** button (⭲) in the lower-right corner of the Ribbon.

Is there another way to hide the Ribbon buttons?
Yes, you can right-click the bottom edge of any group on the Ribbon and, from the menu that appears, click **Unpin the Ribbon.** When the Ribbon buttons are hidden, you can right-click a Ribbon tab to see that a check mark appears beside the Unpin the Ribbon command. You can click the **Unpin the Ribbon** command to permanently redisplay the Ribbon buttons.

Add a Predefined Group to a Ribbon Tab

You can customize the Ribbon to suit your working style. You can work more efficiently if you customize the Ribbon to place the groups of buttons that you use most often on a single Ribbon tab.

For example, suppose that most of the buttons you need appear on the Home tab, but you often use the Page Setup group on the Page Layout tab to change document margins and set up columns. You can add the Page Setup group to the Home tab. That way, you do not need to switch tabs to get to the commands you use most often.

Add a Predefined Group to a Ribbon Tab

1 Click the **File** tab.

Backstage view appears.

2 Click **Options**.

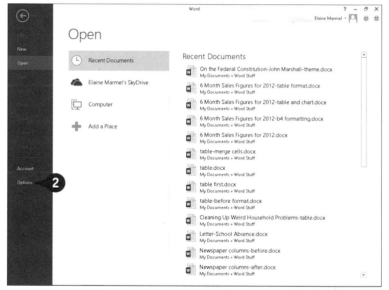

3 In the Word Options dialog box, click **Customize Ribbon**.

4 Click ⌄ and select **Main Tabs**.

5 Click the plus sign (⊞) beside the tab containing the group you want to add (⊞ changes to ⊟).

6 Click the group you want to add.

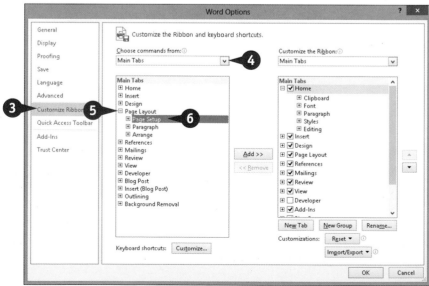

7 Click ⊞ beside the tab where you want to place the group you selected in Step **6** (⊞ changes to ⊟).

8 Click the group you want to appear on the Ribbon to the left of the new group.

9 Click **Add**.

Ⓐ Word adds the group you selected in Step **6** below the group you selected in Step **8**.

10 Repeat Steps **5** to **9** as needed.

11 Click **OK**.

Ⓑ Word adds the group you selected to the appropriate Ribbon tab.

Note: Word might collapse other groups to fit the new group on the tab. In this example, Word collapsed the Editing group.

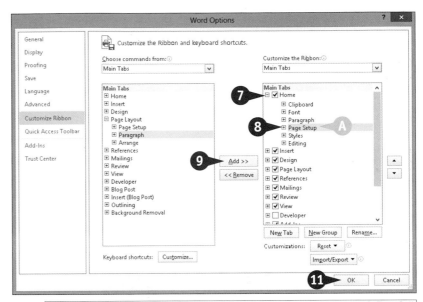

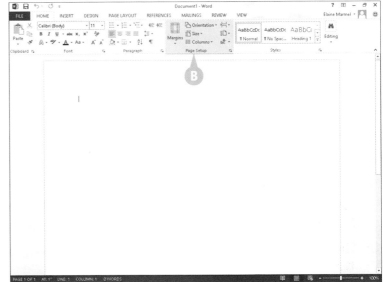

How do I add a single button — instead of a group — to one of the existing groups on the Ribbon?
You cannot modify any of the default groups on the Ribbon. But you can create your own group that contains only those buttons you want to use and then hide the default group that Word displays. See the next section, "Create Your Own Ribbon Group."

If I change my mind, how can I eliminate the changes I made to the Ribbon?
Complete Steps **1** to **3**. In the column on the right, select the Ribbon tab and group you added. Just above the OK button, click **Restore Defaults**, and from the menu that appears, click **Restore only selected Ribbon tab**. Then click **OK**.

Create Your Own Ribbon Group

You cannot add or remove buttons from predefined groups on a Ribbon tab, but you can create your own group and place the buttons you want in the group. Creating your own groups of Ribbon buttons can help you work more efficiently, because you can place all the buttons you use regularly together and save yourself the time of switching groups and even Ribbon tabs.

To create your own Ribbon group, you first make a group, placing it on the tab and in the position where you want it to appear. Then you name it, and finally you add buttons to it.

Create Your Own Ribbon Group

Make a Group

1. Click the **File** tab.

   Backstage view appears.

2. Click **Options**.

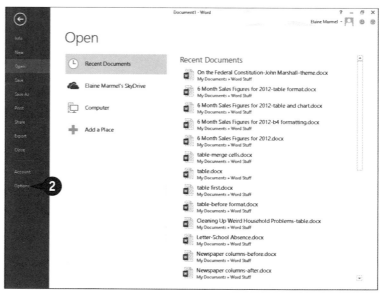

   The Word Options dialog box appears.

3. Click **Customize Ribbon**.

4. Click ⊞ beside the tab to which you want to add a group (⊞ changes to ⊟).

5. Click the group you want to appear on the Ribbon to the left of the new group.

6. Click **New Group**.

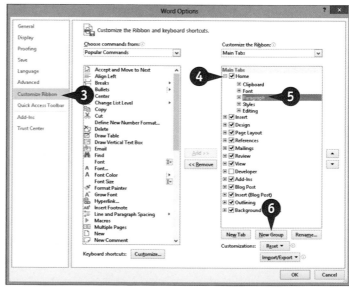

A Word adds a new group to the tab below the group you selected in Step **5** and selects the new group.

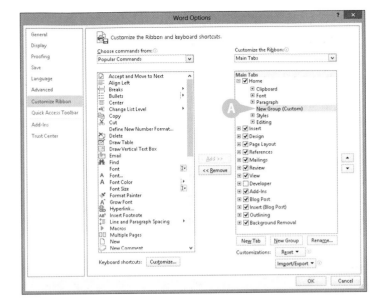

TIP

Can I move the location of my group to another tab?

Yes. Complete Steps **1** to **3**. Then follow these steps:

1 Click ⊞ beside the tab containing the group you want to move and the tab to which you want to move the group to display all groups on both tabs.

2 Click the group you want to move.

3 Click the **Move Up** button (▲) or the **Move Down** button (▼) repeatedly to position the group.

4 Click **OK** to save your changes.

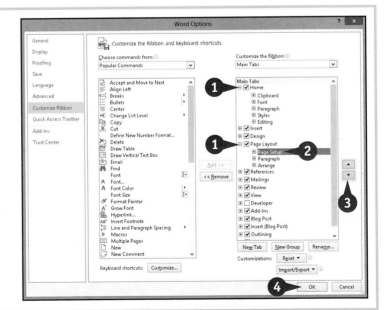

continued ▶

After you add a group to a tab, you can assign a name to it that you find meaningful — for example, something that describes the buttons you intend to include in the group or something that differentiates the group you created from the standard groups on the default Ribbon.

After you name your group, you can then add whatever buttons you need to the group. You are not limited to selecting buttons that appear together on one of the default Ribbon tabs; you can include buttons from any Ribbon tabs and buttons that do not ordinarily appear on the Ribbon.

Create Your Own Ribbon Group (continued)

Assign a Name to the Group

1 Click the group you created in the subsection "Make a Group."

2 Click **Rename**.

The Rename dialog box appears.

3 Type a name for your group.

4 Click **OK**.

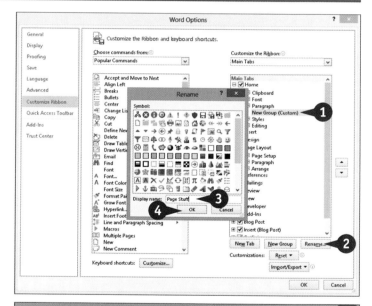

Ⓐ Word assigns the name to your group.

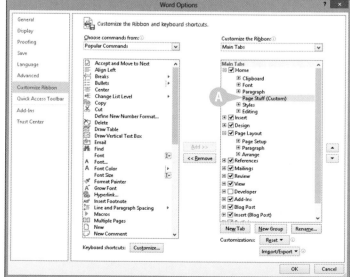

Add Buttons to Your Group

1 Click the group you created.

2 Click a command.

B If the command you want does not appear in the list, click ▾ and select **All Commands**.

3 Click **Add**.

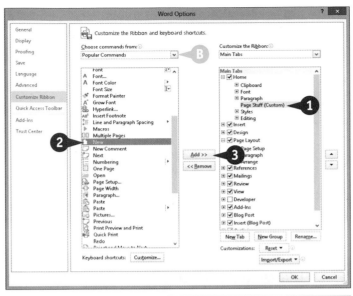

C The command appears below the group you created.

4 Repeat Steps **2** and **3** for each button you want to add to your group.

5 Click **OK** to save your changes.

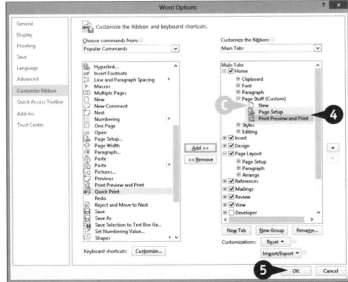

Are there any restrictions for the names I assign to groups I create?

No. In fact, you can even use a name that already appears on the Ribbon, such as Font, and you can place that custom group on the Home tab, where the predefined Font group already exists, or you can place the group on another tab.

Can I assign keyboard shortcuts to the buttons I add to my group?

You do not need to assign keyboard shortcuts; Word assigns them for you, based on the keys already assigned to commands appearing on the tab where you placed your group. If you place the same button on two different tabs, Word assigns different keyboard shortcuts to that button on each tab.

Create Your Own Ribbon Tab

I n addition to creating groups on the Ribbon in which you can place buttons of your choosing, you also can create your own tab on the Ribbon.

Creating your own tab can help you work efficiently; you can store the buttons you use most frequently in groups on your tab. Then you can position your tab on the Ribbon so that it appears by default when you open Word. With all the buttons you use most frequently automatically visible, you save the time of locating the buttons you need on the various Ribbon tabs.

Create Your Own Ribbon Tab

Make a Tab

1 Click the **File** tab.

 Backstage view appears.

2 Click **Options**.

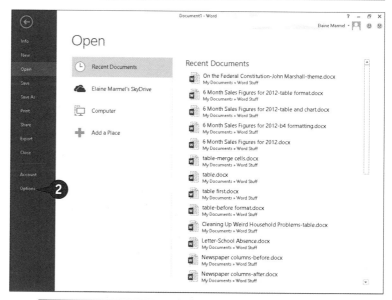

 The Word Options dialog box appears.

3 Click **Customize Ribbon**.

4 Click the tab you want to appear to the left of the new tab.

5 Click **New Tab**.

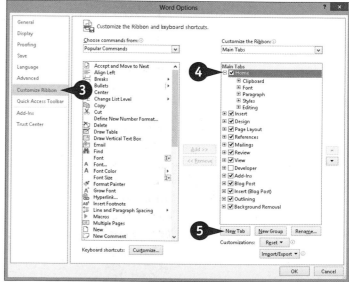

Ⓐ Word creates a new tab below the tab you selected in Step **4**, along with a new group on that tab.

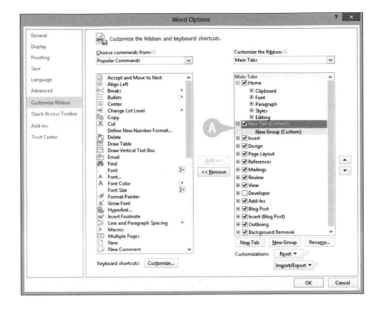

Can I reposition my tab?

Yes. And if you place your tab above the Home tab, it appears as the first tab each time Word opens, giving you instant access to the commands you use most often. Follow these steps:

1 Complete Steps **1** to **3**.

2 Click your tab.

3 Click ▲ or ▼ until your tab appears where you want.

Note: On the Ribbon, Word displays your tab to the right of the tab above it in the Options dialog box.

Ⓐ To make your tab visible immediately every time you open Word, place it above the Home tab.

4 Click **OK** to save your changes.

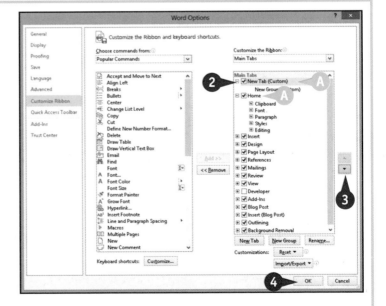

continued ▶

When you create a custom tab, Word automatically creates one group for you so that you can quickly and easily add buttons to the new tab. You can add other groups to the tab and place buttons in them; see the section "Create Your Own Ribbon Group" earlier in this chapter.

You should assign names to both the new tab and the new group that are meaningful to you. For example, you might name your tab to describe its content. Assign group names based on the buttons you intend to place in the group.

Create Your Own Ribbon Tab (continued)

Assign Names

1 Click the group you created, labeled as **New Group (Custom)**.

2 Click **Rename**.

The Rename dialog box appears.

3 Type a name for your group.

4 Click **OK**.

5 Click the new tab you created, labeled as **New Tab (Custom)**.

6 Repeat Steps **2** to **4** to rename your new tab, renamed in this example to File Stuff.

A Word assigns names to your tab and your group.

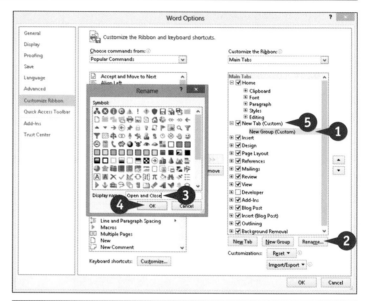

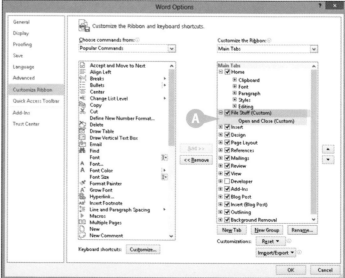

Add Buttons to Your Group

1 Click the group on the tab you created.

2 Click a command.

B If the command you want does not appear in the list, click ⌄ and select **All Commands**.

3 Click **Add**.

C The command appears below the group you created.

4 Repeat Steps **2** and **3** for each button you want to add to the group.

5 Click **OK**.

D The new tab appears on the Ribbon, along with the group containing the buttons you added.

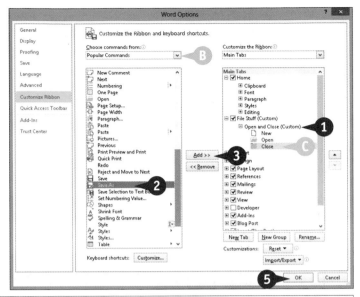

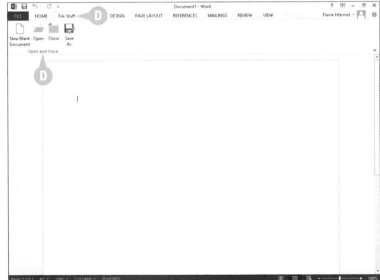

TIP

Is there a way to not display my tab without deleting it?

Yes, you can hide the tab. Complete Steps **1** to **3** in the subsection "Make a Tab." Deselect the tab you want to hide (☑ changes to ☐), and click **OK**. Word redisplays the Ribbon without your custom tab.

Work with the Quick Access Toolbar

You can customize the Quick Access Toolbar (QAT). The QAT is always visible as you work in Word, so, like a customized Ribbon, a customized QAT can help you work more efficiently if you place buttons on it that you use frequently.

By default, the QAT contains three buttons: the Save button, the Undo button, and the Redo button. You can remove any of these buttons as well as quickly and easily add other commonly used commands, and without much additional effort, you can add not-so-commonly used commands. You also can control the position of the QAT, displaying it above or below the Ribbon.

Work with the Quick Access Toolbar

Change Placement

1 Click the **Customize Quick Access Toolbar** ▾.

Word displays a menu of choices.

2 Click **Show Below the Ribbon**.

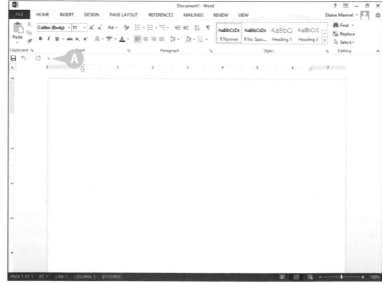

Ⓐ The Quick Access Toolbar (QAT) appears below the Ribbon instead of above it.

You can repeat these steps to move the QAT back above the Ribbon.

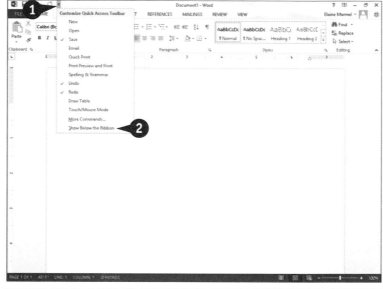

Add Buttons to the QAT

1 Click ⏷.

B A check mark (✓) appears beside commands already on the QAT.

C You can click any command to add it to the QAT and skip the rest of these steps.

2 If you do not see the command you want to add, click **More Commands**.

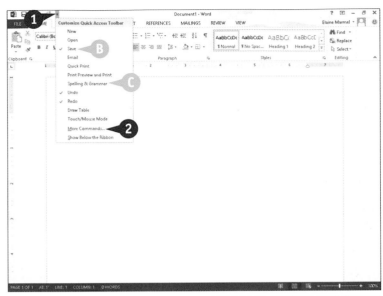

The Word Options dialog box appears, showing the Quick Access Toolbar customization options.

D You can add any of these commands to the QAT.

E If the command you want to add does not appear in the list, click ⏷ and select **All Commands**.

F Commands already on the QAT appear here.

G You can click ⏷ to customize the QAT for all documents or just the current document.

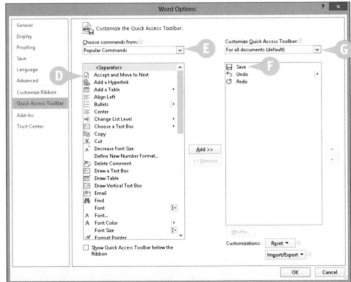

TIP

Is there an easy way to get rid of changes I made to the QAT?
Yes. You can remove an individual button by right-clicking it on the QAT and clicking **Remove from Quick Access Toolbar**. Or, you can reset it by following these steps. Complete Steps **1** and **2** in the subsection "Add Buttons to the QAT." In the Word Options dialog box that appears, click **Reset** and then click **Reset only Quick Access Toolbar**. The Reset Customizations dialog box appears, asking if you are sure of your action. Click **Yes**, and Word resets the QAT. Click **OK** to return to a document.

continued ▶

The buttons on the Quick Access Toolbar are smaller than their counterparts on the Ribbon, but their size should not discourage you from using the QAT. You can always position the mouse pointer over a button to see a tip describing its function.

In addition to repositioning the QAT either below or above the Ribbon and adding buttons to or removing buttons from the QAT, you can reorganize the order in which buttons appear on the QAT. You also can quickly add a button on the Ribbon to the QAT, as described in the tip at the end of this section.

Work with the Quick Access Toolbar (continued)

3 Click ⌄ to display the various categories of commands.

Ⓐ You can select **All Commands** to view all commands in alphabetical order regardless of category.

4 Click a category of commands.

This example uses the Commands Not in the Ribbon category.

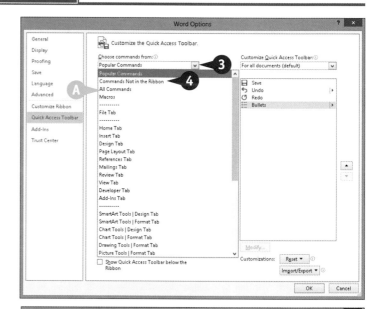

5 Click the command you want to add to the Toolbar.

6 Click **Add**.

Ⓑ Word moves the command from the list on the left to the list on the right.

7 Repeat Steps **3** to **6** for each command you want to add to the Quick Access Toolbar.

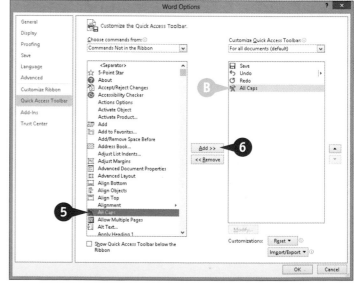

Reorder QAT Buttons

1 While viewing QAT customization options in the Word Options dialog box, click a command in the right column.

Note: Complete Steps **1** and **2** in the subsection "Add Buttons to the QAT" to view QAT customization options.

2 Click ▲ or ▼ to change a command's placement on the Quick Access Toolbar.

3 Repeat Steps **1** and **2** to reorder other commands.

4 Click **OK**.

Ⓒ The updated Quick Access Toolbar appears.

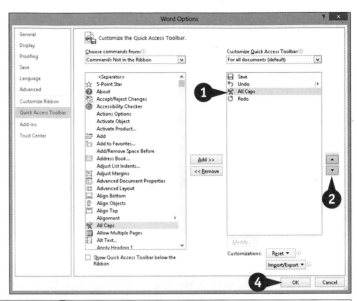

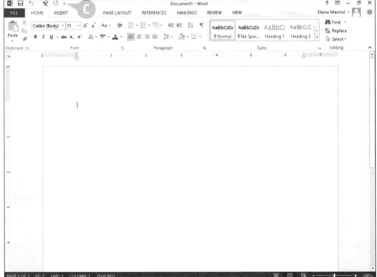

TIP

How do I add a button from the Ribbon to the Quick Access Toolbar?

To add a button from the Ribbon to the Quick Access Toolbar, right-click the button and click **Add to Quick Access Toolbar**. Word adds the button to the QAT.

> Add to Quick Access Toolbar
>
> Customize Quick Access Toolbar...
>
> Show Quick Access Toolbar Below the Ribbon
>
> Customize the Ribbon...
>
> Unpin the ribbon

Add Keyboard Shortcuts

You can add keyboard shortcuts for commands you use frequently. Using a keyboard shortcut can be faster and more efficient than clicking a button on the Ribbon or the QAT because you can keep your hands on your keyboard, increasing typing speed and efficiency.

You might think that a command must appear on either the Ribbon or the Quick Access Toolbar in order to create a keyboard shortcut for it. But, in fact, whether a command appears as a button on the Ribbon does not affect whether you can create a keyboard shortcut. You can, in fact, create keyboard shortcuts for any command.

Add Keyboard Shortcuts

1 Click the **File** tab.

Backstage view appears.

2 Click **Options**.

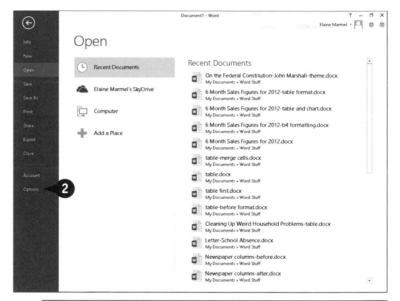

The Word Options dialog box appears.

3 Click **Customize Ribbon**.

4 Click **Customize**.

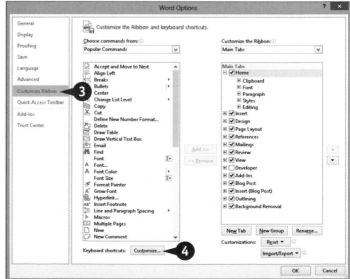

The Customize Keyboard dialog box appears.

Ⓐ Categories of commands appear here.

Ⓑ Commands within a category appear here.

⑤ Click the category containing the command to which you want to assign a keyboard shortcut.

⑥ Click the command.

Ⓒ Any existing shortcut keys for the selected command appear here.

⑦ Click here, and press a keyboard combination.

Ⓓ The keys you press appear here.

Ⓔ The command to which the shortcut is currently assigned appears here.

⑧ Click **Assign**.

⑨ Click **Close**.

⑩ Click **OK**.

Word saves the shortcut.

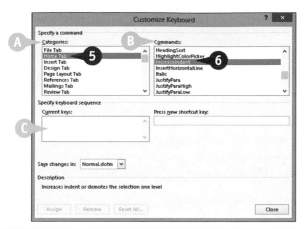

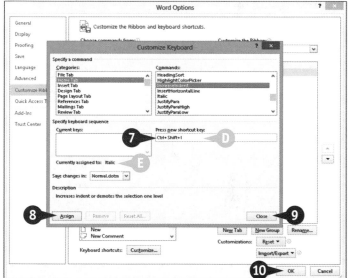

How can I test my shortcut to make sure it works?

You can press the keys you assigned. You also can position the mouse pointer over the tool on the Ribbon; any assigned keyboard shortcut, whether user-assigned or Word-assigned, appears in the ScreenTip. If you do not see keyboard shortcuts in the ScreenTips, open the Word Options dialog box, click **Advanced** on the left, and in the **Display** section, select **Show shortcut keys in ScreenTips** (☐ changes to ☑).

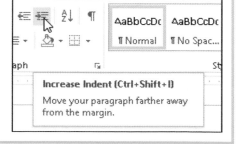

Create a Macro

You can create a macro to save time and repetitive keystrokes. A macro combines a series of actions into a single command. For example, suppose that you often type tables that must fit on the page in landscape orientation. Although you can use commands on the Ribbon to change the page orientation, you can save time and keystrokes if you create a macro that changes the page orientation from portrait to landscape.

Most people find it easiest to create a macro by recording the keystrokes that they use to take the action they want to store in the macro.

Create a Macro

Ⓐ Display the Macro Recording indicator (🖳) on the status bar by right-clicking the status bar and choosing **Macro Recording** from the Customize Status Bar menu.

① Click the **View** tab.

② Click the bottom half of the **Macros** button.

③ Click **Record Macro**.

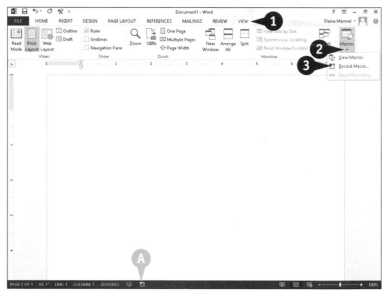

The Record Macro dialog box appears.

④ Type a name for the macro.

Note: Macro names must begin with a letter and contain no spaces.

⑤ Type a description for the macro here.

⑥ Click **OK**.

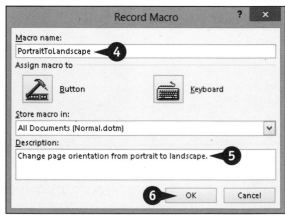

286

B The Macro Recording indicator (⊞) changes to a Stop Recording indicator (◻).

C Stop Recording and Pause Recording buttons appear when you click the bottom half of the **Macros** button.

The mouse pointer changes to ⅍ .

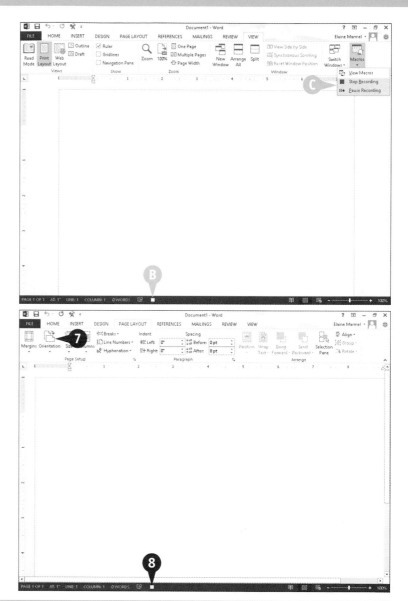

7 Perform the actions you want included in the macro.

Note: Macros can include typing, formatting, and commands. You cannot use the mouse to position the insertion point.

8 When you have taken all the actions you want to include in the macro, click the Stop Recording indicator (◻) on the status bar.

Word saves the macro, and the Macro Recording indicator returns to its original appearance.

TIPS

In the Record Macro dialog box, what do the Button and Keyboard buttons do?

They enable you to assign a macro to a button on the QAT or to a keyboard shortcut at the same time that you create the macro. You can always assign a macro to a QAT button or a keyboard shortcut after you create it. See the next section, "Run a Macro."

Do I need to re-create my macros from Word 2003, Word 2007, or Word 2010?

No. If you upgrade from one of these earlier versions, Word 2013 converts the Normal template you used in those versions. Typically, the converted Normal template contains all your macros, and they should appear in the Macros dialog box and work in Word 2013.

Run a Macro

You can save time by running a macro you created because Word performs whatever actions you stored in the macro. The method you choose to run a macro depends primarily on how often you need to run it. If you use the macro only occasionally, you can run it from the Macros window. If you use it often, you can assign a macro to a keyboard shortcut or a Quick Access Toolbar button.

To record a macro, see the previous section, "Create a Macro."

Run a Macro

Using the Macros Dialog Box

If your macro is dependent upon the position of the insertion point, click in your document where you want the results of the macro to appear.

1 Click the **View** tab.

2 Click **Macros**.

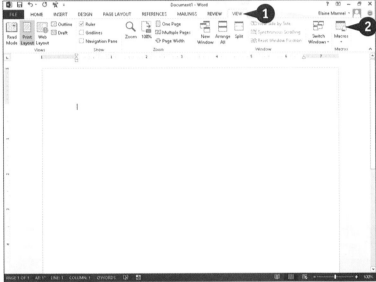

The Macros dialog box appears.

Ⓐ Available macros appear here.

3 Click the macro you want to run.

Ⓑ The selected macro's description appears here.

4 Click **Run**.

Word performs the actions stored in the macro.

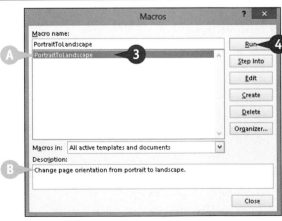

Assign and Use a QAT Button

1 Click the **File** tab.

Backstage view appears.

2 Click **Options**.

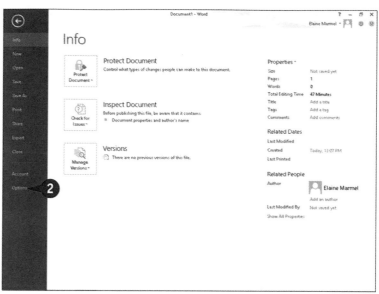

The Word Options dialog box appears.

3 Click **Quick Access Toolbar**.

4 Click ▼ and select **Macros**.

5 Click the macro to add to the QAT.

6 Click **Add**.

C Word adds the macro to the QAT.

7 Click **OK**.

8 Click the macro's button on the QAT to perform the actions stored in the macro.

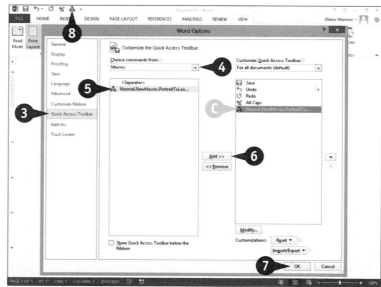

TIPS

How do I assign a keyboard shortcut to a macro?

Follow the steps in the section "Add Keyboard Shortcuts" earlier in this chapter. In Step **5**, scroll to the bottom of the list and select **Macros**. In Step **6**, select the macro.

Can I create a Screen Tip for my QAT button that contains a name I recognize when I point the mouse at the QAT button?

Yes. Complete Steps **1** to **6** in the subsection "Assign and Use a QAT Button." Then in the list on the right, click the macro, and below the list, click **Modify**. In the Modify Button dialog box that appears, type the new name for your macro in the Display Name text box below the button symbols.

CHAPTER 12

Working with Mass Mailing Tools

Why do the work yourself? You can use Word's mass mailing tools to create and mail form letters.

Create Letters to Mass Mail

Using a form letter and a mailing list, you can quickly and easily create a mass mailing that merges the addresses from the mailing list into the form letter. Typically, the only information that changes in the form letter is the addressee information. Wherever changing information appears, you insert a placeholder that Word replaces when you merge.

You can create the mailing list as you create the mass mailing, you can use a mailing list that exists in another Word document or an Excel file, or you can use your Outlook Contact List. This example uses an Excel file.

Create Letters to Mass Mail

Set Up for a Mail Merge

1. Open the Word document that you want to use as the form letter.

Note: The letter should not contain any information that will change from letter to letter, such as the inside address.

2. Click the **Mailings** tab.

3. Click **Start Mail Merge**.

4. Click **Letters**.

The screen flashes, indicating that Word has set up for a mail merge.

Identify Recipients

1. Click **Select Recipients**.

2. Click to identify the type of recipient list you plan to use.

This example uses an existing list in an Excel file.

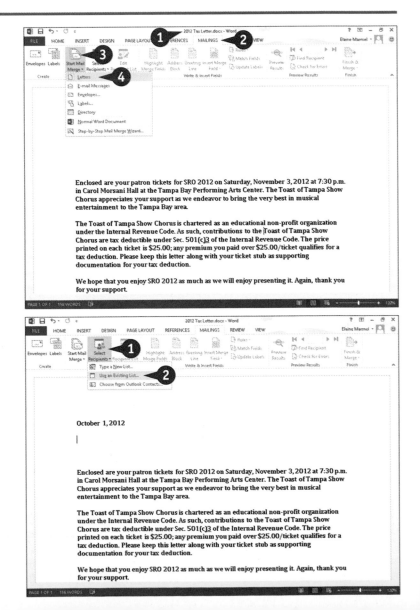

The Select Data Source dialog box appears.

3 Navigate to the folder containing the mailing list file.

4 Click the file containing the mailing list.

5 Click **Open**.

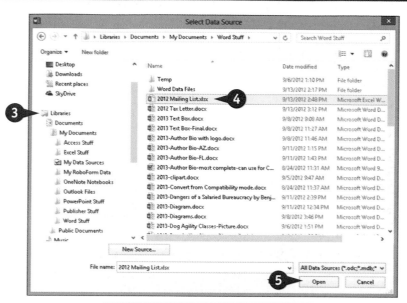

Word links with Excel, and the Select Table dialog box appears.

Note: If the Excel notebook contains multiple sheets, you can select a specific sheet in the Select Table dialog box.

6 If necessary, select a sheet.

7 Click **OK**.

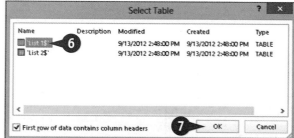

TIP

How do I create a mailing list?

To create a mailing list, perform the steps that follow. In Step **2** in the subsection "Identify Recipients," click **Type New List**. In the New Address List dialog box, type recipient information for each addressee (**A**), and click **OK**. Save the file in the Save Address List dialog box that appears. Skip to the subsection "Create the Address Block" to finish the steps.

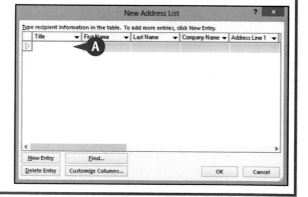

continued ▶

You are not limited to sending letters to all recipients in a list; you can select specific recipients from the mailing list to receive the form letter.

You use merge fields, which are placeholders, to identify the location in your document where the recipient's address and greeting should appear. You can modify the appearance of both the recipient's address and the greeting line. For example, in the address block, you can include or exclude titles such as "Mr." in the recipient's name, and in the greeting line, you can address the recipient formally, using a title and last name, or informally, using a first name.

Create Letters to Mass Mail (continued)

⑧ Click **Edit Recipient List**.

The Mail Merge Recipients window appears.

Ⓐ A check box (☑) appears beside each person's name, identifying the recipients of the form letter.

⑨ Deselect any addressee for whom you do not want to prepare a form letter (☑ changes to ☐).

⑩ Click **OK**.

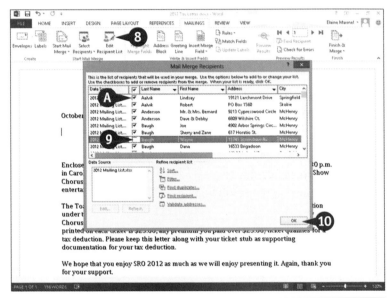

Create the Address Block

① Click the location where you want the inside address to appear in the form letter.

② Click **Address Block**.

The Insert Address Block dialog box appears.

③ Click a format for each recipient's name.

Ⓑ You can preview the format here.

④ Click **OK**.

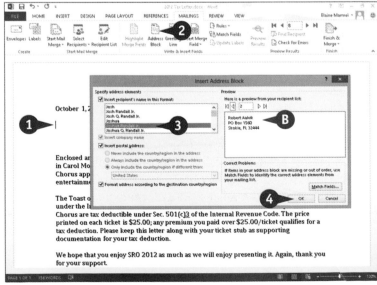

C The <<Address Block>> merge field appears in the letter.

Create a Greeting

1 Click at the location where you want the greeting to appear.

2 Click **Greeting Line**.

The Insert Greeting Line dialog box appears.

3 Click these (⌄) to select the greeting format.

D A preview of the greeting appears here.

4 Click **OK**.

E The <<Greeting Line>> merge field appears in the letter.

Preview and Merge

1 Click **Preview Results** to preview your merge results.

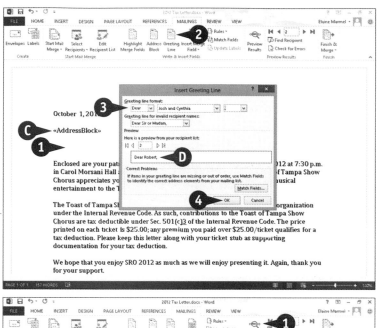

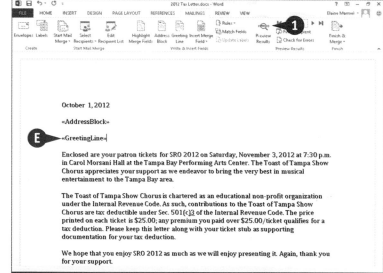

TIP

What should I do if the preview in the Insert Address Block dialog box is blank or incorrect?

Perform the steps that follow. After you complete Step **3** in the subsection "Create the Address Block," click **Match Fields**. The Match Fields dialog box appears. Beside each field you use in your merge, click ⌄ and select the corresponding field name in your mailing list file. Click **OK** and continue with Step **4** in the subsection "Create the Address Block." Word matches your fields.

continued ▶

You can preview the letters; information from your mailing list replaces the merge fields that were acting as placeholders. Word gives you another opportunity to select specific recipients before creating individual letters.

After you review the letters, you can print them. Or, if your mailing list contains e-mail addresses, you can send the letters as e-mail messages; Word prompts you for a subject line and a format — HTML, plain text, or an attachment — and then places the message in the Outlook outbox. You must finish by opening Outlook and sending the messages.

Create Letters to Mass Mail (continued)

Ⓐ Word displays a preview of the merged letter, using the unchanging content of the letter and changing information from the address file.

Ⓑ You can click the **Next Record** button (▶) to preview the next letter and the **Previous Record** button (◀) to move back and preview the previous letter.

Ⓒ You can click **Preview Results** to redisplay merge fields.

② Click **Finish & Merge**.

③ Click **Edit Individual Documents**.

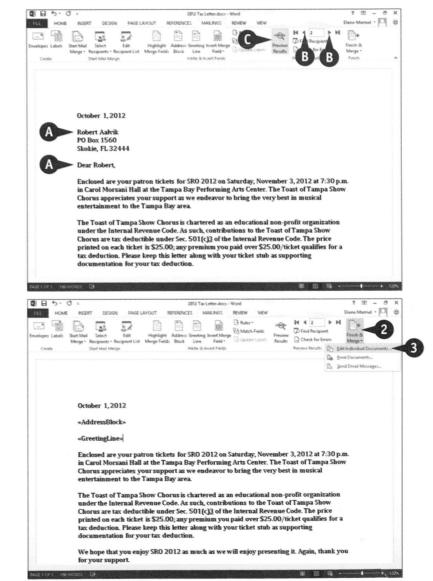

The Merge to New Document dialog box appears.

④ Select an option to identify the recipients of the letter (○ changes to ◉).

The **All** option creates a letter for all entries on the mailing list; the **Current record** option creates only one letter for the recipient whose letter you are previewing; and the **From** and **To** option creates letters for recipients you identify by their numeric position in the address list, not by their names.

⑤ Click **OK**.

Ⓓ Word merges the form letter information with the mailing list information, placing the results in a new document named Letters1.

Ⓔ The new document contains individual letters for each mailing list recipient.

⑥ Click ▾.

⑦ Click **Quick Print**.

Ⓕ You can click the **Save** button (💾) on the Quick Access Toolbar (QAT) and assign a new name to save the merged letters.

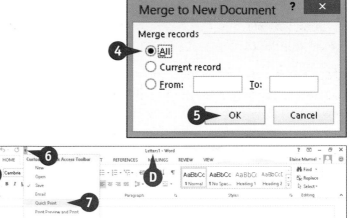

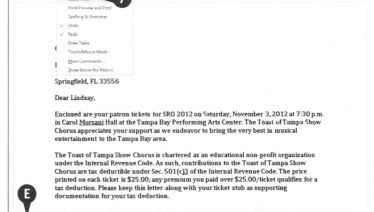

TIP

Can I create envelopes to go with my form letter?
Yes. Display the form letter containing merge fields. Click **Envelopes** to display the Envelopes and Labels dialog box. Click **Add to Document** to place an envelope in your document. You can type a return address in the upper-left corner of the envelope. Click in the lower center of the envelope to locate the address box; dotted lines surround it. Complete the steps in the subsections "Create the Address Block" and "Preview and Merge."

Create Labels for a Mass Mailing

In addition to creating personalized form letters for a mass mailing, you can use the merge feature to create mailing labels for mass mailing recipients. Mailing labels can be useful when you do not want to use your printer to print separate envelopes for your letters. For example, your mailing might include more than a letter so that you must use larger envelopes than your printer can print. By creating mailing labels, you can automate the process of addressing your larger envelopes.

Word's mass mailing feature enables you to select from a wide variety of commonly used labels from various manufacturers.

Create Labels for a Mass Mailing

Select a Label Format

① Start a new blank document.

Note: See Chapter 2 for details on starting a new document.

② Click the **Mailings** tab.

③ Click **Start Mail Merge**.

④ Click **Labels**.

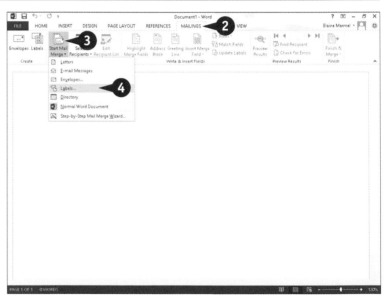

The Label Options dialog box appears.

⑤ Select a printer option (○ changes to ●).

⑥ Click ⌄ to select a label vendor.

⑦ Use the scroll arrows (⌃ and ⌄) to find and click the label's product number.

Ⓐ Information about the label dimensions appears here.

⑧ Click **OK**.

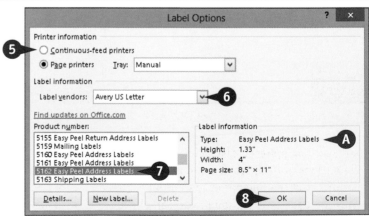

Word sets up the document for the labels you selected.

Note: If gridlines identifying individual labels do not appear, click the **Layout** tab and then click **View Gridlines**.

Identify Recipients

1 Click **Select Recipients**.

2 Click to identify the type of recipient list you plan to use.

In this example, an existing list in an Excel file is used.

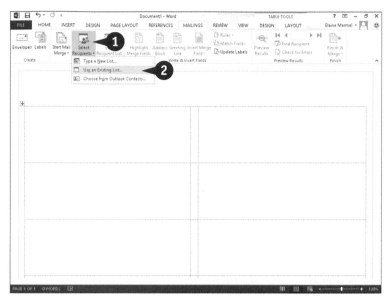

The Select Data Source dialog box appears.

3 Navigate to the folder containing the mailing list file.

4 Click the file containing the mailing list.

5 Click **Open**.

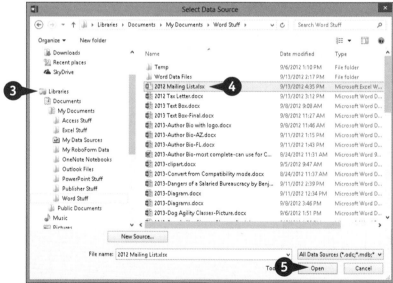

TIPS

What happens if I click Details in the Label Options dialog box?

A dialog box appears, displaying the margins and dimensions of each label, the number of labels per row, and the number of rows of labels, along with the page size. Although you can change these dimensions, you run the risk of having label information print incorrectly if you do.

What happens if I click New Label in the Label Options dialog box?

A dialog box appears that you can use to create your own custom label. Word bases the appearance of this dialog box on the settings selected in the Label Options dialog box. Type a name for the label, and then adjust the margins, height and width, number across or down, vertical or horizontal pitch, and page size as needed.

continued ▶ 299

Create Labels for a Mass Mailing (continued)

Using your label options, Word sets up a document of labels to which you attach a file containing recipient information. You can use an existing file or your Outlook contacts, or you can create a new recipient list. You also can select specific recipients from the mailing list for whom to create labels.

You use a merge field, which serves as a placeholder, to identify the location in the label document where the recipient's address should appear. You can modify the appearance of the recipient's address to, for example, include or exclude titles such as "Mr."

This example uses addresses stored in an Excel file.

Create Labels for a Mass Mailing (continued)

Word links with Excel, and the Select Table dialog box appears.

Note: If the Excel notebook contains multiple sheets, you can select a specific sheet in the Select Table dialog box.

6 If necessary, select a sheet.

7 Click **OK**.

A Word inserts a <<Next Record>> field in each label except the first one.

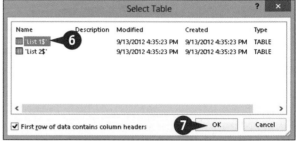

Add a Merge Field

1 Click the first label to place the insertion point in it.

2 Click **Address Block**.

The Insert Address Block dialog box appears.

3 Click a format for each recipient's name.

B You can preview the format here.

4 Click **OK**.

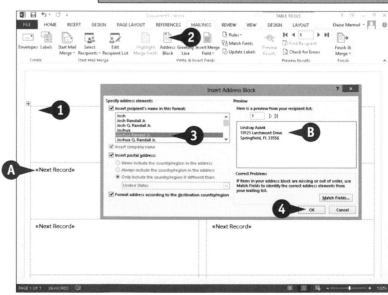

C Word adds the <<Address Block>> merge field to the first label.

Note: When you merge the information, Word replaces the merge field with information from the mailing address file.

5 Click **Update Labels**.

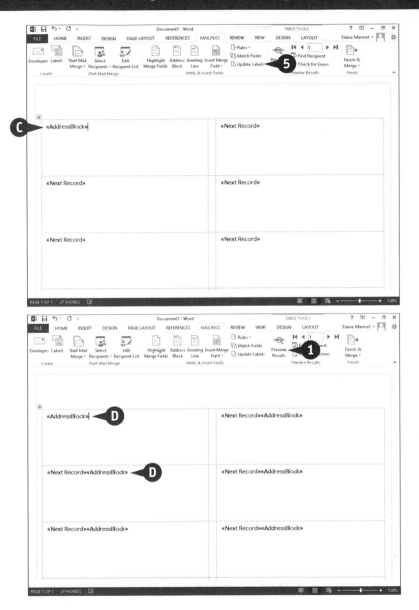

D Word adds the <<Address Block>> merge field to every label.

Preview and Print

1 You can click **Preview Results** to preview your merged results.

TIP

Can I selectively create labels using an existing file?
Yes. Perform the steps that follow. Click **Edit Recipient List**. The Mail Merge Recipients dialog box appears. Deselect any addressee for whom you do not want to create a mailing label (☑ changes to ☐), and click **OK**.

continued ▶

Create Labels for a Mass Mailing (continued)

You can preview the labels before you print them. Information from your mailing list replaces the placeholder merge field. Word gives you another opportunity to select specific recipients before creating sheets of labels.

After you review the labels, you can print the label document, or you can remerge the label sheets directly to your printer. Although you can send a label as an e-mail message, it probably will not mean much to the recipient because the e-mail body contains the recipient address only. You might consider this option if you need to confirm physical addresses.

Create Labels for a Mass Mailing (continued)

Word displays a preview of your labels, replacing the merge field with information from the mailing list file.

Ⓐ You can click ▶ to preview the next label and ◀ to move back and preview the previous label.

② Click **Preview Results** to redisplay merge fields.

③ Click **Finish & Merge**.

④ Click **Edit Individual Documents**.

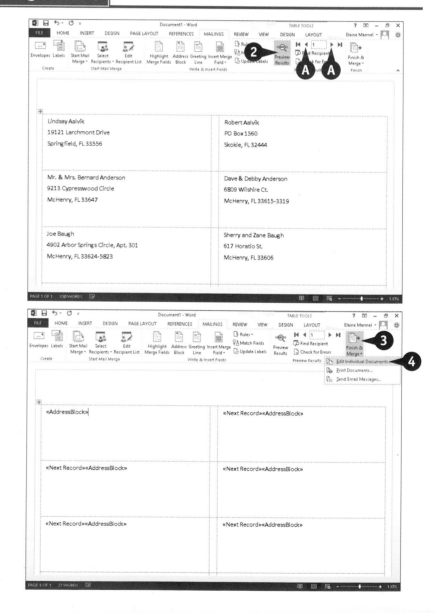

The Merge to New Document dialog box appears.

⑤ Select an option to identify the recipients of the letter (○ changes to ◉).

The **All** option creates a label for all entries on the mailing list, the **Current record** option creates only one label for the recipient you are previewing, and the **From** option creates labels for recipients you specify.

⑥ Click **OK**.

Ⓑ Word creates the labels in a new Word document named Labels1.

The new document contains individual labels for each mailing list recipient.

⑦ Click ⊟.

⑧ Click **Quick Print**.

The labels print.

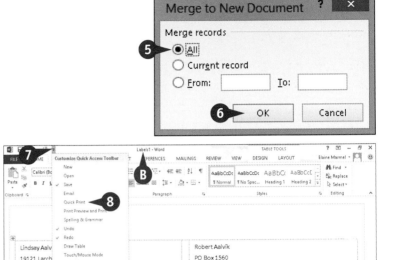

What does the Check for Errors button on the Ribbon do?
When you click this button, Word gives you the opportunity to determine whether you have correctly set up the merge. In the Checking and Reporting Errors dialog box that appears, select an option (○ changes to ◉) and click **OK**. Depending on the option you choose, Word reports errors as they occur or in a new document.

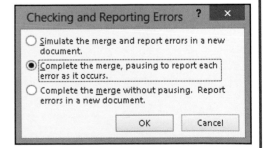

CHAPTER 13

Word and the World beyond Your Desktop

You can use Word to reach beyond your desktop. You can e-mail a document, post to your blog, or work with your SkyDrive cloud storage.

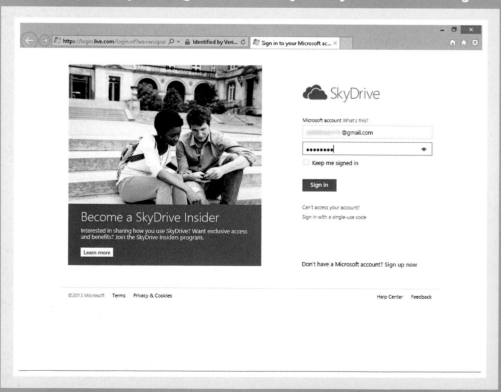

E-Mail a Document

Y ou can share a Word document with others via e-mail. Although you could create a new e-mail message in your e-mail program and add the file as an attachment, you really do not need to go to the extra trouble. Instead, you can e-mail a Word document from Word. Word sends the document as an attachment in a variety of formats.

Although you do not need to send the document from your e-mail program, your e-mail program must be set up on your computer. Note that, to open the file, recipients must have the appropriate software on their computer.

E-Mail a Document

1. Open the document you want to send by e-mail.

2. Click the **File** tab.

   Backstage view appears.

3. Click **Share**.

4. Click **Email**.

5. Click a method to send the document.

   This example sends the document as an attachment.

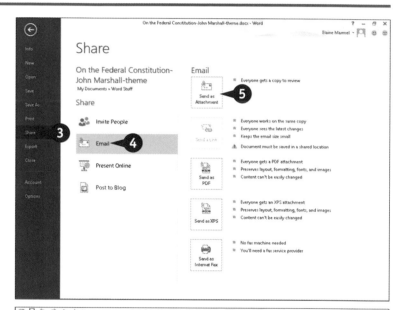

An e-mail message window appears.

Ⓐ The e-mail attachment appears here; in this example, the attachment is a Word document.

6. Click here to type the e-mail address of the recipient.

Ⓑ You also can type the e-mail address of someone to whom you want to send a copy of the message.

Note: To send to multiple recipients, separate the e-mail addresses with a semicolon (;) and a space.

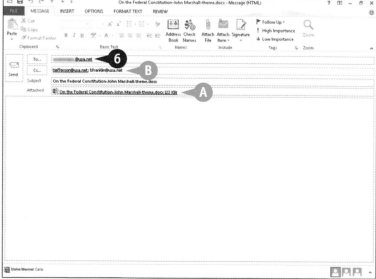

7 Click here to type a subject for the e-mail message.

Note: Subjects are not required, but including one is considerate. Word automatically supplies the document name for the subject; you can replace the document name with anything you want.

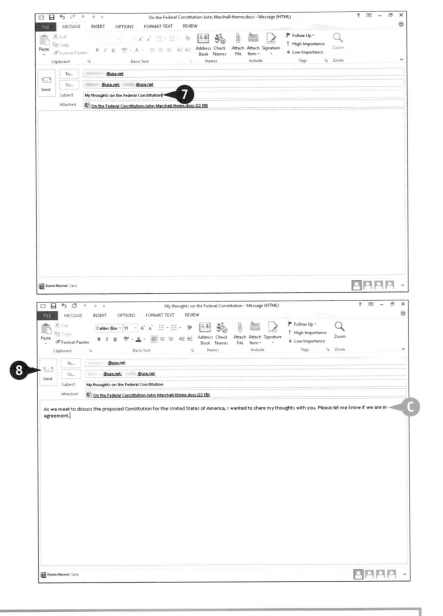

C You can type a message here.

8 Click **Send**.

Word places the message in your e-mail program's Outbox and closes the e-mail message window.

Note: You must open your e-mail program and, if your e-mail program does not automatically send and receive periodically, send the message.

What should I do if I change my mind about sending the e-mail message while viewing the e-mail message window?

Click ✕ in the e-mail message window. A message appears, asking if you want to save the message. Click **No**.

What happens if I choose Send as PDF in Step 5?

Word creates a PDF version of the document and attaches the PDF version to the e-mail message instead of attaching the Word file. The recipient cannot edit the PDF file with Word; to edit the document, the recipient would need special software, such as Adobe Acrobat Pro.

Create a Hyperlink

You can create a hyperlink in your Word document. You use hyperlinks to connect a word, phrase, or graphic image in a Word document to another document on your computer or in your company's network or to a web page on the Internet. Hyperlinks are useful when you want to refer, in your Word document, to other information that you want the reader to be able to view quickly and easily.

The hyperlink you create in a Word document works just like the ones you use on web pages you browse. Clicking a hyperlink takes you to a new location.

Create a Hyperlink

1 Select the text or graphic you want to use to create a hyperlink.

2 Click the **Insert** tab.

3 Click **Links**.

4 Click **Hyperlink**.

You can right-click the selection and click **Hyperlink** instead of performing Steps **2** and **3**.

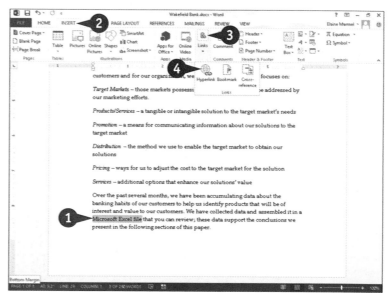

The Insert Hyperlink dialog box appears.

5 Click **Existing File or Web Page**.

Ⓐ Files in the current folder appear here.

6 Click ▾, and navigate to the folder containing the document to which you want to link.

7 Click the file to select it.

8 Click **ScreenTip**.

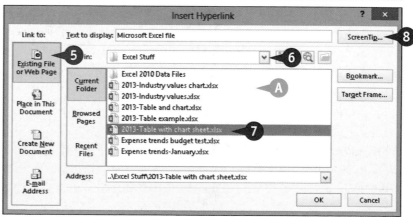

The Set Hyperlink ScreenTip dialog box appears.

9 Type text that should appear when a user positions the mouse pointer over the hyperlink.

10 Click **OK**.

11 Click **OK** in the Insert Hyperlink dialog box.

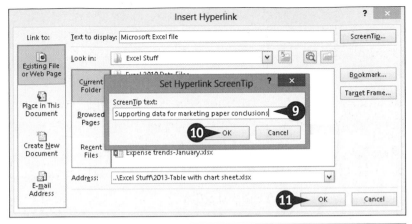

B Word creates a hyperlink shown as blue, underlined text in your document.

12 Slide the mouse pointer over the hyperlink.

C The screen tip text you provided in Step **9** appears, along with instructions to the reader on how to use the hyperlink.

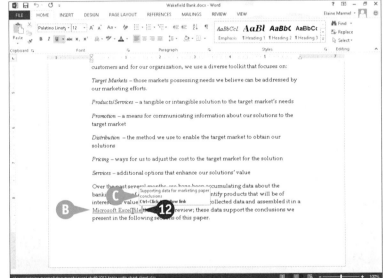

TIPS

How do I use a hyperlink that appears in a Word document?

Press and hold Ctrl as you click the hyperlink. The linked document or web page will appear.

My hyperlink to a file does not work anymore. Why not?

In all likelihood, the file no longer exists at the location you selected in Step **6**. If you moved the file to a new folder, edit the hyperlink to update the file location. To edit the hyperlink, slide the mouse pointer over it and right-click. From the menu that appears, click **Edit Hyperlink**. Then follow Steps **5** to **7**.

Post to Your Blog

If you keep an online blog, you can use Word to create a document to post on it. This enables you to take advantage of Word's many proofing and formatting tools. You can then post the blog entry directly from Word.

To post your blog entry, you must first set up Word to communicate with the Internet server that hosts your online blog; the first time you post a blog entry from Word, the program prompts you to register your blog account. Click **Register Now**, choose your blog provider in the dialog box that appears, and follow the on-screen prompts.

Post to Your Blog

Note: You must be connected to the Internet to complete this section.

1. Click the **File** tab.

2. Click **New**.

3. Click **Blog post**.

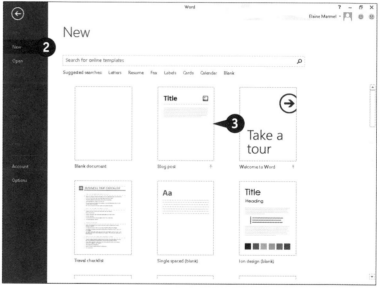

Word opens the blog post document.

Note: The first time you use the blog feature, Word prompts you to register your blog account. Click **Register Now**, choose your blog provider in the dialog box that appears, and follow the on-screen prompts.

Ⓐ You can use the buttons in the Blog group to manage blog entries. For example, you can click Manage Accounts to set up blog accounts.

Ⓑ You can use these tools to format text as you type.

4. Click the **Insert** tab.

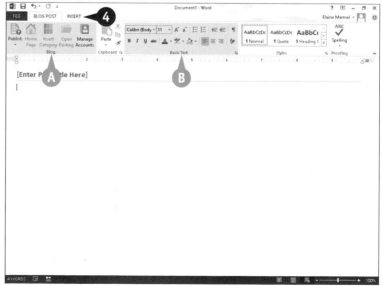

C Use these buttons to incorporate tables, pictures, clip art, shapes, graphics, screenshots, WordArt, symbols, and hyperlinks in a blog entry.

5 Click here, and type a title for your blog entry.

6 Click here, and type your entry.

7 Click the **Blog Post** tab.

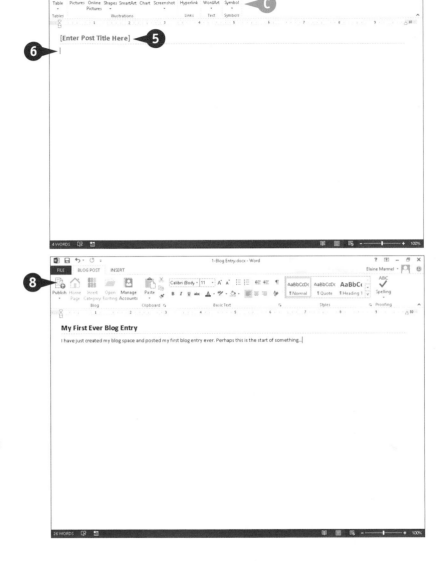

Note: You can save your blog entry on your hard drive the same way you save any document.

8 Click **Publish**.

Word connects to the Internet, prompts you for your blog username and password, and posts your entry.

A message appears above the blog entry title, identifying when the entry was posted.

TIPS

Can I edit my blog accounts from within Word?
Yes. Click the **Manage Accounts** button on the Blog Post tab when viewing a blog page in Word to open the Blog Accounts dialog box. Here, you can edit an existing account, add a new account, or delete an account that you no longer use.

Can I post entries as drafts to review them before making them visible to the public?
Yes. Click ▼ on the bottom half of the **Publish** button, and click **Publish as Draft**. When you are ready to let the public review your entry, open it in Word and click **Publish**.

Word and the Cloud

Word 2013 offers a completely new experience when it comes to working in a mobile environment. Today, people are on the go but often want to take work with them to do while sitting in the doctor's office waiting room, the airport, or a hotel room. Word 2013 was designed to help you work from anywhere using almost any device available because, among other reasons, it works with SkyDrive, Microsoft's cloud space. From SkyDrive, you can log into cloud space and, using the Word Web App — essentially, a tool with which you are already familiar — get to work.

Sign In to Office Online

Office Online connects your Microsoft Word to the world beyond your computer. When you sign in on any device and launch Word, the program Start screen and the program window show that you are signed in. Signing in gives you access to online pictures and clip art stored at Office.com and enables Word to synchronize documents between your computer, SkyDrive, and SharePoint.

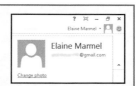

SkyDrive and Office 2013

The SkyDrive app, Microsoft's cloud storage service, comes with Word 2013; 7GB are free, and you can rent additional space. Word 2013 saves all documents by default to your SkyDrive so that your documents are always available to you.

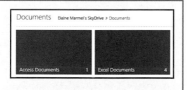

Using the Word Web App

You can use the appropriate Web App to open and edit Word, Excel, OneNote, and PowerPoint documents from your SkyDrive. The Office Web Apps are scaled-down editions of Office programs that you can use to easily review documents and make minor changes.

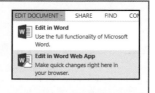

Take Your Personal Settings with You Everywhere

Word 2013 keeps track of personal settings like your recently used files and favorite templates and makes them available from any computer. Word and PowerPoint also remember the paragraph and slide you were viewing when you close a document, and they display that location when you open the document on another machine, making it easy for you to get back to work when you move from one work location to another.

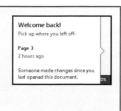

Your Documents Are Always Up to Date

Word 2013 saves your documents by default in the SkyDrive folder that installs along with Word. In the background as you work, Word synchronizes files with changes to your SkyDrive. And the technology will not bog down your work environment because Word uploads only changes, not entire documents, saving bandwidth and battery life as you work from wireless devices.

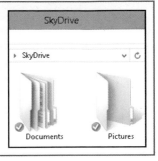

Share Your Documents from Anywhere

You can share your documents both from within Word and from your SkyDrive. And from either location, you can e-mail the document to recipients you choose, post a document at a social media site, or create a link to the document that you can provide to users so that they can view the document in a browser. You also can use Microsoft's free online presentation service to present Word and PowerPoint documents online.

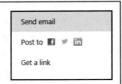

Take Advantage of the Office Store

The Office Store contains add-in applications that work with Microsoft Word 2013. For example, the dictionary you use to look up words in Word does not automatically install when you install the program. But when you need an add-on for Word, you can download it from the Office Store.

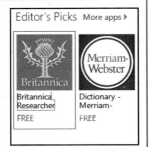

Office 2013 On Demand

Office 2013 comes in three "traditional" editions, where you buy the program; you can install any traditional edition on one machine. Office 2013 also comes in two "subscription" editions; essentially, you pay an annual rental fee to use the software on five PCs or Macs.

Subscription editions include the Office On Demand feature; subscribers can run temporary instances of Word on computers where they normally would not be able to install software. To keep the process fast, only parts of the application actually download as needed, and it runs locally. When you close Word, it uninstalls itself.

Subscribers must be online and logged in to validate their right to use Office On Demand.

Sign In to Office Online

You can use Office Online to work from anywhere. Sign in to Office Online using any of your devices, and then go to work using the Word Web App. Word remembers some of your personal settings such as your Recent Documents list so that you always have access to them.

When you work offline, Word creates, saves, and opens your files from the local SkyDrive folder. Notifications appear periodically, reminding you that you are working offline. Occasionally, Word alerts you if changed files are pending upload to the cloud. Whenever you reconnect, Word uploads your changes to the cloud automatically.

Sign In to Office Online

1 Open Word.

The Word Start screen appears.

2 Click here.

Note: If you are viewing a document, click the Sign in link in the upper-right corner of the screen.

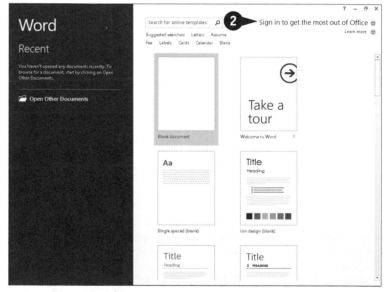

The Sign in to Office window appears.

3 Click **Microsoft account** or **Organizational account**, depending on the user ID you use with Office.

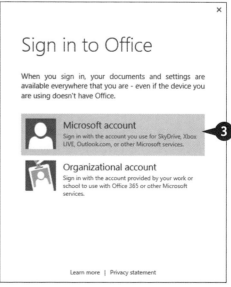

The Microsoft account sign-in window appears.

4 Type your Microsoft Account e-mail address here.

5 Type your Microsoft Account password here.

Ⓐ If you do not have a Microsoft account, you can click here to sign up for one. You can establish any existing e-mail address as your Microsoft Account address.

6 Click **Sign in**.

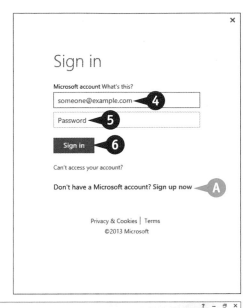

Ⓑ This area indicates that you have signed in to Office Online.

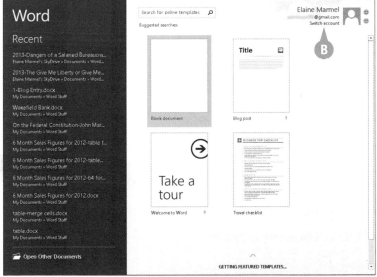

How do I sign out of Office Online?

Sign in to Windows 8 using a local account, and perform the steps that follow. Click the **File** tab, **Account**, and **Sign out** (Ⓐ). The Remove Account dialog box appears to warn you that continuing removes all customizations and synchronization might stop. In most cases, it is perfectly safe to click **Yes**. If you are unsure, check with your system administrator.

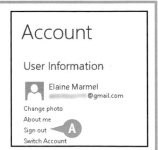

Open a Cloud Document

You can open and edit a document stored in the cloud. The process is quite similar to opening any document as described in Chapter 2. To open a document stored in the cloud, you use your local SkyDrive folder.

Documents stored in the local SkyDrive folder are automatically synchronized with your cloud storage so that all versions are up to date. Further, the synchronization technology ensures that synchronization occurs quickly because only changes are synchronized, which is particularly useful if your Internet connection bandwidth is not particularly good or if you are working on a wireless device with low battery life.

Open a Cloud Document

1 Make sure you are signed in to Office Online by looking for your name here.

Note: See the section "Sign In to Office Online" if your name does not appear.

2 Click the **File** tab.

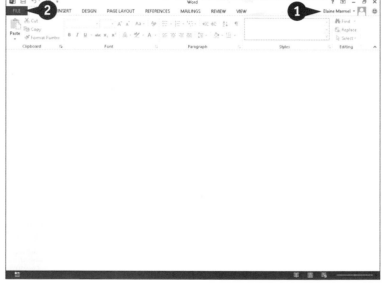

Backstage view appears.

3 Click **Open**.

Note: If you are viewing the Word Start screen, click **Open Other Documents**.

4 Click your SkyDrive.

5 Click **Browse**.

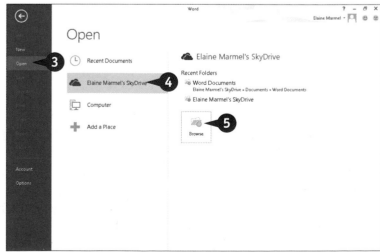

6 In the Open dialog box that appears, navigate to and click the SkyDrive folder.

7 Click the file you want to open.

8 Click **Open**.

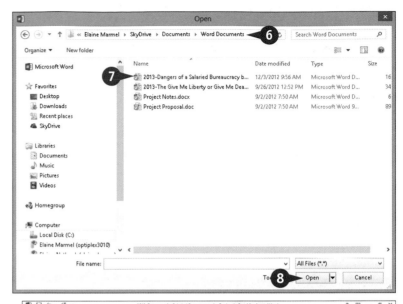

The document stored in the cloud appears.

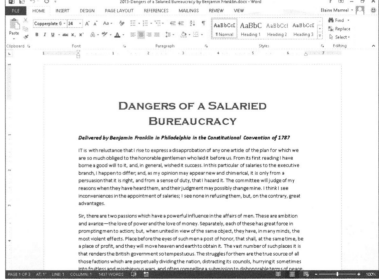

TIP

What happens if I am not signed in to Office Online?

When you choose SkyDrive under Places, you can click the **Sign in** button and supply your ID and password as described in the section "Sign In to Office Online."

Be aware that, instead of signing in to Office Online, you can open and edit the local version of the cloud document from the SkyDrive folder. You will see notifications letting you know that you are working offline. If you save the local version of the cloud document to your SkyDrive folder, Word will alert you that the changes to your file are pending upload to the cloud.

Save a Document to the Cloud

By default, Word 2013 saves all your documents to the local SkyDrive folder. Installing Word 2013 automatically gives you 7GB of cloud storage space for free, and you can rent additional space.

The first time you save a document to your SkyDrive, Word sets up automatic synchronization for you. So each time you subsequently save changes to the document, synchronization between the local file and the file stored in your cloud storage space at SkyDrive happens automatically. If you do not want your files automatically saved to your SkyDrive, you can change that option.

Save a Document to the Cloud

1 With the document that you want to save to your SkyDrive open, click the **File** tab.

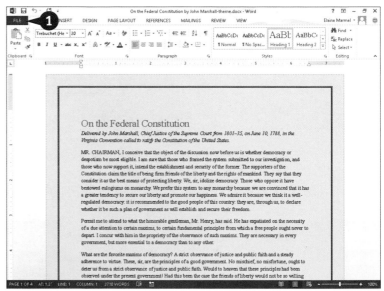

Backstage view appears.

2 Click **Save As**.

3 Click your SkyDrive.

4 If the folder where you want to save the document appears in the Current Folder or Recent Folders lists, click that folder; otherwise, click **Browse**.

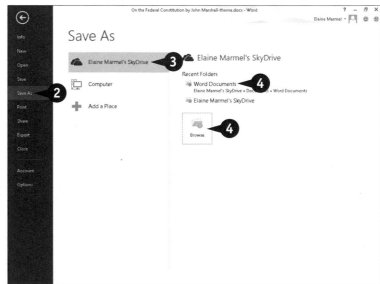

The Save As dialog box appears.

5 Click here to navigate to your SkyDrive.

6 Open the SkyDrive folder where you want to place the document.

7 Provide a filename.

8 Click **Save**.

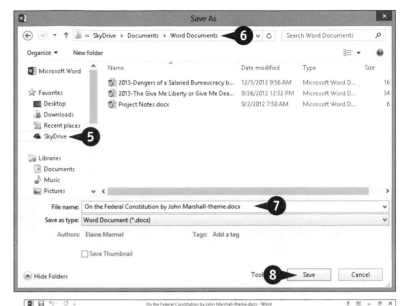

A Your document uploads to your SkyDrive.

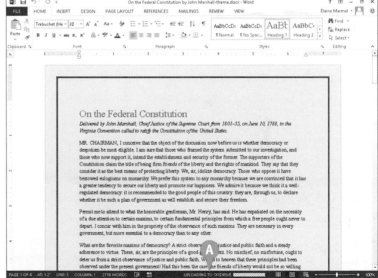

Share a Document from Word

You can easily share documents using Office Online. You can share an Office document by posting it using a social network or to a blog or sending a document as an e-mail attachment. You also can take advantage of a free online presentation service Microsoft offers and share your document by presenting it online. Or, as shown in this section, you can send a link to your SkyDrive — as part of Office 2013, you receive free cloud space at SkyDrive — where the recipient can view and even work on only the shared document. When you finish, you can stop sharing the document.

Share a Document from Word

Share a Document

1 With the document you want to share on-screen, click the **File** tab.

Backstage view appears.

2 Click **Share**.

3 Click **Invite People**.

4 Type e-mail addresses of people with whom you want to share here.

Note: If you enter multiple addresses, Office separates them with a semicolon (;).

5 Click ▼ and decide whether these people can edit or simply view the document.

A You can type a personal message to include with the invitation.

6 Click **Share**.

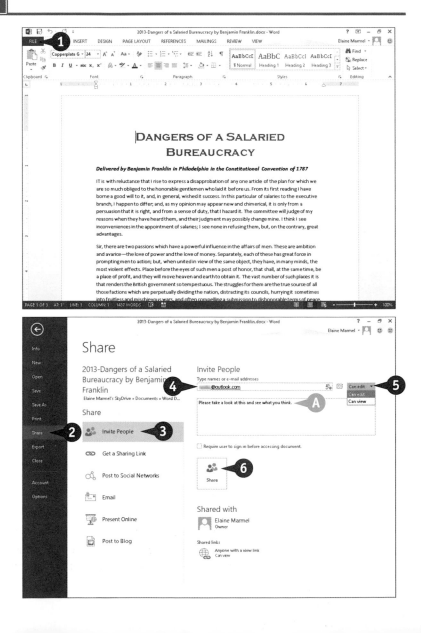

Office sends e-mail messages to the people you listed.

B Recipients with whom you shared the document appear here.

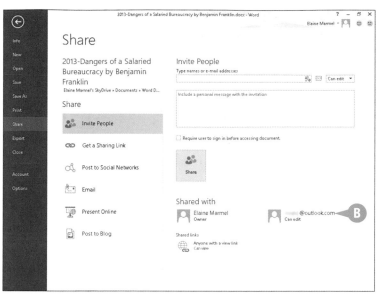

Stop Sharing

1 Open the document you want to stop sharing, and click the **File** tab to display Backstage view.

2 Click **Share**.

3 Click **Invite People**.

4 Right-click the recipient with whom you no longer wish to share.

5 Click **Remove User**.

The program updates document permissions and removes the user from the screen.

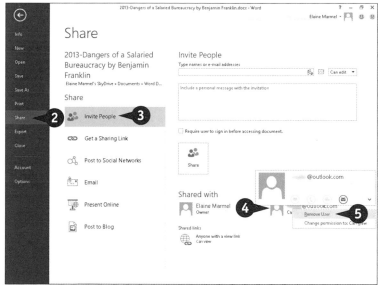

TIP

Why do I see a screen indicating I must save my document before sharing it?

If you have not previously saved your document to your SkyDrive, Word will prompt you to do so before starting the Share process. By default, Word saves all your documents to your SkyDrive, but if you changed that option, click the **Save to Cloud** button that appears. The program displays the Save As pane of Backstage view; click your SkyDrive and then click a folder in the Recent Folders list, or click **Browse** to navigate to the SkyDrive folder where you want to place the document.

Download Apps from the Office Store

You can use the Office Store to download add-on applications, or *apps*, for Word. Unlike its predecessors, Word 2013 does not include applications like the dictionary you use to look up definitions of words. But when you need to use one of these features, you can download it as an app from the Office Store.

In addition to add-on apps you have used in the past, the Office Store also contains add-on apps created by developers outside of Microsoft — apps that work with Word. The developer can choose to charge for an app or make it available for free.

Download Apps from the Office Store

Install an App

① Click the **Insert** tab.

② Click the top half of **Apps for Office**.

The Insert App dialog box appears, displaying featured apps.

Ⓐ You can click here to view all apps in the Office Store.

③ Click an app to download.

Note: This section adds the Merriam-Webster Dictionary to Word as an example.

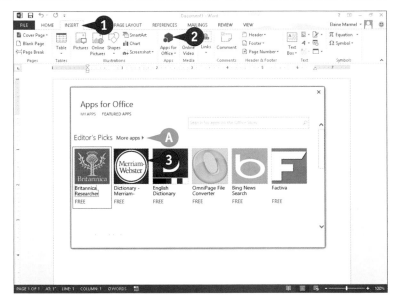

The web page for the app appears.

Ⓑ You can read the information about the app.

Note: Additional apps you might like appear at the bottom of the page.

④ Click **Add**.

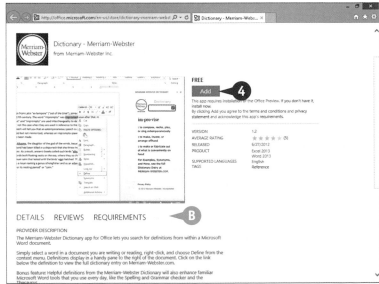

A web page appears, asking you to sign into the Office Store using your Microsoft account.

5 Fill in the login information.

6 Click **Sign in**.

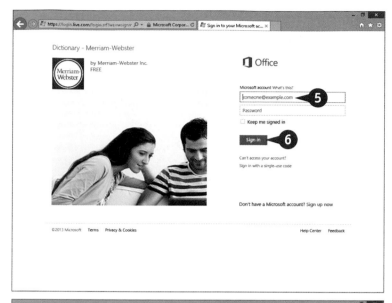

A web page appears, asking you to confirm that you want to add the app; click **Continue**.

C A web page appears, providing directions to activate the app.

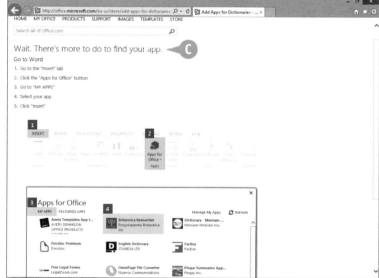

TIP

How do I get a Microsoft Account?

You can establish any valid e-mail address as your Microsoft account; if you have an existing Hotmail or Windows Live ID, you can use those as your Microsoft account. Using your browser, visit http://account.live.com. On the sign-in page that appears, click the **Sign up now** link. You will be redirected to a page where you supply some information about yourself and the e-mail address you want to use. Complete the page, and accept the terms of agreement. You might receive a verification e-mail; follow its instructions to complete the sign-up process.

Download Apps from the Office Store (continued)

When you need an app for Microsoft Word 2013, you go to the Office Store. You visit the Office Store from within the program to review available apps. You then choose, buy if necessary, download, and install apps in which you are interested.

After you finish installing an app that you download from the Office Store, you must, in most cases, activate the app so that you can use it in Microsoft Word. This section describes how to activate the Merriam-Webster Dictionary in Word. See Chapter 4 for details on using the dictionary in Word.

Download Apps from the Office Store (continued)

Activate the Dictionary App

1 In Word, click the **Insert** tab.

2 Click the top half of **Apps for Office**.

Note: If you click the bottom half of the **Apps for Office** button, click **See All**.

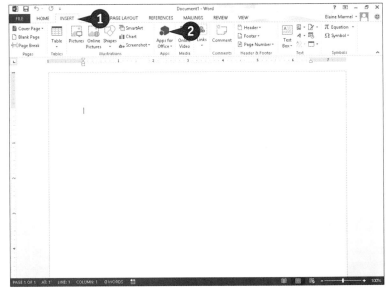

The Insert App dialog box appears.

3 Click **Refresh**.

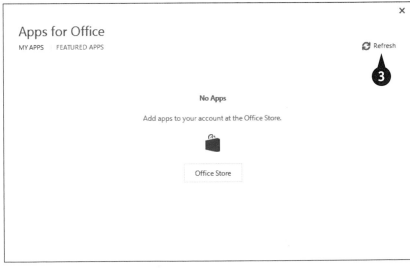

The app you downloaded appears.

4 Click the app.

5 Click **Insert**.

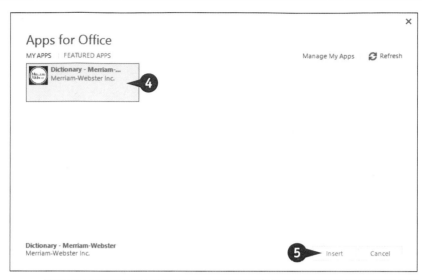

Ⓐ The app loads. For the Merriam-Webster Dictionary, a pane opens on the right side of the Word screen.

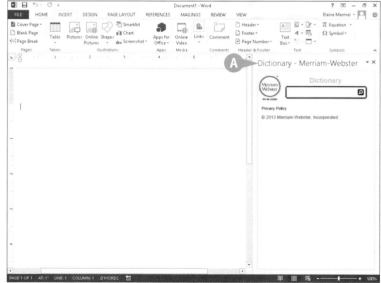

TIP

Do I need to keep the Merriam-Webster Dictionary pane open all the time to use the dictionary?
No. Click ✕ in the pane to close it. See Chapter 4 to learn how to use the dictionary.

Using the Word Web App in SkyDrive

From SkyDrive, you can use the Word Web App to open and edit Word documents with the same basic editing tools you use in Microsoft Word.

Do not let the limitation of "basic editing tools" stop you; although you cannot perform advanced functions like creating or using macros, you can perform basic functions. For example, in the Word Web App, you can apply character and paragraph formatting, such as bold or italics, align text, change margins, insert a table or a picture stored on the local drive, and add clip art available from Microsoft's clip art collection.

Using the Word Web App in SkyDrive

1 Use your browser to go to https://skydrive.live.com.

2 Type the e-mail address and password associated with your Microsoft Account.

3 Click **Sign in**.

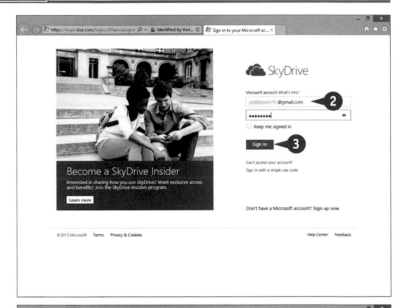

Your SkyDrive appears.

4 Click to navigate to the folder containing the document you want to open.

5 Click the document you want to open.

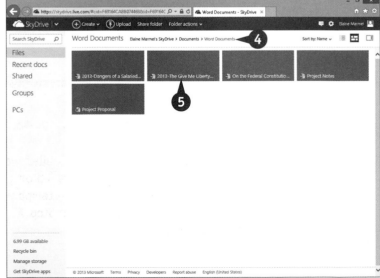

The document appears for viewing only.

6 Click **Edit Document**.

7 Click **Edit in Word Web App**.

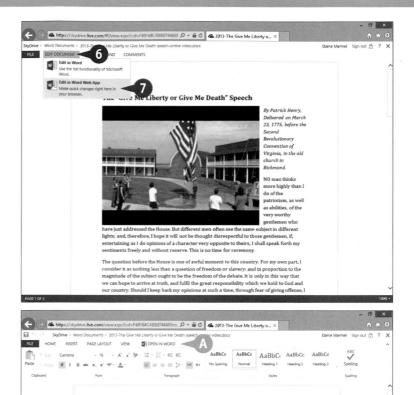

The document appears in the Word Web App, where you can make quick changes.

A The Ribbon contains only a few tabs.

What should I do if I need features not available in the Word Web App?

If the computer on which you are working has Word installed, you can choose **Edit in Word** in Step **7**. If Word is not installed on your computer but you have a subscription to Word, you can temporarily install and use the program by clicking **Edit in Word** in Step **7**. When you close Word, it will uninstall itself.

How do I sign out of SkyDrive?

Save and close the Word Web App by clicking **File, Save** followed by **File, Exit**. In the upper-right corner of the SkyDrive window, click your name and then click **Sign Out**.

Index

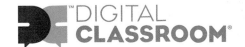

There's a Visual book
for every learning level...

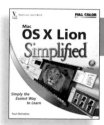

Simplified®

The place to start if you're new to computers. Full color.

- Computers
- Creating Web Pages
- Digital Photography
- Internet
- Mac OS
- Office
- Windows

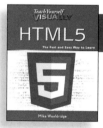

Teach Yourself VISUALLY™

Get beginning to intermediate-level training in a variety of topics. Full color.

- Access
- Computers
- Digital Photography
- Dreamweaver
- Excel
- Flash
- HTML
- iLife
- iPhoto
- Mac OS
- Office
- Photoshop
- Photoshop Elements
- PowerPoint
- Windows
- Wireless Networking
- Word
- iPad
- iPhone
- Wordpress
- Muse

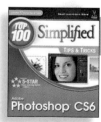

Top 100 Simplified® Tips & Tricks

Tips and techniques to take your skills beyond the basics. Full color.

- Digital Photography
- eBay
- Excel
- Google
- Internet
- Mac OS
- Office
- Photoshop
- Photoshop Elements
- PowerPoint
- Windows